Manual Therapy for the Low Back and Pelvis
A Clinical Orthopedic Approach

Joseph E. Muscolino, BA, DC

Chiropractor

Adjunct Professor of Anatomy, Physiology, and Kinesiology
at Purchase College, State University of New York

Owner of *The Art and Science of Kinesiology*

. Wolters Kluwer
Health

Philadelphia · Baltimore · New York · London
Buenos Aires · Hong Kong · Sydney · Tokyo

Acquisitions Editor: Jonathan Joyce
Supervisor, Product Development: Eve Malakoff-Klein
Product Development Editor: Linda Francis
Production Project Manager: David Orzechowski
Marketing Manager: Leah Thomson
Design Coordinator: Terry Mallon
Illustrations: Lightbox Visuals, Inc.
Photographs: Yanik Chauvin Photography
Compositor: Absolute Service, Inc.

First Edition

351 West Camden Street   Two Commerce Square
Baltimore, MD 21201   2001 Market Street
                                Philadelphia, PA 19103

Printed in China

9   8   7   6   5   4   3   2   1

Library of Congress Cataloging-in-Publication Data

Muscolino, Joseph E., author.
  Manual therapy for the low back and pelvis : a clinical orthopedic approach / Joseph E. Muscolino. — First edition.
       p. ; cm.
  Includes bibliographical references and index.
  ISBN 978-1-58255-880-6 (alk. paper)
  I. Title.
  [DNLM: 1. Musculoskeletal Diseases—diagnosis. 2. Musculoskeletal Diseases—therapy. 3. Low Back Pain—therapy. 4. Lumbosacral Region. 5. Manipulation, Orthopedic—methods. 6. Massage—methods. 7. Pelvic Pain—therapy. 8. Pelvis. WE 750]
  RD771.B217
  617.5'6406—dc23
                                                                    2013049086

DISCLAIMER

Care has been taken to confirm the accuracy of the information present and to describe generally accepted practices. However, the authors, editors, and publisher are not responsible for errors or omissions or for any consequences from application of the information in this book and make no warranty, expressed or implied, with respect to the currency, completeness, or accuracy of the contents of the publication. Application of this information in a particular situation remains the professional responsibility of the practitioner; the clinical treatments described and recommended may not be considered absolute and universal recommendations.

The authors, editors, and publisher have exerted every effort to ensure that drug selection and dosage set forth in this text are in accordance with the current recommendations and practice at the time of publication. However, in view of ongoing research, changes in government regulations, and the constant flow of information relating to drug therapy and drug reactions, the reader is urged to check the package insert for each drug for any change in indications and dosage and for added warnings and precautions. This is particularly important when the recommended agent is a new or infrequently employed drug.

Some drugs and medical devices presented in this publication have Food and Drug Administration (FDA) clearance for limited use in restricted research settings. It is the responsibility of the health care providers to ascertain the FDA status of each drug or device planned for use in their clinical practice.

To purchase additional copies of this book, call our customer service department at (800) 638-3030 or fax orders to (301) 223-2320. International customers should call (301) 223-2300.

Visit Lippincott Williams & Wilkins on the Internet: http://www.lww.com. Lippincott Williams & Wilkins customer service representatives are available from 8:30 am to 6:00 pm, EST.

This book is lovingly dedicated
to my son, Joseph C. Muscolino

REVIEWERS

The author and the Wolters Kluwer Health team would like to extend our sincere thanks to those who offered feedback and reviews throughout the development of this book:

Karen Casciato, LMT
Portland, OR

Lisa Krause, MS, CMT
Instructor, Wisconsin School of Massage Therapy
Germantown, WI

Karen Lilly, AAS
Wichita, KS

Jeffrey Lutz, CMTPT
The Pain Treatment and Wellness Center
Greensburg, PA

Lou Peters, LMT, CNMT, BS
Instructor, American Institute of Alternative Medicine
Columbus, OH

Antonella Sena, DC
Chiropractor, Academy of Massage Therapy
Hackensack, NJ

PREFACE

As the field of massage therapy has gained greater acceptance, its role within the health field has increased commensurately. For this reason, there is a growing need for treatment techniques that are oriented toward clinical orthopedic rehabilitation of clients who present with musculoskeletal conditions. The purpose of this book is to present an array of these treatment techniques that can be used by the massage therapist and other manual therapists.

Manual Therapy for the Low Back and Pelvis: A Clinical Orthopedic Approach is designed to be used by the practicing therapist who wants to learn techniques that likely were not taught during his or her training at school. This book is also designed to comfortably fit into the curriculum of a massage therapy or other manual or movement therapy school that desires to teach these techniques, whether it is within the core curriculum or within the continuing education offerings. Note that what is and what is not within the scope of practice of a massage therapist or other manual therapist varies from state to state, and occasionally varies from one town, city, county, or province to another. It is the responsibility of the practicing therapist to make sure that he or she is practicing legally and employing treatment techniques that are within the scope of his or her license or certification.

ORGANIZATION

The content of this book is divided into three parts.

- Part 1 addresses the foundational information necessary to be able to understand the client's low back/pelvis condition, assess it, and determine the appropriate options.
- Part 2 covers the actual low back/pelvis treatment techniques. Each chapter covers a specific technique.
- Part 3 covers the use of hydrotherapy and postural self-care for the client and therapist. Part 3 chapters are available online at thepoint.lww.com/MuscolinoLowBack.

Every effort has been made to make this book as user friendly and as accessible as possible. Each chapter contains a simplified outline, learning objectives, and a list of key terms. Technique chapters located in Part 2 also contain a list of the treatment routines that will be covered in that chapter, along with case studies, Think-It-Through questions, precautions, and practical applications. Furthermore, every chapter concludes with a brief review of the chapter's content and provides 20 chapter review questions online.

Part 1: Anatomy, Pathology, and Assessment

Of course, proper treatment can only be applied if the foundational anatomy, physiology, and kinesiology are first understood. To this end, Chapter 1 provides a review of the anatomy and physiology of the low back and pelvis. This review is just that—a review. It is not meant to replace the entire science curriculum of a massage school training. Rather, it covers the essential elements of the anatomy and physiology of the lumbar spine and sacroiliac joints so that the treatment principals presented in later chapters can be more easily understood, learned, and applied. I recommend that readers begin with this chapter before continuing on to technique chapters.

Applying the proper treatment techniques also requires a clear understanding of the anatomy and physiology of the pathologic condition that the client is experiencing. Therefore, Chapters 2 and 3 discuss the most common musculoskeletal conditions that affect the lumbar spine and pelvis. Chapter 2 addresses the presentation and causes of these conditions; Chapter 3 addresses their assessment.

Part 2: Treatment Techniques

There are a number of therapeutic techniques that are available to the practicing massage and manual therapist. Principal among these is Swedish-based massage. Although any Swedish-based massage application is therapeutic in nature due to its effect on the parasympathetic branch of the nervous system and on the circulatory system, deeper tissue techniques often offer the advantage of further clinical benefit. Chapter 4 of this book offers technique strategies for working the musculature of the low back and pelvis more efficiently with less effort. I like to think of it as showing you how to work smart, not hard. Due to the unique anatomy of the musculature of the abdominal wall, Chapter 5 specifically addresses massage treatment of this region.

However, massage is not the only therapeutic tool available to the massage and manual therapist. Stretching is another effective treatment option. Unfortunately, stretching is often only lightly covered in massage therapy curricula and therefore underutilized by most practicing massage therapists. Chapters 6 through 9 of this book review basic stretching and present a number of advanced stretching techniques for the lumbar spine and pelvis that can be used effectively for the treatment of our clients.

Joint mobilization is even more underutilized than stretching within the scope of practice of most massage therapists. When performed appropriately and with skill, joint mobilization can be an extremely powerful tool for the treatment of lumbar spine and sacroiliac joint problems. However, it must be done carefully and judiciously. Chapter 10 of this book presents a number of joint mobilization techniques that can be used by massage therapists for the safe and effective treatment of their client's lumbar spinal and sacroiliac joint problems.

Part 3: Self-Care for the Client and Therapist

The critical subject of self-care for the client and for the therapist is covered in two additional chapters, available online at thepoint.lww.com/MuscolinoLowBack. Online Chapter 11 discusses the use of hydrotherapy and proper instruction to our clients for home care. Hydrotherapy, or using water to transmit heat and/or cold to the client, can be a very helpful adjunct to our treatment sessions. This chapter also looks at knowing when to use heat versus cold, as well as the specific application of these various therapies. And, given that no client treatment plan strategy is complete without the proper instruction to the client on what he or she can do at home between massage sessions, self-care is also discussed.

Online Chapter 12 addresses self-care for the therapist. Massage and other manual therapies can be physically demanding, and maintaining our bodies in good physical shape is of paramount importance. To that end, Chapter 12 offers self-care exercises for the therapist to perform to stay strong and healthy and help assure career longevity.

ANCILLARIES

Given the dynamic nature of the treatment techniques presented in this book, depending on still photos and text description alone is difficult. For this reason, *Manual Therapy for the Low Back and Pelvis: A Clinical Orthopedic Approach* also provides access to a companion website at thepoint.lww.com/MuscolinoLowBack, with videos that demonstrate many of the assessment and treatment techniques covered in this book being performed on clients, along with a complete image bank.

In addition to the videos and to the self-care chapters described earlier, this book's companion website provides chapter review questions and answers, and answers to the case studies that begin in Chapter 3.

As massage and other forms of manual and movement therapy take their rightful place within the world of complementary and alternative medicine, the need for increased education grows. This book offers a number of treatment techniques that empower manual therapists to be able to better work with and help clients who present with musculoskeletal conditions. Along with *its companion* website, *Manual Therapy for the Low Back and Pelvis: A Clinical Orthopedic Approach* will be an invaluable asset to your practice.

ACKNOWLEDGMENTS

Because my name is the only name on the front cover of this book, the reader could incorrectly assume that I am the only person responsible for its creation. This is far from the truth. Many people helped create the book that you are holding. This is my opportunity to both directly thank them and to acknowledge them to you, the readers.

Much of the beauty of this book lies in its artwork. I am lucky to have worked for many years with an amazing team. Yanik Chauvin is the principal photographer and videographer. His eye for the best angle to portray motion and the best lighting to focus the viewer is unsurpassed. He is also one of the most enjoyable people to work with! The principal illustrator is Giovanni Rimasti of LightBox Visuals. Under the extremely competent direction of Jodie Bernard (owner of LightBox Visuals), he provided clear and crisply drawn illustrations that ably convey to the reader both the underlying anatomy and the motion of the body. And of course, I was fortunate to have a wonderful group of models: Hyesun Bowman, Vaughn Bowman, Victoria Caligiuri, Simona Cipriani, Emilie Miller, Joseph C. Muscolino, Maryanne Peterson, Jintina Sundarabhaya, and Kei Tsuruharatani. Thank you to all for contributing to the beauty of this book!

Editing and production are especially invisible parts of the creation of a book. But anyone who has ever had the opportunity to see the first draft of a book and compare it to its final publication knows how invaluable editing and production are. Many thanks to everyone on the Wolters Kluwer Health team who helped to create this book and bring it to fruition: Eve Malakoff-Klein, who supervised the project; Jonathan Joyce, acquisitions editor; David Orzechowski and Harold Medina who coordinated the production; Linda Francis, who handled development and manuscript preparation; and Jen Clements, who assisted with the art.

Particular thanks are owed to Brett M. Carr, MS, DC, for writing the online chapter on *Self-Care for the Therapist* (Chapter 12). His expertise was invaluable and helped to round out and strengthen the content of this book.

As usual, a special thank you to a former student, now instructor, William Courtland, who first spurred me to become a textbook author with the simple words: "You should write a book."

And, finally, most important of all, thank you to my entire family, especially my wife, Simona Cipriani, for all of your love, understanding, support, and encouragement. You make it all worthwhile!

Joseph E. Muscolino

Joseph E. Muscolino, BA, DC, has been teaching core curriculum and continuing education musculoskeletal anatomy, physiology, kinesiology, assessment, and treatment courses to manual and movement therapists for more than 25 years. He was an instructor at the Connecticut Center for Massage Therapy from 1986 to 2010 and is presently an adjunct professor at Purchase College, State University of New York (SUNY).

Dr. Muscolino is the author of numerous other manual and movement therapy textbooks, covering musculoskeletal anatomy and physiology, kinesiology, musculoskeletal pathology, palpation and orthopedic assessment, and hands-on treatment techniques. In addition, he has authored many assessment and treatment DVDs for manual and movement therapists. He also writes the column "Body Mechanics" in the *Massage Therapy Journal*, and has written for numerous other journals in the United States and internationally.

Dr. Muscolino teaches continuing education (CE) workshops around the globe on such topics as body mechanics, deep tissue massage, stretching, advanced stretching, joint mobilization, muscle palpation, joint motion palpation, orthopedic assessment, musculoskeletal pathologic conditions, kinesiology, and cadaver workshops. Through The Art and Science of Kinesiology, Dr. Muscolino offers a Certification in Clinical Orthopedic Manual Therapy (COMT). He also runs instructor in-services for kinesiology and hands-on treatment instructors. He is an approved provider of continuing education; credit is available through the National Certification Board for Therapeutic Massage and Bodywork (NCBTMB) toward certification renewal for massage therapists and bodyworkers.

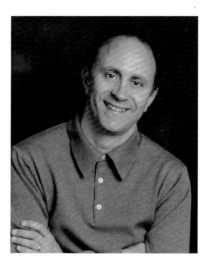

Dr. Muscolino holds a Bachelor of Arts in Biology from SUNY at Binghamton, Harpur College, and a Doctor of Chiropractic from Western States Chiropractic College in Portland, Oregon. He has been in private practice in Connecticut for more than 28 years and incorporates soft tissue work into his chiropractic practice for all his patients.

For further information regarding *Manual Therapy for the Low Back and Pelvis: A Clinical Orthopedic Approach*, please visit thepoint.lww.com/MuscolinoLowBack. For information on Dr. Muscolino's other publications, DVDs, and workshops, or to contact Dr. Muscolino directly, please visit his website, www.learnmuscles.com, or follow him on Facebook at The Art and Science of Kinesiology.

CONTENTS

The chapters and materials listed below are located online at thePoint.lww.com/MuscolinoLowBack

PART ONE

Anatomy, Pathology, and Assessment

CHAPTER **1** ## Anatomy and Physiology Review

CHAPTER OUTLINE

OBJECTIVES

After completing this chapter, the student should be able to:

1. Describe the structure of the lumbar spine and pelvis.
2. Discuss the importance and implications of the lumbar spinous processes to assessment and treatment.
3. Discuss the importance and implications of the posterior superior iliac spine (PSIS) and anterior superior iliac spine (ASIS) to assessment and treatment.
4. Describe the structure and function of the lumbar spinal, sacroiliac, and hip joints.
5. Describe the motions of the lumbar spinal, sacroiliac, and hip joints.
6. List the attachments and actions of the muscles of the lumbar spine and pelvis.
7. Classify the muscles of the lumbar spine and hip joints into their major structural and functional groups.
8. Explain why knowing the actions of a muscle can facilitate palpating and stretching it.
9. List and describe the structure and function of the ligaments of the lumbar spine and pelvis.
10. Explain how ligaments and antagonist muscles are similar in function.
11. Describe the major precautions and contraindications when working on the low back and pelvis.
12. Define each key term in this chapter.

KEY TERMS

abdominal aorta
abdominal aponeurosis
annulus fibrosus
anterior longitudinal ligament
anterior sacroiliac ligaments
anterior superior iliac spine
  (ASIS)
cardinal planes
central canal
circumduction
closed chain
coccyx
contralateral muscles

contralateral rotation
counternutation
disc joint
facet joints
femoral artery
femoral nerve
femoral triangle
femoral vein
femoropelvic rhythm
glide
hyperlordotic
hypolordotic
iliac crest

iliofemoral ligament
iliolumbar ligaments
ilium
interspinous ligaments
intertransverse ligaments
intervertebral foramina
intrapelvic motion
ipsilateral rotation
ischiofemoral ligament
ischium
lamina
laminar groove
ligamentum flavum

ligamentum teres
lordotic curve (lordosis)
lumbar spine
lumbosacral joint
nucleus pulposus
nutation
open chain
pars interarticularis
pelvic bones
posterior longitudinal ligament
posterior sacroiliac ligaments
posterior superior iliac spine
  (PSIS)

pubis	sacroiliac joint (SIJ)	segmental joint level	vertebral foramina
pubofemoral ligament	sacrospinous ligament	spinous process	zona orbicularis
reverse actions	sacrotuberous ligament	supraspinous ligament	zygapophyseal joints (Z joints)
sacral base	sacrum	thoracolumbar fascia	
sacral tubercles	sciatic nerve	translation	

INTRODUCTION

This chapter is an overview of the anatomy and physiology of the low back and pelvis. Having a solid foundation in the structure and function of a region allows you to understand and better apply treatment techniques to that region. For more complete coverage of the structure and function of the low back and pelvis, anatomy, physiology, and kinesiology textbooks should be consulted.

THE LUMBAR SPINE AND PELVIS

The low back is defined by the **lumbar spine**, and the pelvis is defined by the bones of the pelvic girdle. The lumbar spine is composed of five vertebrae, named L1 to L5 from superior to inferior. The pelvis is composed of the two pelvic bones and the sacrum and coccyx (the pelvic bones are also known as the coxal, innominate, or hip bones) (Fig. 1-1).

Lumbar Spine

From a lateral view, the healthy lumbar spine can be seen to have a **lordotic curve (lordosis)**, which is defined as being concave posteriorly and convex anteriorly (Fig. 1-2). (The terms *lordotic* and *lordosis* are often used to denote an excessive and unhealthy lordotic curve. However, these terms are also used to refer to the healthy and normal curve of the low back and neck.) All lumbar vertebrae have a **spinous process** that extends posteriorly and can usually be palpated. How easy or difficult it is to palpate the lumbar spinous processes depends largely on the degree of the client's lordotic curve. Because the lumbar curve is lordotic, the spinous processes are recessed and not as superficial for palpation as are the spinous processes of the thoracic spine. However, some clients' lumbar curves are decreased or even straight; a decreased or absent lordotic curve is termed **hypolordotic**, making palpation of the spinous processes much easier. If, on the other hand, the client's lumbar curve is excessive, it is termed **hyperlordotic**; the spinous processes of a hyperlordotic lumbar spine are more difficult to palpate. Other prominent lumbar bony landmarks are the **lamina**, **laminar groove**, mammillary process, transverse process, facets, **pars interarticularis**, and vertebral body. The spinal cord travels through the **central canal** formed by the **vertebral foramina** (singular: foramen), and the lumbar spinal nerves travel through the **intervertebral foramina** between adjacent vertebrae (Fig. 1-3).

Because of the lordotic curve and the thick musculature that overlies the lumbar spine, the only easily palpable bony landmark is the spinous process. Therefore, the spinous processes (and laminae) are used when contacting the lumbar spine for motion palpation assessment and joint mobilization treatment.

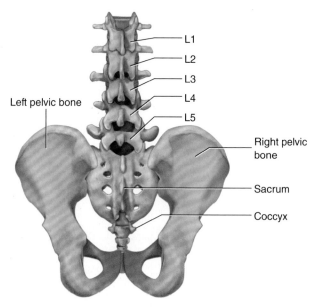

Figure 1-1 Posterior view of the lumbar spine and pelvis. The lumbar spine is composed of five vertebrae, named L1 to L5 from superior to inferior. The pelvis is composed of the two pelvic bones and the sacrum and coccyx.

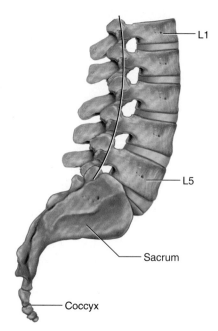

Figure 1-2 Right lateral view of the lumbar spine. The lumbar spine's curve is described as lordotic, with its concavity facing posteriorly and its convexity facing anteriorly.

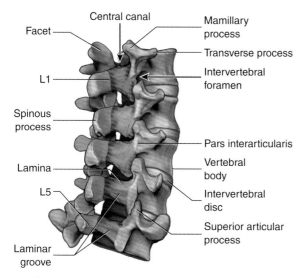

Figure 1-3 Right posterolateral view of the lumbar spine. Prominent bony landmarks are labeled.

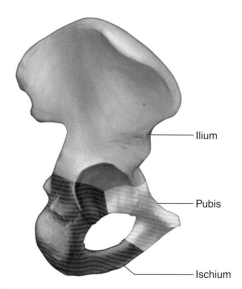

Figure 1-4 Lateral view of the right pelvic bone. The ilium, ischium, and pubis have been colored to discern their borders: The ilium is blue, the ischium is pink, and the pubis is yellow.

Pelvic Girdle

The bones of the pelvic girdle are the two **pelvic bones** and the **sacrum** and **coccyx** (see Fig. 1-1). Each pelvic bone is composed of three bones—the **ilium**, **ischium**, and **pubis**—that fuse together embryologically (Fig. 1-4). The sacrum is composed of five vertebrae that did not fully form and fused together to create a triangular-shaped bone. The triangular-shaped sacrum is upside down, with the **sacral base** located superiorly and the apex located inferiorly. Between the sacrum and iliac portion of the pelvic bone on each side of the body is a **sacroiliac joint (SIJ)**. The coccyx, usually considered to be the evolutionary remnant of a tail, is composed of four poorly formed vertebral segments that often fuse as a person ages. There are a number of important bony landmarks of the pelvis. On the posterior side are the **posterior superior iliac spine (PSIS)**, posterior inferior iliac spine (PIIS), greater sciatic notch, ischial tuberosity, ischial spine, and **sacral tubercles** (Fig. 1-5A). A dimple in the skin of the client can usually be seen where the skin falls in on the medial side of the PSIS (Fig. 1-5B). Locating this dimple is helpful when palpating for the PSIS. On the anterior side are the **anterior superior iliac spine (ASIS)**, anterior inferior iliac spine (AIIS), and pubic tubercle (Fig. 1-6). The **iliac crest** is located laterally between the PSIS and ASIS (see Figs. 1-5A and 1-6). The PSIS and ASIS are easily palpable and important contacts for stabilization of the pelvis when stretching the client. The PSIS and sacral tubercles are also important when performing motion palpation assessment of the SIJs of the pelvis,

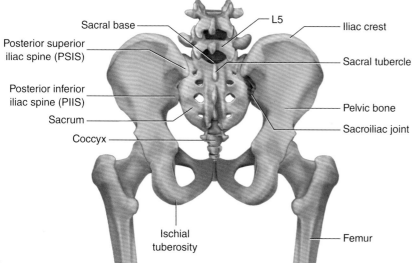

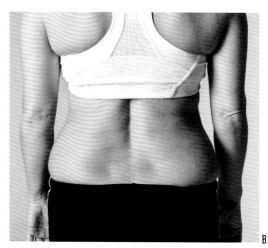

Figure 1-5 Posterior views of the lumbar spine and pelvis. **(A)** View of bones and bony landmarks. **(B)** Dimples are usually visible immediately medial to the PSISs.

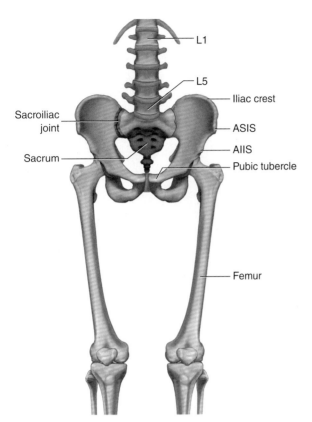

Figure 1-6 Anterior view of the lumbar spine and pelvis. The prominent bones and bony landmarks have been labeled. *AIIS,* anterior inferior iliac spine; *ASIS,* anterior superior iliac spine.

and the PSIS is an important contact point when mobilizing the SIJ.

LUMBAR SPINAL JOINTS AND PELVIC JOINTS

Lumbar Spinal Joints

In the lumbar spine, three joints are located between each two adjacent vertebrae: one **disc joint** (intervertebral disc joint) and two paired (left and right) **facet joints**. The disc joint is located anteriorly, and the facet joints are located posterolaterally (Fig. 1-7A).

The disc joint is a cartilaginous joint composed of outer fibers called the **annulus fibrosus** that encircle the inner **nucleus pulposus**. The annulus fibrosus is composed of 10 to 20 layers of fibrocartilaginous fibers that attach along the periphery of the bodies of the two adjacent vertebrae. The annular fibers provide a strong and stable enclosure for the nucleus pulposus.

The nucleus pulposus is a thick jellylike substance located within the disc joint (Fig. 1-7B). It has two main functions:

1. It holds the two vertebral bodies apart, which not only creates a larger intervertebral foramen where the spinal nerve enters and exits the spine but also allows the disc joint a greater range of motion.
2. It provides cushioning to the spine.

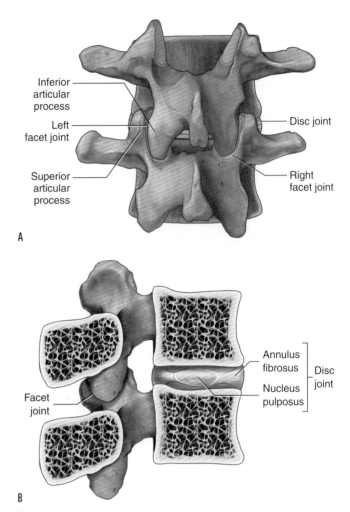

Figure 1-7 The disc and facet joints of the spine. (**A**) Posterior view. The disc joint is located anteriorly; the paired facet joints are located posterolaterally. (**B**) Right lateral view of a sagittal plane cross section. The disc joint is composed of the outer annulus fibrosus fibers and an inner nucleus pulposus. (Courtesy of Joseph E. Muscolino.)

As a whole, the disc joint itself has three major functions:

1. The disc joint bears the weight of the body above it. The increasing size of the vertebral bodies and discs descending the spine helps the disc joints bear the increasing weight of the body above it.
2. The disc joint's thickness allows for a great deal of motion. Overall, the intervertebral discs comprise 25% of the height of the entire spine. The greater the relative height of the discs compared to vertebral body height, the greater the possible range of motion at that region of the spine.
3. The intervertebral discs help to absorb shock.

Each facet joint is a synovial joint that is located between the inferior vertebra's superior articular process and the superior vertebra's inferior articular process (see Fig. 1-7). It is called a facet joint because the joint surface of each of the articular processes has a facet (a smooth flat surface) on it. The scientific name for facet joints is **zygapophyseal joints**,

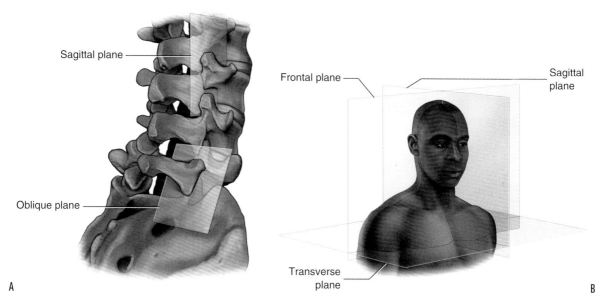

Figure 1-8 Plane of the facet joints of the lumbar spine. (**A**) The plane of the lumbar facets is oriented in the sagittal plane, except for the facet plane of the lumbosacral joint, which is oriented in an oblique plane that is close to the frontal plane. Right posterolateral oblique view. (**B**) Review of all three cardinal (major) planes of the body. ([**B**] Reproduced with permission from Muscolino JE. *Advanced Treatment Techniques for the Manual Therapist: Neck.* Baltimore, MD: Lippincott Williams & Wilkins; 2013.)

hence they are also often known as **Z joints**. Facet joints function to guide motion at that segmental joint level of the spine. The term **segmental joint level** refers to a specific joint level of the spine that includes the disc and facet joints at that level. For example, the joint between L3 and L4, known as the L3-L4 joint, is a segmental level; the L4-L5 joint is another segmental level. The joint between L5 and the base of the sacrum is known as the L5-S1 joint, or simply the **lumbosacral joint**. An understanding of the posture of the lumbosacral joint is extremely important toward understanding pelvic tilt posture and its effect on the lumbar lordotic curve.

The disc joint determines how much vertebral motion is possible at a particular segmental level, and the facet joints determine the type of motion (i.e., the direction of motion) that can occur there. In the lumbar spine, the plane of the facets is vertically oriented in the sagittal plane. An exception to this is at the L5-S1 level where the facet plane is oriented in an oblique plane that is very close to the frontal plane (Fig. 1-8A). *Note*: Figure 1-8B is a review of the three cardinal (major) planes of the body. The three **cardinal planes** are the sagittal, frontal (also known as coronal), and transverse. Any plane that is not perfectly sagittal, frontal, or transverse is an oblique plane.

Because of the sagittal plane orientation of the lumbar facets, the lumbar spine moves extremely well in flexion and extension (sagittal plane motions). Because the facets of the lumbosacral joint are oriented approximately within the frontal plane, right and left lateral flexion motions occur more freely at that level. It is important to be aware of the type of motion that each level of the spine allows when performing joint mobilization (discussed in Chapter 10).

Pelvic Joints

Pelvic joints can be divided into two categories: joints between the pelvis and adjacent body parts and joints located within the pelvis. The lumbosacral joint is located between the pelvis and trunk (more specifically, between the sacrum of the pelvis and L5 of the lumbar spine) (see Fig. 1-2), and the hip joints are located between the pelvis and the thighs (more specifically, the femurs of the thighs) (see Fig. 1-6). Within the pelvis, there are two SIJs and one symphysis pubis joint. Each SIJ is located posteriorly between the sacrum and the iliac portion of the pelvic bone on that side (see Figs. 1-5A and 1-6). The symphysis pubis joint is located anteriorly between the two pubic bone portions of the pelvic bones (see Fig. 1-6).

MOTIONS OF THE LUMBAR SPINE AND PELVIS

Lumbar Spine Motions

The lumbar spine can move axially and nonaxially in all three cardinal planes (sagittal, frontal, and transverse). The axial motions, shown in Figure 1-9, are as follows:

- Extension and flexion in the sagittal plane
- Left lateral flexion and right lateral flexion in the frontal plane
- Right rotation and left rotation in the transverse plane

The term **ipsilateral rotation** is used to describe the motion created by a muscle that rotates the trunk to the same side

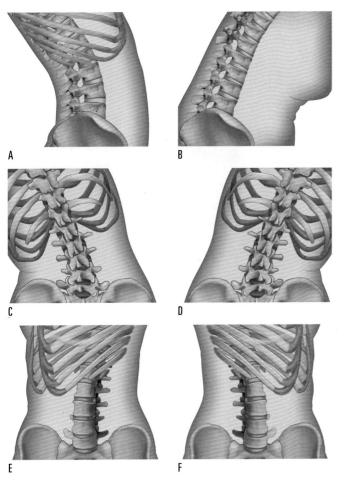

Figure 1-9 Six axial cardinal plane motions of the lumbar spine. **(A, B)** Extension and flexion in the sagittal plane respectively; lateral views. **(C, D)** Left lateral flexion and right lateral flexion in the frontal plane respectively; posterior views. **(E, F)** Right rotation and left rotation in the transverse plane respectively; anterior views.

as where the muscle is located—in other words, a left-sided muscle that rotates the trunk to the left side is performing ipsilateral rotation, as is a right-sided muscle that rotates the trunk to the right side. The term **contralateral rotation** is used to describe the motion created by a muscle that rotates the trunk to the opposite side from where it is located—in other words, a left-sided muscle that rotates the trunk to the right side is performing contralateral rotation, as is a right-sided muscle that rotates the trunk to the left side.

The spinal joints of the trunk can also circumduct. **Circumduction** is not a joint action but a series of four joint actions performed in sequence: left lateral flexion, flexion, right lateral flexion, and extension. If these joint actions are carried out sequentially, one at a time, the trunk will transcribe a square shape. However, if these joint actions are performed smoothly, as is usually done, with the "corners" of the joint actions rounded off, then the trunk moves in a cone shape (Fig. 1-10) that leads many therapists to describe the motion as rotation. However, circumduction is not rotation—in fact, no transverse plane rotation occurs with circumduction. All four joint actions of circumduction occur in the sagittal and frontal planes.

Table 1-1 shows average healthy ranges of axial motion for the lumbar spine as well as the thoracic spine and the thoracolumbar spine. It is important to keep in mind that not every client will necessarily have these ranges. Ranges such as those shown in Table 1-1 are averages across the entire population. Elderly people usually have a smaller range of motion than do younger people, and people with chronic injuries may also have decreased ranges of motion.

The lumbar spine can also move nonaxially. Nonaxial joint motion is known as **translation**, or **glide**. The lumbar spine can translate/glide anteriorly and posteriorly, laterally to the right and left, and superiorly and inferiorly. Anterior translation is

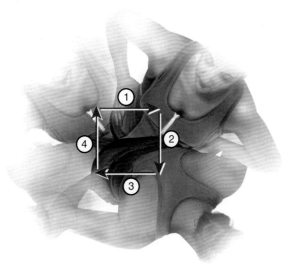

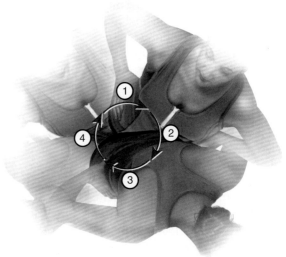

A B

Figure 1-10 Circumduction of the trunk at the spinal joints. Circumduction is a series of four joint actions (left lateral flexion, flexion, right lateral flexion, and extension) carried out one after the other. **(A)** Joint actions shown sequentially. **(B)** Joint actions with the corners "rounded off."

TABLE 1-1 Lumbar, Thoracic, and Thoracolumbar Spine Ranges of Motion			
Average Healthy Ranges of Motion Measured from Anatomic Position			
	Lumbar Spine (L1-L2 to L5-S1)	**Thoracic Spine (T1-T2 to T12-L1)**	**Thoracolumbar Spine (T1-T2 to L5-S1)**
Flexion	50 degrees	35 degrees	85 degrees
Extension	15 degrees	25 degrees	40 degrees
Right lateral flexion	20 degrees	25 degrees	45 degrees
Left lateral flexion	20 degrees	25 degrees	45 degrees
Right rotation	5 degrees	30 degrees	35 degrees
Left rotation	5 degrees	30 degrees	35 degrees

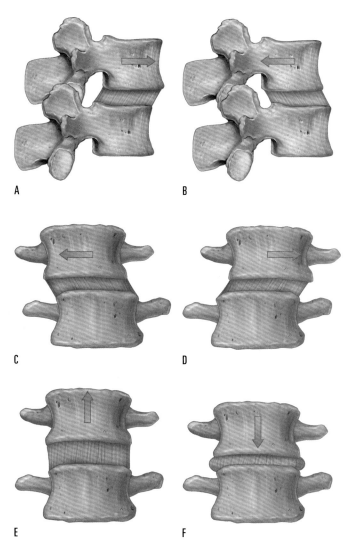

A   B

C   D

E   F

Figure 1-11 Nonaxial motions of the lumbar spine. **(A, B)** Anterior glide (protraction) and posterior glide (retraction), respectively; right lateral views. **(C, D)** Right lateral glide and left lateral glide, respectively; anterior views. **(E, F)** Superior glide (also known as distraction or traction) and inferior glide (also known as compression), respectively; anterior views. (Courtesy of Joseph E. Muscolino.)

also called protraction, and posterior translation is also called retraction. Superior translation is also called distraction or traction, and inferior translation is also called compression (Fig. 1-11). Nonaxial glide motions of the lumbar spine are not as large in excursion as in other regions of the spine but should be considered. Superior glide/traction is especially important because it helps to decompress the joints of the spine.

Pelvic Motions

Pelvic motion can be considered in two ways. The pelvis can move as a unit relative to adjacent body parts. Motion can also occur within the pelvis; this is called intrapelvic motion.

Motion of the Pelvis as a Unit at the Hip Joint(s)

When the pelvis moves as a unit, it can move relative to both thighs at the hip joints or relative to one thigh at the hip joint on that side. These motions are anterior and posterior tilt in the sagittal plane, depression and elevation in the frontal plane (depression is also known as lateral tilt; elevation is also known as hip hiking), and left rotation and right rotation in the transverse plane. It is helpful to understand that motions of the pelvis at the hip joint are **reverse actions** of standard action motions of the thigh at the hip joint. In other words, the same functional group of muscles that moves the thigh at the hip joint when the pelvis is stabilized/fixed also moves the pelvis at the hip joint when the thigh is stabilized/fixed. The thigh moves at the hip joint when the distal end of the lower extremity kinematic chain is free to move, in other words, **open chain** kinematics; the pelvis tends to move at the hip joint when the distal end of the lower extremity kinematic chain is stabilized/fixed, in other words, **closed chain** kinematics. Specific pelvic reverse actions relative to the same-side thigh are as follows: pelvic anterior tilt is the reverse action of thigh flexion, pelvic posterior tilt is the reverse action of thigh extension, pelvic depression is the reverse action of thigh abduction, pelvic elevation is the reverse action of thigh adduction, pelvic contralateral rotation is the reverse action of thigh lateral rotation, and pelvic ipsilateral rotation is the reverse action of thigh medial rotation (Fig. 1-12 and Table 1-2).

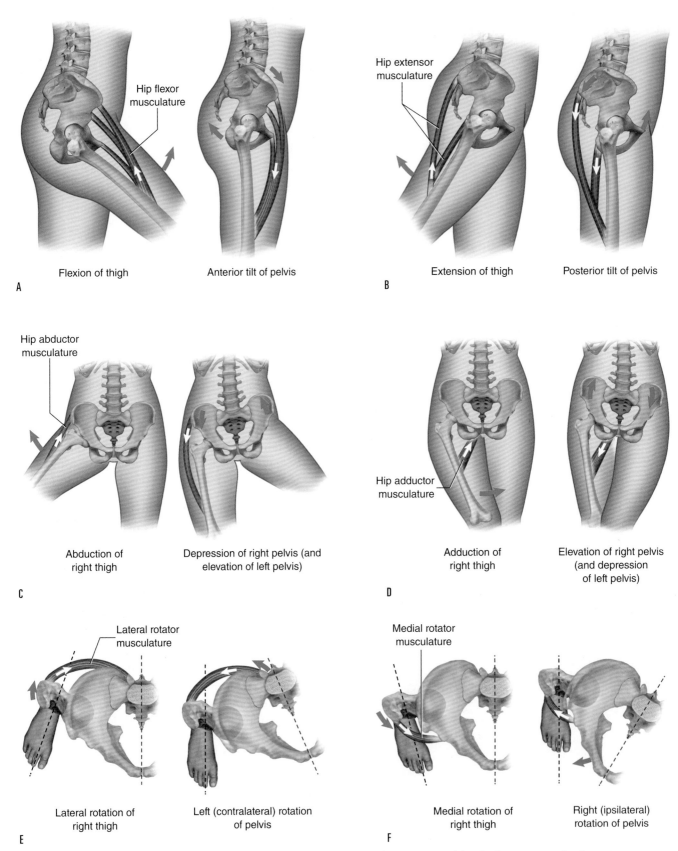

Figure 1-12 Joint actions of the pelvis at the hip joint are the reverse actions of the thigh moving at that hip joint. (**A, B**) Pelvic anterior tilt is the reverse action of thigh flexion; pelvic posterior tilt is the reverse action of thigh extension. (**C, D**) Pelvic depression is the reverse action of thigh abduction; pelvic elevation is the reverse action of thigh adduction. (**E, F**) Pelvic contralateral rotation is the reverse action of thigh lateral rotation; pelvic ipsilateral rotation is the reverse action of thigh medial rotation.

TABLE 1-2	Standard and Reverse Actions at the Hip Joint
Standard Open Chain Thigh Actions	**Reverse Closed Chain Pelvic Actions**
Flexion	Anterior tilt
Extension	Posterior tilt
Abduction	Depression
Adduction	Elevation
Lateral rotation	Contralateral rotation
Medial rotation	Ipsilateral rotation

BOX 1.1

Horizontal Flexion and Extension

Two other motions of the thigh at the hip joint are named. They are horizontal flexion (also known as horizontal adduction) and horizontal extension (also known as horizontal abduction) (see accompanying figures). Horizontal abduction is a posterior/lateral motion of the thigh at the hip joint when the thigh is already flexed to 90 degrees (**Fig. A**); horizontal adduction is an anterior/medial motion of the thigh at the hip joint when the thigh is already flexed to 90 degrees (**Fig. B**). Horizontal adduction is useful when stretching the musculature of the posterior pelvis.

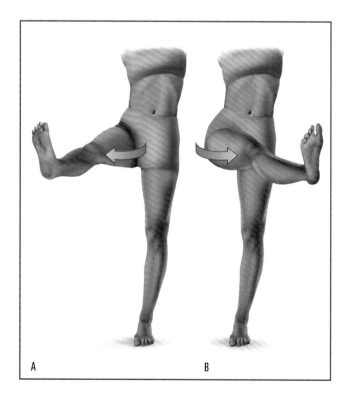

A   B

Motion of the Pelvis as a Unit Relative to the Lumbosacral Joint

The pelvis can also move relative to the trunk at the lumbosacral joint. These are the same named actions as when the pelvis moves at the hip joint: anterior and posterior tilt in the sagittal plane, elevation and depression in the frontal plane, and right rotation and left rotation in the transverse plane. Similar to pelvic motion being reverse actions of the thigh at the hip joint, pelvic actions can also be reverse actions of the trunk at the lumbosacral joint. When the inferior end of the body (the pelvis) is stabilized/fixed and the superior end of the body (the trunk) is free to move, the trunk moves at the lumbosacral joint (this could be looked at as open chain kinematics); when the superior end of the body (the trunk) is stabilized/fixed and the inferior end of the body (the pelvis) is free to move, the pelvis moves at the lumbosacral joint (this could be looked at as closed chain kinematics). Specifically, pelvic anterior tilt is the reverse action of trunk extension, pelvic posterior tilt is the reverse action of trunk flexion, elevation of the right side of the pelvis is the reverse action of trunk right lateral flexion, elevation of the left side of the pelvis is the reverse action of trunk left lateral flexion, pelvic rotation to the right is the reverse action of trunk rotation to the left, and pelvic rotation to the left is the reverse action of trunk rotation to the right (Fig. 1-13 and Table 1-3).

BOX 1.2

Pelvic Posture and the Spine

The base (superior surface) of the sacrum forms the base upon which the spine sits. Therefore, if the posture of the pelvis changes, the posture of the sacral base changes, and the posture of the spine changes. For this reason, pelvic posture is critically important to the posture of the spine, and it is important for the therapist to be aware of all muscular, ligamentous, and other fascial structures that can affect the posture of the pelvis. See Chapter 2 for more details.

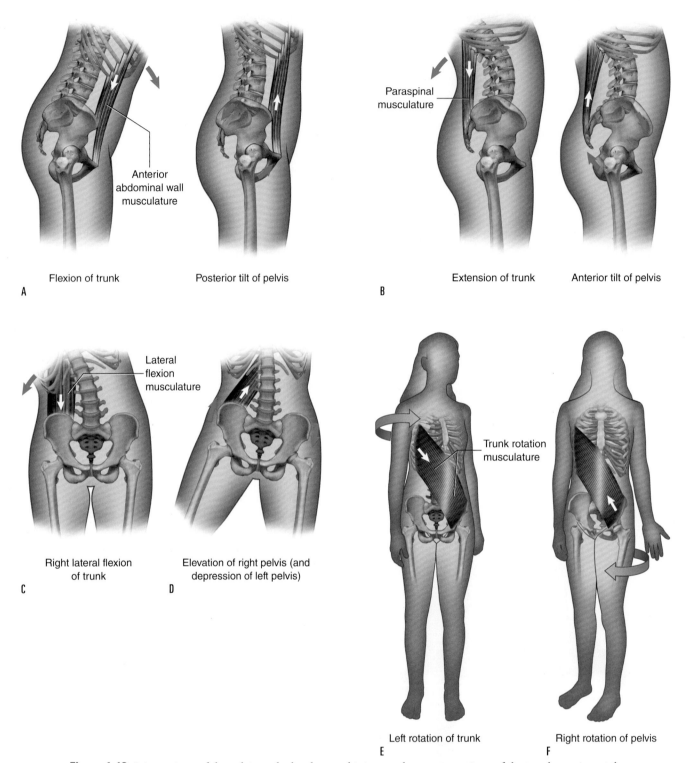

Figure 1-13 Joint actions of the pelvis at the lumbosacral joint are the reverse actions of the trunk moving at the lumbosacral joint. **(A, B)** Pelvic posterior tilt is the reverse action of trunk flexion; pelvic anterior tilt is the reverse action of trunk extension. **(C, D)** Pelvic right side elevation is the reverse action of trunk right lateral flexion (pelvic left side elevation is the reverse action of trunk left lateral flexion). **(E, F)** Pelvic right rotation is the reverse action of trunk left rotation (pelvic left rotation is the reverse action of trunk right rotation).

TABLE 1-3	Standard and Reverse Actions at the Lumbosacral Joint
Standard Open Chain Trunk Actions	**Reverse Closed Chain Pelvis Actions**
Extension	Anterior tilt
Flexion	Posterior tilt
Right lateral flexion	Right side elevation*
Left lateral flexion	Left side elevation*
Left rotation	Right rotation
Right rotation	Left rotation

*When one side of the pelvis elevates, the other side of the pelvis depresses.

Even though the pelvis can move at the hip joint(s) and the lumbosacral joint, pelvic motion at the hip joints is functionally more important, both from the standpoint of posture and motion.

Intrapelvic Motion

Motion can also occur within the pelvis; this is termed as **intrapelvic motion**. Intrapelvic motion involves motion of a pelvic bone relative to the sacrum or motion of the sacrum relative to the pelvic bone at the SIJ located between them (this also involves motion between the pelvic bones at the symphysis pubis joint anteriorly). These motions can be named for the sacral motion that occurs or for the motion of the pelvic bone.

When describing the sacral motion within the sagittal plane (or near sagittal plane), the terms **nutation** and **counternutation** are used. When the sacral base drops anteriorly, it is called nutation; when the sacral base moves in the posterior direction, it is called counternutation (Fig. 1-14). Nutation can also be described as anterior tilt; counternutation can also be described as posterior tilt.

When describing motion of the pelvic bone at the SIJ in the sagittal plane (or near sagittal plane), the terms *posterior tilt* and *anterior tilt* are used. In effect, posterior tilt of the pelvic bone is the reverse action of nutation of the sacrum at the SIJ, and anterior tilt of the pelvic bone is the reverse action of counternutation of the sacrum at the SIJ. The pelvic bone can also be described as moving in the transverse plane. The term *internal (or medial) rotation* describes the anterior surface of the pelvic bone orienting medially (in effect, toward the opposite side of the body). This motion gaps (opens) the posterior aspect of the SIJ (and approximates [closes] the anterior aspect of the SIJ). The term *external (or lateral) rotation* describes the anterior surface of the pelvic bone orienting more laterally (toward the same side of the body). This motion gaps the anterior aspect of the SIJ (and approximates the posterior aspect of the SIJ) (Fig. 1-15). In effect, intrapelvic motion involves one side of the pelvis moving relative to the other side. SIJ motions are small but are very important. An understanding of this motion is critically important when performing joint mobilization technique.

Figure 1-14 Right lateral view of nutation and counternutation of the sacrum. (**A**) Nutation. (**B**) Counternutation.

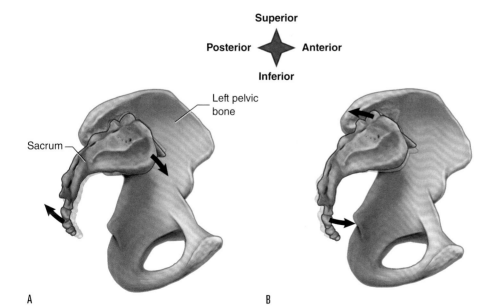

Superior

Posterior ◄✦► Anterior

Inferior

Left pelvic bone

Sacrum

A   B

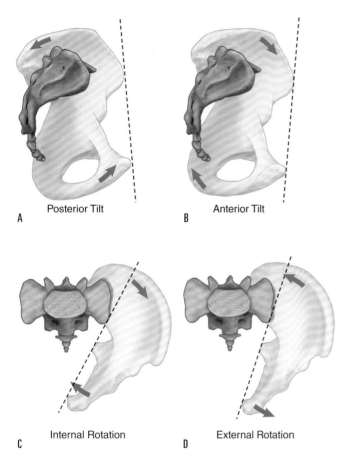

Figure 1-15 Motion of the pelvic bone at the SIJ. **(A, B)** Right lateral view of posterior tilt and anterior tilt, respectively. **(C, D)** Superior view of internal rotation and external rotation of the pelvic bone, respectively.

MUSCULATURE OF THE LUMBAR SPINE AND PELVIS

To perform clinical low back and pelvis treatment that is accurate and specific, the therapist needs to know the attachments and actions of the muscles of the region. For example, to know where to place the palpating hand when applying deep tissue work into the low back and pelvis, the manual therapist must know the attachments of the target muscle to be worked to be able to locate the target muscle accurately.

Furthermore, the therapist needs to know the target muscle's mover actions. Knowing the mover actions allows the therapist to ask the client to contract and engage the target muscle so that it palpably hardens. This hardening helps to distinguish the target muscle from the adjacent soft tissues, thereby alerting the therapist to its exact position and depth. Knowing a target muscle's mover actions is also important when stretching the client, regardless of the stretching technique that is employed. Stretching a muscle is accomplished by lengthening it, which involves doing the opposite of the muscle's mover actions. For example, if the target muscle is a trunk extensor, it is stretched by flexing the client's trunk; if the target muscle is an anterior tilter of the pelvis, it is stretched by posteriorly tilting the client's pelvis, and so on.

Before memorizing the detailed actions of each muscle of the trunk or pelvis, it is helpful first to visualize each muscle within its larger structural and functional groups. Figures 1-16 through 1-18 display the muscles of the trunk and pelvis.

Muscles of the Trunk

The muscles of the trunk can be divided into posterior and anterior groups. Although this division is not perfect (e.g., the external and internal abdominal oblique muscles of the anterior abdominal wall attach all the way around to the posterior abdominal wall), it is a good beginning framework. It is also helpful to view the muscles as being located either on the right side or the left side of the trunk. Therefore, for this book's purposes, the trunk muscles may be divided into four major structural groups, each in its own quadrant:

- Anterior right side
- Anterior left side
- Posterior right side
- Posterior left side

Viewing the muscles as part of these larger structural groups enhances the therapist's understanding of the *functional groups* of muscle movers. This is so because structural groups largely determine functional groups—that is, the structural location of a muscle largely determines its mover function of the trunk. There are six major functional groups of muscles of the trunk: flexors and extensors in the sagittal plane, right lateral flexors and left lateral flexors in the frontal plane, and right rotators and left rotators in the transverse plane (alternatively, their reverse pelvic actions could be named and considered instead; see Table 1-3).

Knowing the structural location of a muscle helps make it possible to understand its action and place it into its functional group for standard and reverse actions without having to memorize this information. For example, all muscles that cross the spinal joints anteriorly are flexors of the trunk at the spinal joints and posterior tilters of the pelvis at the lumbosacral joint. Similarly, all muscles that cross the spinal joints posteriorly are extensors of the trunk at the spinal joints and anterior tilters of the pelvis at the lumbosacral joint. Whether anterior or posterior, if the muscle is located to the right side of the trunk, it can right laterally flex the trunk at the spinal joints and elevate the pelvis on the right side (and consequently depress the pelvis on the left side). Similarly, muscles on the left side can left laterally flex the trunk and elevate the left side of the pelvis (and consequently depress the right side of the pelvis).

It is also important to know the rotation action of the target muscle when treating it. The rotation component of a muscle's actions is more challenging to visualize immediately because it is less dependent on the muscle's structural location, as noted in the previous paragraph. As with all muscles, the direction of the muscle's line of pull determines the muscle's action, and the direction of the muscle's fibers essentially determines the line of pull. Muscles that perform flexion, extension, right lateral flexion, and/or left lateral

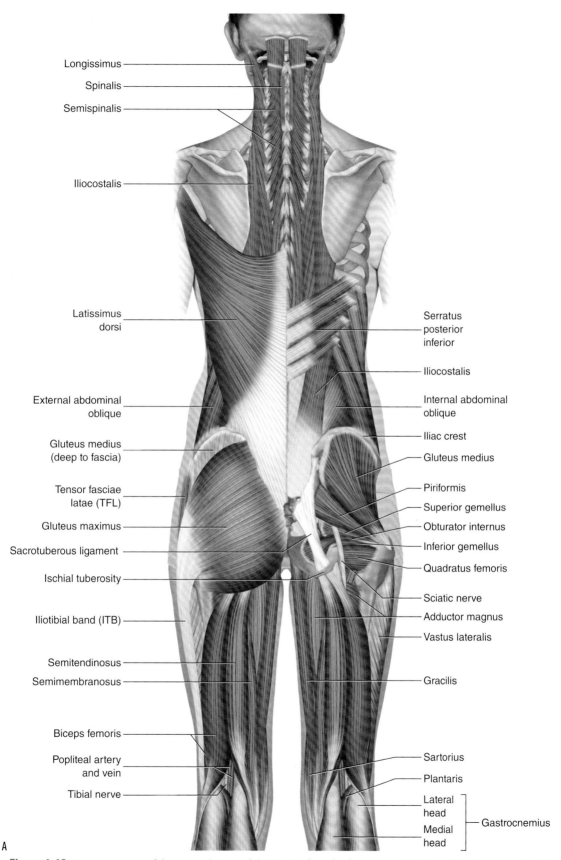

Longissimus

Spinalis

Semispinalis

Iliocostalis

Latissimus dorsi

External abdominal oblique

Gluteus medius (deep to fascia)

Tensor fasciae latae (TFL)

Gluteus maximus

Sacrotuberous ligament

Ischial tuberosity

Iliotibial band (ITB)

Semitendinosus

Semimembranosus

Biceps femoris

Popliteal artery and vein

Tibial nerve

Serratus posterior inferior

Iliocostalis

Internal abdominal oblique

Iliac crest

Gluteus medius

Piriformis

Superior gemellus

Obturator internus

Inferior gemellus

Quadratus femoris

Sciatic nerve

Adductor magnus

Vastus lateralis

Gracilis

Sartorius

Plantaris

Lateral head
Medial head
Gastrocnemius

A

Figure 1-16 Posterior view of the musculature of the low back and pelvis region. **(A)** Superficial view on the left with an intermediate view on the right. *(continued)*

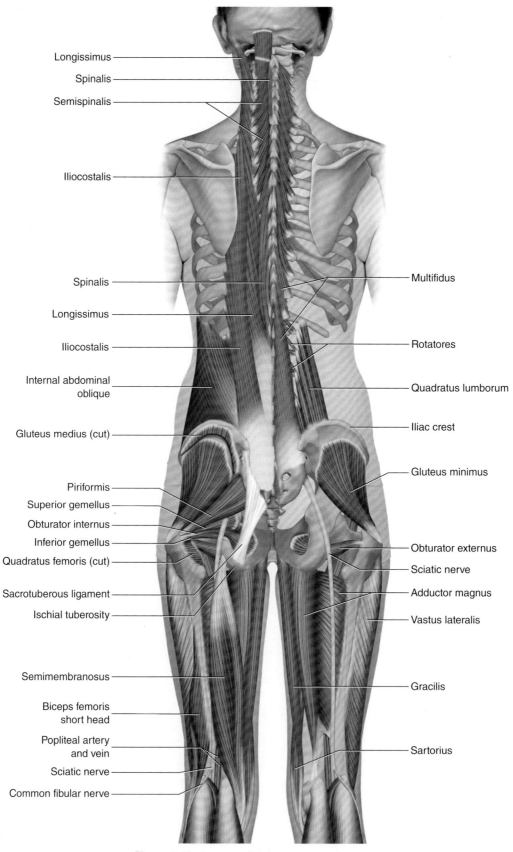

Longissimus

Spinalis

Semispinalis

Iliocostalis

Spinalis

Longissimus

Iliocostalis

Internal abdominal oblique

Gluteus medius (cut)

Piriformis

Superior gemellus

Obturator internus

Inferior gemellus

Quadratus femoris (cut)

Sacrotuberous ligament

Ischial tuberosity

Semimembranosus

Biceps femoris short head

Popliteal artery and vein

Sciatic nerve

Common fibular nerve

Multifidus

Rotatores

Quadratus lumborum

Iliac crest

Gluteus minimus

Obturator externus

Sciatic nerve

Adductor magnus

Vastus lateralis

Gracilis

Sartorius

B

Figure 1-16 *(continued)* **(B)** Deeper set of views.

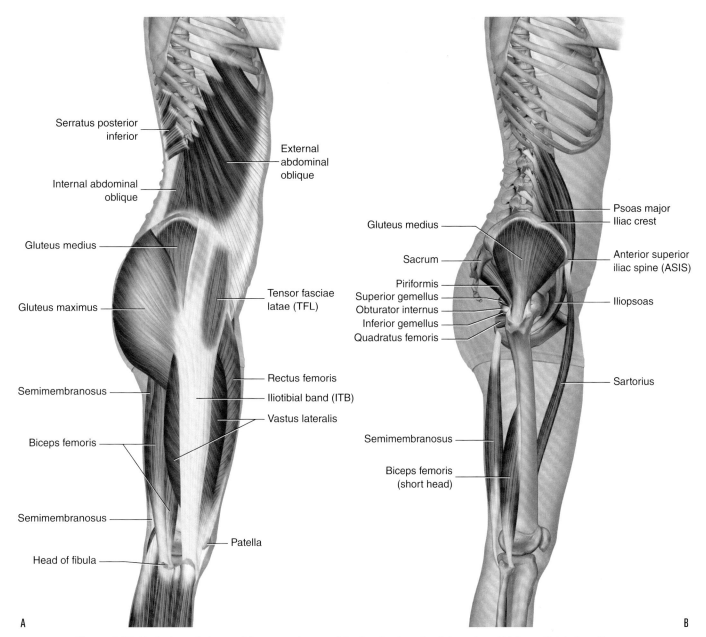

Figure 1-17 Right lateral views of the musculature of the low back and pelvis region. (**A**) Superficial view. Deeper view.

flexion must have a vertical component to their fiber direction. Muscles that perform right or left rotation must have a horizontal component to their fiber direction; in fact, it can be helpful to view them as partially "wrapping" horizontally around the trunk. Thus, considering the fiber direction of a trunk muscle is important when determining its rotational ability.

These six major functional groups are not mutually exclusive. A muscle can be a member of more than one functional group. For example, the right external abdominal oblique can flex, right laterally flex, and left (contralaterally) rotate the trunk at the spinal joints. Knowledge of the functional group actions of musculature is critically important when learning to perform multiplane stretching, which is presented in Chapter 6.

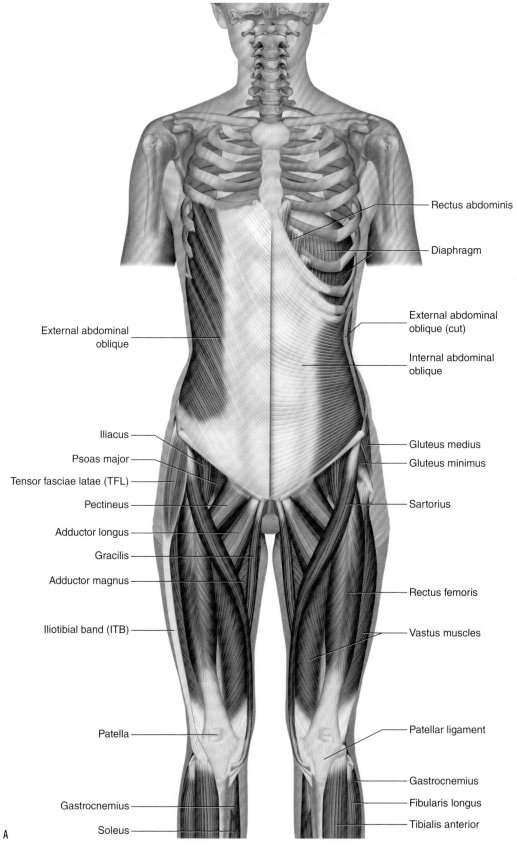

Figure 1-18 Anterior views of the musculature of the low back and pelvis region. **(A)** Superficial view on the right with an intermediate view on the left. *(continued)*

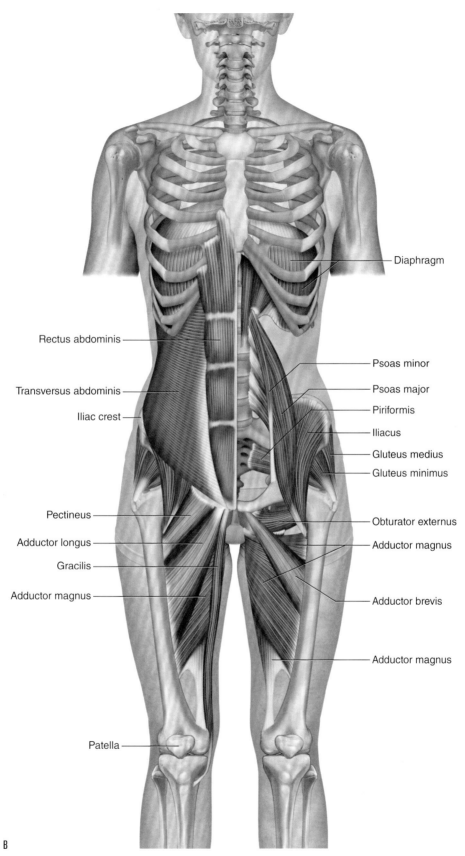

Figure 1-18 *(continued)* (**B**) Deeper set of views.

Figures 1-19 through 1-29 (in the following Attachments and Actions boxes) illustrate the individual muscles and muscle groups of the trunk along with their specific attachment and action information.

| 1.1 | **ATTACHMENTS AND ACTIONS** |

Erector Spinae Group

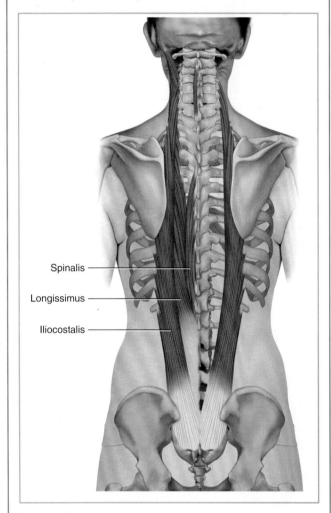

Figure 1-19 Posterior view of the erector spinae musculature of the low back. The erector spinae is composed of three subgroups: iliocostalis, longissimus, and spinalis. All three subgroups are shown on the left side; only the iliocostalis is shown on the right side.

■ The erector spinae in the trunk and pelvis attaches from the sacrum, medial iliac crest, vertebral transverse and spinous processes, and angles of ribs *to* angles of ribs and transverse and spinous processes of vertebrae above.

■ As a group, the erector spinae extends, laterally flexes, and ipsilatcrally rotates the trunk at the spinal joints. It also anteriorly tilts and contralaterally rotates the pelvis and elevates the same-side pelvis at the lumbosacral joint.

| 1.2 | **ATTACHMENTS AND ACTIONS** |

Transversospinalis Group

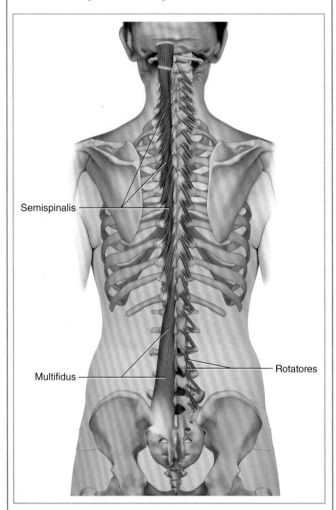

Figure 1-20 Posterior view of the transversospinalis musculature. The transversospinalis is composed of three groups: semispinalis, multifidus, and rotatores (the semispinalis does not attach into the lumbar spine). The multifidus and semispinalis are shown on the left side, and the rotatores are shown on the right side. *Note:* The multifidus is the largest muscle of the lumbar spine.

■ The multifidus and rotatores of the transversospinalis group in the trunk lie within the laminar groove of the lumbar and thoracic spine. The multifidus attaches from the sacrum and PSIS and the mammillary processes of the lumbar spine and transverse processes of the thoracic spine *to the* spinous processes of vertebral segments three to four levels superior to the inferior attachment. The rotatores attach from transverse processes of the lumbar and thoracic spine to vertebral segments one to two levels superior to the inferior attachment.

■ As a group, the transversospinalis extends, laterally flexes, and contralaterally rotates the trunk at the spinal joints. It also anteriorly tilts and ipsilaterally rotates the pelvis and elevates the same-side pelvis at the lumbosacral joint.

| **1.3** | **ATTACHMENTS AND ACTIONS** |

Quadratus Lumborum

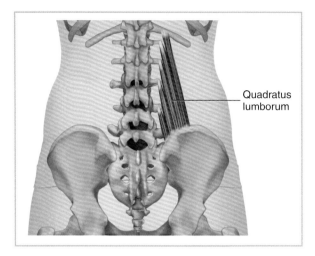

Figure 1-21 Posterior view of the right quadratus lumborum.

■ The quadratus lumborum attaches from the inferomedial border of the 12th rib and the transverse processes of L1-L4 *to the* posteromedial iliac crest.

■ The quadratus lumborum elevates the same-side pelvis and anteriorly tilts the pelvis at the lumbosacral joint and extends and laterally flexes the trunk at the spinal joints. It also depresses the 12th rib at the costovertebral joint.

| **1.4** | **ATTACHMENTS AND ACTIONS** |

Serratus Posterior Inferior

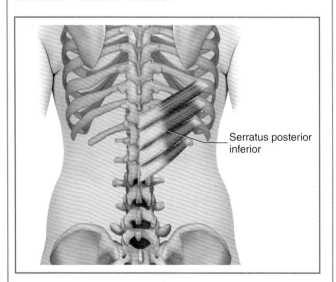

Figure 1-22 Posterior view of the right serratus posterior inferior.

■ The serratus posterior inferior attaches from the spinous processes of T11-L2 *to* ribs 9 through 12.

■ The serratus posterior inferior depresses ribs 9 through 12 at the sternocostal and costospinal joints.

| **1.5** | **ATTACHMENTS AND ACTIONS** |

Latissimus Dorsi

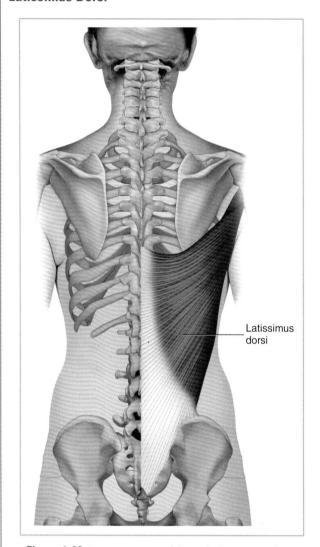

Figure 1-23 Posterior view of the right latissimus dorsi.

■ The latissimus dorsi attaches from the spinous processes of T7-L5, the posterior sacrum, and the posterior iliac crest (via the thoracolumbar fascia) *to the* lowest three or four ribs and the inferior angle of the scapula *to the* medial lip of the bicipital groove of the humerus.

■ The latissimus dorsi extends, medially rotates, and adducts the arm at the glenohumeral joint. It also anteriorly tilts the pelvis at the lumbosacral joint. Via its attachment to the scapula, it can also depress the scapula (shoulder girdle) at the scapulocostal joint.

1.6	**ATTACHMENTS AND ACTIONS**

Rectus Abdominis

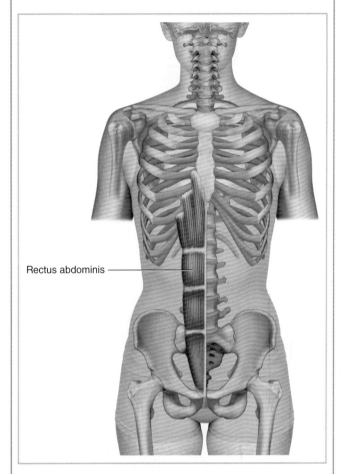

Figure 1-24 Anterior view of the right rectus abdominis.

- The rectus abdominis attaches from the crest and symphysis of the pubic bone *to the* xiphoid process of the sternum and the costal cartilages of ribs 5 through 7.
- The rectus abdominis flexes and laterally flexes the trunk at the spinal joints and posteriorly tilts the pelvis at the lumbosacral joint. The rectus abdominis also compresses the abdominal contents.

1.7	**ATTACHMENTS AND ACTIONS**

External Abdominal Oblique

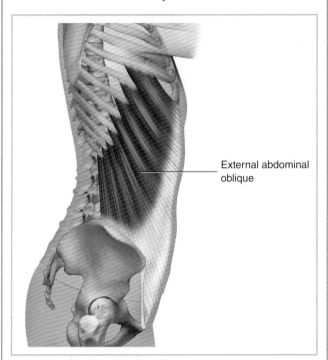

External abdominal oblique

Figure 1-25 Lateral view of the right external abdominal oblique.

- The external abdominal oblique attaches from the abdominal aponeurosis, pubic bone, inguinal ligament, and the anterior iliac crest *to the* lower eight ribs.
- The external abdominal oblique flexes, laterally flexes, and contralaterally rotates the trunk at the spinal joints. It also posteriorly tilts and ipsilaterally rotates the pelvis and elevates the same-side pelvis at the lumbosacral joint. The external abdominal oblique also compresses the abdominal contents.

1.8	**ATTACHMENTS AND ACTIONS**

Internal Abdominal Oblique

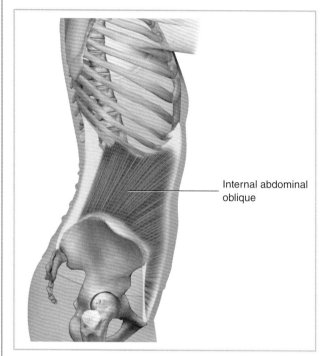

Internal abdominal oblique

Figure 1-26 Lateral view of the right internal abdominal oblique.

- The internal abdominal oblique attaches from the inguinal ligament, iliac crest, and thoracolumbar fascia *to the* lower three ribs and the abdominal aponeurosis.
- The internal abdominal oblique flexes, laterally flexes, and ipsilaterally rotates the trunk at the spinal joints. It also posteriorly tilts and contralaterally rotates the pelvis and elevates the same-side pelvis at the lumbosacral joint. The internal abdominal oblique also compresses the abdominal contents.

1.9	**ATTACHMENTS AND ACTIONS**

Transversus Abdominis

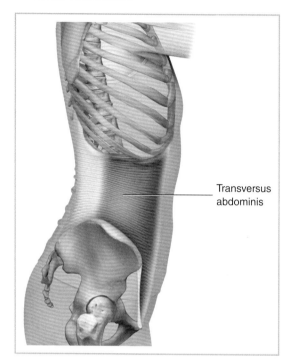

Transversus abdominis

Figure 1-27 Lateral view of the right transversus abdominis.

- The transversus abdominis attaches from the inguinal ligament, iliac crest, thoracolumbar fascia, and the costal cartilages of ribs 7 through 12 *to the* abdominal aponeurosis.
- The transversus abdominis compresses the abdominal contents.

1.10	ATTACHMENTS AND ACTIONS

Psoas Minor

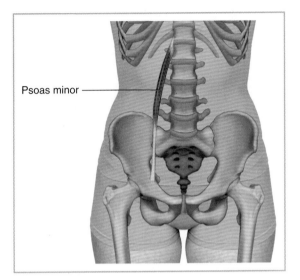

Figure 1-28 Anterior view of the right psoas minor.

- The psoas minor attaches from the anterolateral bodies of T12 and L1 *to the* pelvic bone.
- The psoas minor flexes the trunk at the spinal joints and posteriorly tilts the pelvis at the lumbosacral joint.

1.11	ATTACHMENTS AND ACTIONS

Diaphragm

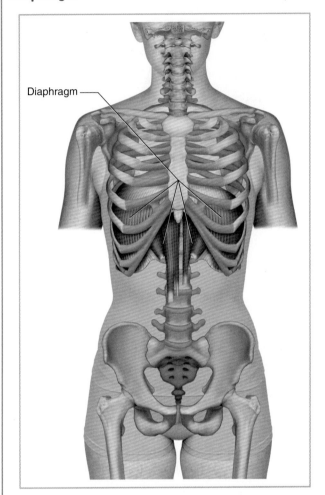

Figure 1-29 Anterior view of the diaphragm.

- The diaphragm attaches to the internal surfaces of the sternum, the lower six ribs and their costal cartilages, and L1-L3.
- The diaphragm increases the volume of the thoracic cavity by its central dome dropping down and/or by pulling the rib cage attachment up.

Muscles of the Pelvis

Similar to learning the muscles of the trunk, it can be helpful to first look at the functional groups of muscles of the pelvis when learning or reviewing them. Before doing that, it is important to first place muscles of the pelvis into their three major categories. They are

- Muscles that attach from the pelvis to the trunk and cross the lumbosacral joint
- Muscles that attach from the pelvis to the thigh/leg and cross the hip joint
- Pelvic floor muscles that are located wholly within the pelvis

Pelvic Muscles that Cross the Lumbosacral Joint and Attach onto the Trunk

Muscles of the pelvis that cross the lumbosacral joint to attach onto the trunk were described in the previous section on "Muscles of the Trunk." Their reverse action pelvic motions occur when their superior trunk attachment is fixed, and the pelvic attachment moves instead. Given that they are the same trunk muscle groups simply looked at from the perspective of their pelvic action, they can also be divided into the same four quadrants. The anterior muscles posteriorly tilt the pelvis, the posterior muscles anteriorly tilt the pelvis, the muscles on the right side elevate the right side of the pelvis (and therefore depress the left side of the pelvis), and the muscles on the left side elevate the left side of the pelvis (and therefore depress the right side of the pelvis).

As with the discussion of these muscles from the perspective of the trunk, understanding pelvic rotation motions by these muscles requires visualizing the horizontal component to the fiber direction of the muscles. Alternately, you simply realize that because these are reverse actions, if a muscle rotates the trunk in one direction, it must rotate the pelvis in the opposite (reverse) direction. See Table 1-3 for more information on this.

Pelvic Muscles that Cross the Hip Joint and Attach onto the Thigh/Leg

Muscles that cross the hip joint are usually thought of with respect to their open chain motion of the thigh relative to the pelvis at the hip joint. As such, you can also divide the musculature that moves the thigh at the hip joint into quadrants. The flexors are located anteriorly, extensors posteriorly, abductors laterally, and adductors medially. Rotation musculature is not as easily equated with location; however, as a general rule, lateral rotators are located posteriorly and medial rotators are located anteriorly. However, looking at these muscles' open chain actions on the thigh is not as important as understanding their closed chain actions on the pelvis. This is crucially important because the foot is so often on the ground, causing closed chain kinematic pelvic motion.

Posture and motion of the pelvis then have repercussions on spinal posture and motion (see Chapter 2). See Table 1-2 for more information on the standard/reverse actions of the thigh and pelvis at the hip joint for these muscles. Following are hip joint muscles of the pelvis.

Figures 1-30 through 1-39 (in the following Attachments and Actions boxes) illustrate the individual muscles and muscle groups of the pelvis at the hip joint along with their specific attachment and action information.

1.12 ATTACHMENTS AND ACTIONS

Tensor Fasciae Latae

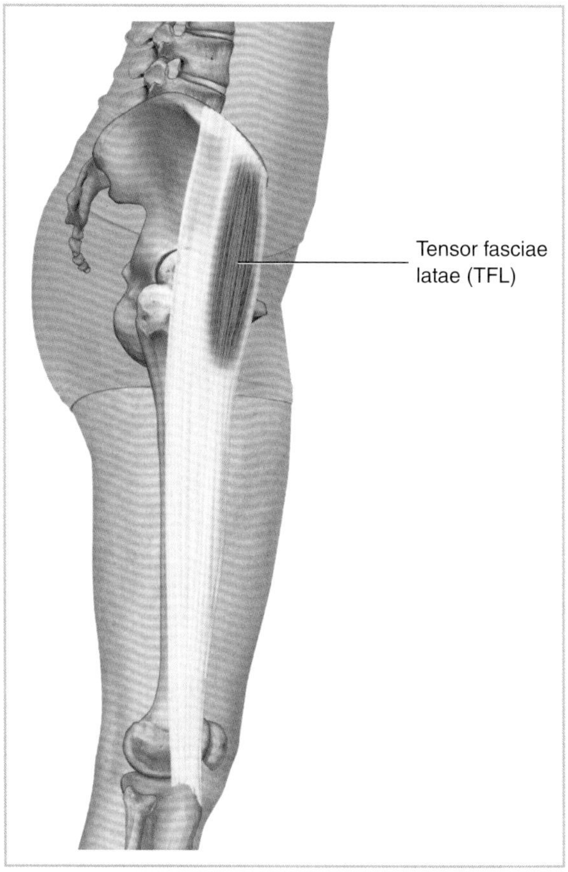

Tensor fasciae latae (TFL)

Figure 1-30 Lateral view of the right TFL.

- The tensor fasciae latae (TFL) attaches from the ASIS and anterior iliac crest *to the* iliotibial band (ITB), one-third of the way down the thigh.
- The TFL flexes, abducts, and medially rotates the thigh at the hip joint and anteriorly tilts and depresses the same-side pelvis at the hip joint.

1.13	**ATTACHMENTS AND ACTIONS**

Rectus Femoris

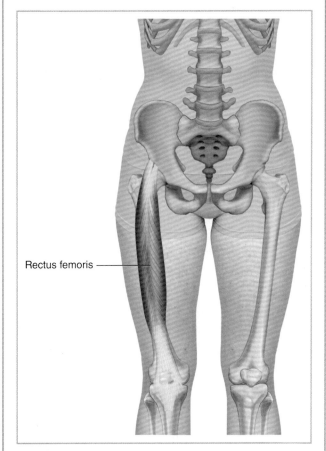

Figure 1-31 Anterior view of the right rectus femoris of the quadriceps femoris group.

- The rectus femoris of the quadriceps femoris group attaches from the AIIS *to the* patella and then onto the tibial tuberosity via the patella ligament.
- The rectus femoris flexes the thigh at the hip joint and anteriorly tilts the pelvis at the hip joint. It also extends the leg (and/or thigh) at the knee joint.

1.14	**ATTACHMENTS AND ACTIONS**

Sartorius

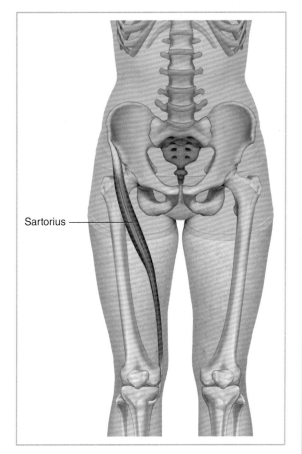

Figure 1-32 Anterior view of the right sartorius.

- The sartorius attaches from the ASIS *to the* pes anserine tendon at the proximal anteromedial tibia.
- The sartorius flexes, abducts, and laterally rotates the thigh at the hip joint and anteriorly tilts the pelvis and depresses the same-side pelvis at the hip joint. It also flexes the leg (and/or thigh) at the knee joint.

| 1.15 | **ATTACHMENTS AND ACTIONS** |

Iliopsoas

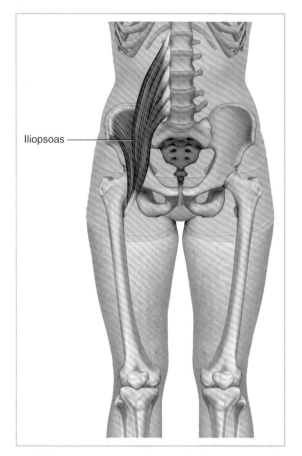

Figure 1-33 Anterior view of the right iliopsoas muscle. The iliopsoas is composed of the iliacus and psoas major muscles.

- The psoas major of the iliopsoas attaches from the anterolateral bodies and discs of T12-L5 and transverse processes of L1-L5 *to the* lesser trochanter of the femur. The iliacus of the iliopsoas attaches from the internal surface of the ilium *to the* lesser trochanter of the femur.
- Both the psoas major and iliacus flex and laterally rotate the thigh at the hip joint and anteriorly tilt the pelvis at the hip joint. The psoas major also flexes, laterally flexes, and contralaterally rotates the trunk at the spinal joints.

| 1.16 | **ATTACHMENTS AND ACTIONS** |

Adductor Group

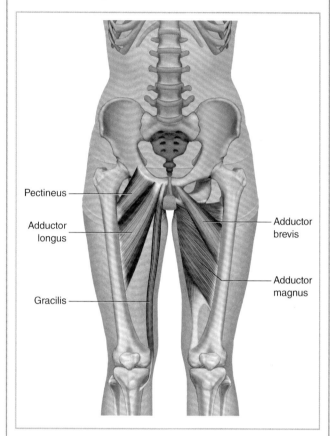

Figure 1-34 Anterior view of the adductor group. The adductor group is composed of the pectineus, adductor longus, adductor brevis, adductor magnus, and gracilis. The pectineus, adductor longus, and gracilis are shown on the client's right side (left side of figure); the adductor brevis and adductor magnus are shown on the client's left side (right side of figure).

- The adductor group attaches from the pubic bone and ischium *to the* linea aspera, pectineal line, adductor tubercle of the femur, and the pes anserine tendon at the proximal anteromedial tibia.
- As a group, the adductors adduct, flex, and medially rotate the thigh at the hip joint and anteriorly tilt and ipsilaterally rotate (and elevate the same-side) pelvis at the hip joint. The gracilis can also flex the leg (and/or thigh) at the knee joint. The adductor magnus extends the thigh and posteriorly tilts the pelvis at the hip joint.

1.17	**ATTACHMENTS AND ACTIONS**

Hamstring Group

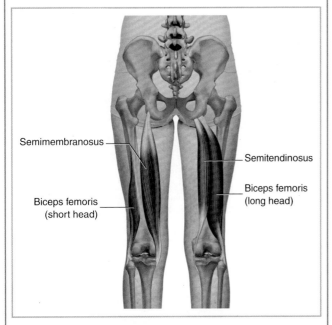

Figure 1-35 Posterior view of the hamstring group. The hamstring group is composed of the semitendinosus and semimembranosus medially and the biceps femoris laterally. The semitendinosus and long head of the biceps femoris are shown on the right side; the deeper semimembranosus and short head of the biceps femoris are shown on the left side.

- The biceps femoris attaches from the ischial tuberosity (long head) and linea aspera of the femur (short head) *to the* head of the fibula. The semitendinosus attaches from the ischial tuberosity *to the* pes anserine tendon at the proximal anteromedial tibia. The semimembranosus attaches from the ischial tuberosity *to the* posterior surface of the medial condyle of the tibia.
- As a group, the hamstrings extend the thigh and posteriorly tilt the pelvis at the hip joint. They also flex the leg (and/or thigh) at the knee joint. (*Note:* The short head of the biceps femoris does not cross the hip joint and therefore has no action at that joint.)

1.18	**ATTACHMENTS AND ACTIONS**

Gluteus Maximus

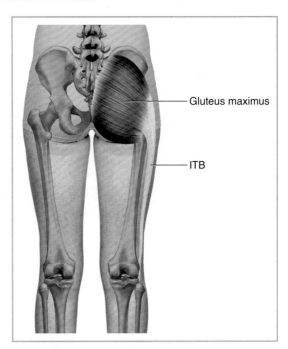

Figure 1-36 Posterior view of the right gluteus maximus. *ITB,* iliotibial band.

- The gluteus maximus attaches from the posterior iliac crest, posterolateral sacrum, and coccyx *to the* gluteal tuberosity and ITB.
- The gluteus maximus extends, laterally rotates, abducts (upper fibers), and adducts (lower fibers) the thigh at the hip joint. It also posteriorly tilts and contralaterally rotates the pelvis at the hip joint.

1.19   ATTACHMENTS AND ACTIONS

Gluteus Medius

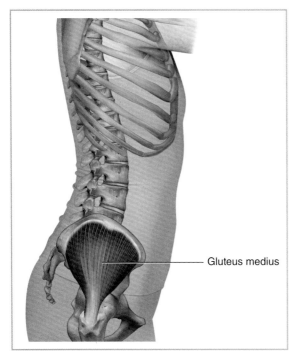

Figure 1-37 Lateral view of the right gluteus medius.

- The gluteus medius attaches from the external ilium *to the* greater trochanter of the femur.
- The entire gluteus medius abducts the thigh at the hip joint and depresses the same-side pelvis at the hip joint. The anterior fibers also flex and medially rotate the thigh and anteriorly tilt and ipsilaterally rotate the pelvis at the hip joint; the posterior fibers also extend and laterally rotate the thigh and posteriorly tilt and contralaterally rotate the pelvis at the hip joint.

1.20   ATTACHMENTS AND ACTIONS

Gluteus Minimus

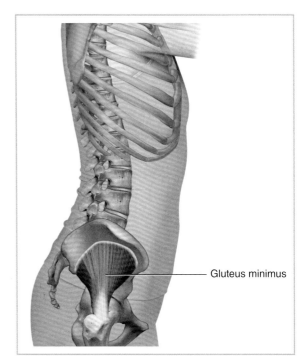

Figure 1-38 Lateral view of the right gluteus minimus.

- The gluteus minimus attaches from the external ilium *to the* greater trochanter of the femur (*Note*: The gluteus minimus is located deep to the gluteus medius).
- The entire gluteus minimus abducts the thigh at the hip joint and depresses the same-side pelvis at the hip joint. The anterior fibers also flex and medially rotate the thigh and anteriorly tilt and ipsilaterally rotate the pelvis at the hip joint; the posterior fibers also extend and laterally rotate the thigh and posteriorly tilt and contralaterally rotate the pelvis at the hip joint.

1.21   ATTACHMENTS AND ACTIONS

Deep Lateral Rotator Group

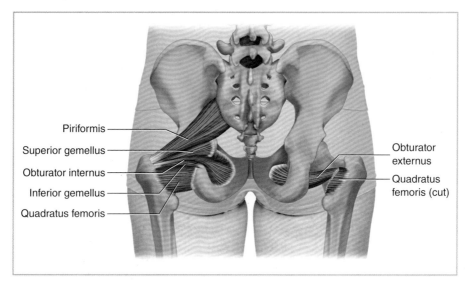

Figure 1-39 Posterior view of the deep lateral rotator group. All muscles of the group are drawn on the left side (the obturator externus is not seen). The quadratus femoris has been cut on the right side to visualize the obturator externus.

- The deep lateral rotator group attaches from the sacrum (piriformis) and the pelvic bone (the rest of the group) *to the* (or nearby the) greater trochanter of the femur.
- As a group, the deep lateral rotators laterally rotate the thigh at the hip joint and contralaterally rotate the pelvis at the hip joint. If the thigh is first flexed to 90 degrees, the deep lateral rotators can horizontally extend (horizontally abduct) the thigh at the hip joint. *Note*: If the thigh is first flexed (approximately 60 degrees or more), the piriformis changes to become a medial rotator of the thigh at the hip joint instead of a lateral rotator.

BOX 1.3

Femoropelvic Rhythm

The term **femoropelvic rhythm** is used to describe the coordinated rhythm to how the femur and pelvis move. For example, when flexing the thigh at the hip joint to lift the foot up into the air anteriorly, the brain usually co-orders the pelvis to drop into posterior tilt because this facilitates bringing the foot even higher. Therefore, by femoropelvic rhythm, thigh flexion couples with pelvic posterior tilt. Similarly, thigh extension couples with pelvic anterior tilt. (*Note*: Femoropelvic rhythm is not the same as reverse actions at the hip joint. For example, the reverse action of thigh flexion at the hip joint is anterior pelvic tilt [not posterior pelvic tilt as with femoropelvic rhythm] at the hip joint).

Pelvic Floor Muscles Wholly Located Within the Pelvis

Muscles of the pelvic floor do not cross from the pelvis to another body part; therefore, they do not move the pelvis as a unit relative to the trunk or thighs. Rather, their function is primarily to stabilize the sacroiliac and symphysis pubis joints as well as to create a stable floor for the visceral contents of the abdominopelvic cavity.

Figure 1-40 (in the following Attachments and Actions boxes) illustrates the muscles of the pelvic floor along with their specific attachment and action information. Pelvic floor work is often performed intrarectally or intravaginally and is therefore usually beyond the scope of practice for most manual therapists. However, some pelvic floor musculature (coccygeus and levator ani) are partially accessible from the outside, inferior to the piriformis.

1.22   **ATTACHMENTS AND ACTIONS**

Pelvic Floor Musculature

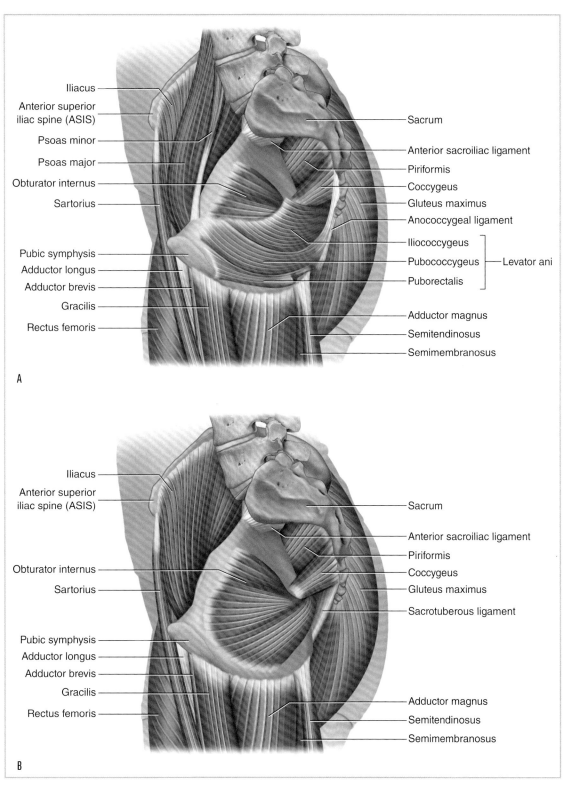

Figure 1-40 The muscles of the pelvic floor. (**A, B**) Medial views of the right side of the pelvis. (**A**) Superficial. (**B**) Deep. *(continued)*

1.22 **ATTACHMENTS AND ACTIONS** *(continued)*

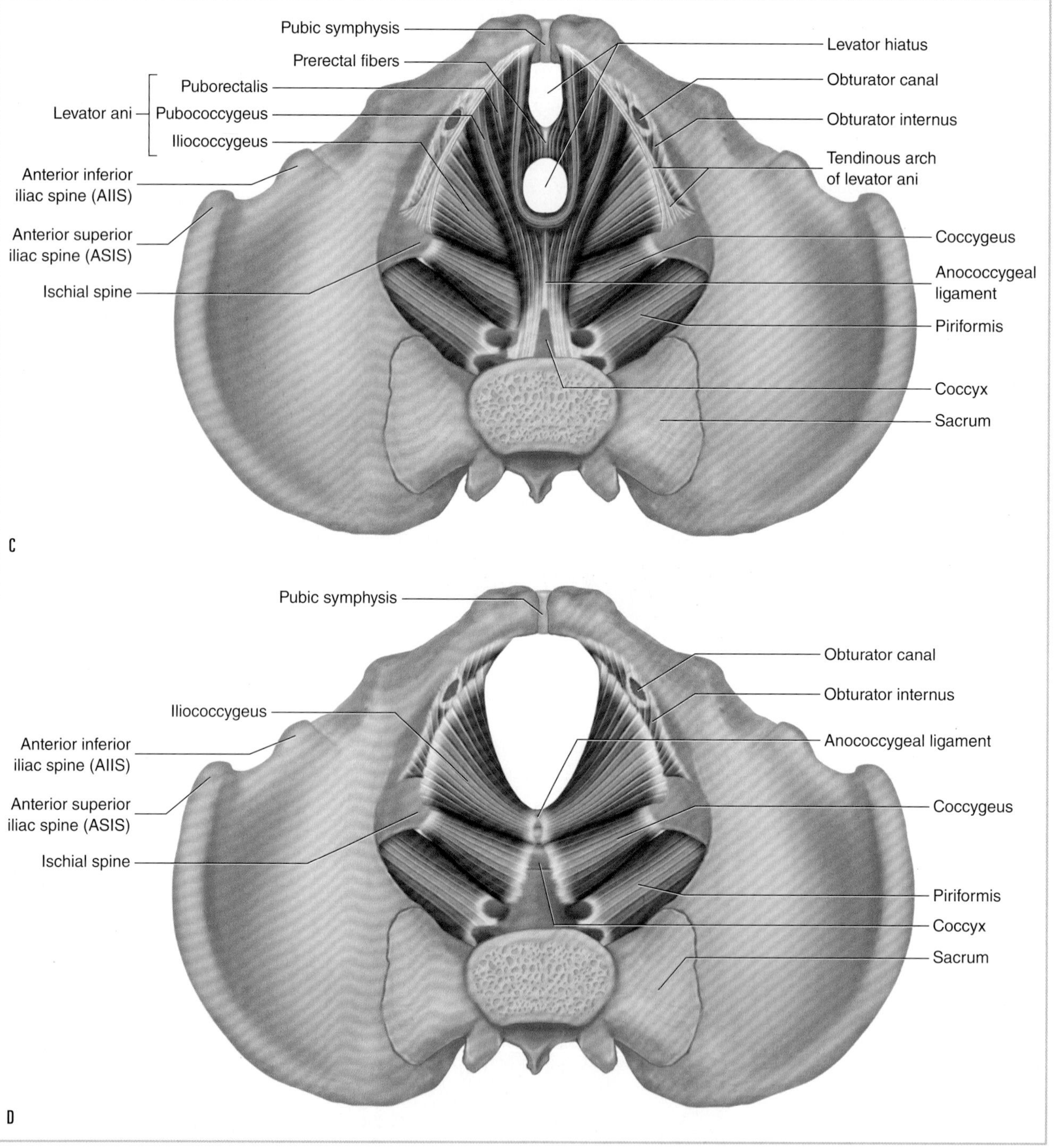

Pubic symphysis

Prerectal fibers

Levator ani
— Puborectalis
— Pubococcygeus
— Iliococcygeus

Anterior inferior iliac spine (AIIS)

Anterior superior iliac spine (ASIS)

Ischial spine

Levator hiatus

Obturator canal

Obturator internus

Tendinous arch of levator ani

Coccygeus

Anococcygeal ligament

Piriformis

Coccyx

Sacrum

C

Pubic symphysis

Iliococcygeus

Anterior inferior iliac spine (AIIS)

Anterior superior iliac spine (ASIS)

Ischial spine

Obturator canal

Obturator internus

Anococcygeal ligament

Coccygeus

Piriformis

Coccyx

Sacrum

D

Figure 1-40 *(continued)* **(C, D)** Superior views of the muscles of the female pelvic floor. **(C)** Superficial. **(D)** Deep.

LIGAMENTS OF THE LUMBAR SPINE AND PELVIS

As with the muscles, it is also helpful to know the ligaments of the lumbar spine and pelvis to be able to effectively stretch the client. Whatever technique is used, the purpose of stretching is to loosen all soft tissues that are taut and restricting joint motion. Even though the function of a ligament is to stabilize and limit motion of the bones to which it attaches, a taut ligament can be just as culpable as a tight muscle in excessively restricting the motion of a joint. Therefore, when a client presents with a tight low back, a basic knowledge of the ligaments of the lumbar spine and pelvis is valuable.

The "action" of a ligament is similar to that of an antagonist muscle. If an antagonist muscle is tight, it restricts motion that is opposite that of its mover action(s). For example, if a trunk extensor (located posteriorly) is tight, it restricts motion of the trunk anteriorly into flexion. Because the limited motion is usually to the side of the body opposite the side on which the muscle is located, antagonist muscles are sometimes called **contralateral muscles**; *contralateral* literally means *opposite side*. Similarly, ligaments tend to be located contralaterally, on the other side of the joint from the motion that they limit. For example, if the trunk resists moving into flexion, the taut ligaments that would restrict this motion are located posteriorly (where antagonist trunk extensor muscles are located). If the motion that is limited is right lateral flexion of the trunk, the taut ligaments limiting this motion would be located in the left side of the trunk (where antagonist left lateral flexor muscles are located) (Fig. 1-41).

As is typically the case, rotation is a bit trickier. Just as muscles that perform rotation may be on either side of the body in relation to the rotation they create, ligaments that restrict right or left rotation can also be located on either side of the body. Similar to musculature, determining a ligament's role in restricting rotation can best be seen by looking at how the ligament (partially) "wraps" around the body part in the transverse plane.

Ligaments of the Lumbar Spine

The major ligaments of the lumbar spine are shown in Figure 1-42. The **supraspinous ligament, interspinous ligaments**, fibrous capsules of the facet joints (which are ligamentous in structure and therefore also function to limit motion), **ligamentum flavum**, and **posterior longitudinal ligament** are all located posterior to the axis of motion for flexion and extension of the spine; therefore, they all limit flexion. The **anterior longitudinal ligament** is located anterior to the axis of motion for flexion and extension of the spine; therefore, it limits extension. The **intertransverse ligaments** are located laterally. They limit lateral flexion to the opposite side of the body (contralateral lateral flexion) from where they are located. Many of these ligaments also act to limit rotation of the lumbar spine to one side or the other.

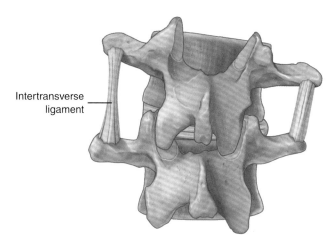

Figure 1-41 Ligament function. Posterior view of two vertebrae that illustrates how a ligament becomes taut and limits motion of the bones of a joint in the direction opposite the ligament's location. In this example, when the superior vertebra right laterally flexes, the intertransverse ligament located on the left side becomes taut and limits this motion. (Courtesy of Joseph E. Muscolino.)

Ligaments of the Pelvis

The bones of the pelvic girdle are well supplied with ligaments for stabilization (Fig. 1-43). Most lumbar spinal ligaments continue down to connect the lumbar spine to the sacrum and pelvic bones. The **iliolumbar ligaments** can be viewed as extensions of the intertransverse ligaments between L4 and the pelvis and L5 and the pelvis. Within the pelvis itself, copious ligaments provide stabilization to the SIJ, both posteriorly and anteriorly. Besides the **posterior sacroiliac ligaments** and **anterior sacroiliac ligaments** that attach directly from the sacrum to the pelvic bone on each side, note the strong and powerful **sacrotuberous ligament** and **sacrospinous ligament** posteriorly.

Ligaments of the Hip Joint

Connecting the pelvic bone to the femur on each side are the ligaments of the hip joint. The fibrous capsule of the hip joint is reinforced by three capsular ligaments: the **iliofemoral ligament** anteriorly, the **ischiofemoral ligament** posteriorly, and the **pubofemoral ligament** medially (Fig. 1-44). The iliofemoral ligament primarily limits extension of the thigh and posterior tilt of the pelvis at the hip joint. The ischiofemoral ligament, due to its horizontal wrapping around the joint, primarily limits medial rotation of the thigh and ipsilateral rotation of the pelvis at the hip joint. The pubofemoral ligament primarily limits abduction of the thigh and depression (lateral tilt) of the same-side pelvis at the hip joint. The joint capsule is reinforced near the neck of the femur; this area is termed the **zona orbicularis**. Internal within the joint is the **ligamentum teres** that connects the head of the femur to the acetabulum and limits axial distraction (traction) of the joint (see Fig. 1-44).

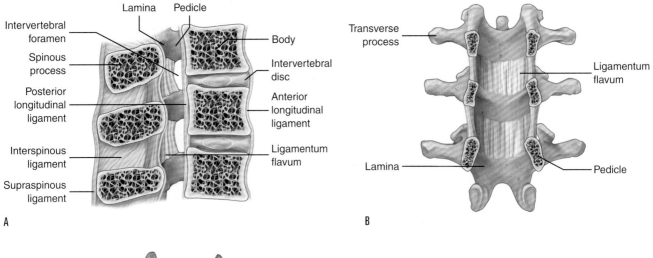

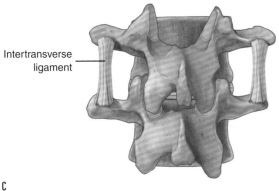

Figure 1-42 Ligaments of the spine. (**A**) Right lateral view of a sagittal plane cross section through the spine. (**B**) Anterior view of a frontal plane section through the pedicles of the spine in which the ligamentum flavum inside the spinal canal can be seen. (**C**) Posterior view depicting the intertransverse ligaments. (Courtesy of Joseph E. Muscolino.)

BOX 1.4

Thoracolumbar Fascia and Abdominal Aponeurosis

In addition to the fibrous fascial ligaments and joint capsules of the lumbosacral and sacroiliac region, further stabilization is provided by the **thoracolumbar fascia** posteriorly and the **abdominal aponeurosis** anteriorly. The thoracolumbar fascia is well developed in the lumbar region where it divides to form three layers: a posterior layer superficially, a middle layer between the erector spinae and transversospinalis musculature and the quadratus lumborum, and a deep anterior layer between the quadratus lumborum and psoas major (**see Figs. A and B**). The abdominal aponeurosis is created by the anterior aponeuroses of the external and internal abdominal obliques (EAO and IAO) and transversus abdominis (TA) muscles and forms a sheath around the rectus abdominis musculature (**see Figs. C and D**). (*Note*: The abdominal aponeurosis does not totally ensheathe the rectus abdominis at its inferior end, as seen in the lower figure of D.)

continued

BOX 1.4 *(continued)*

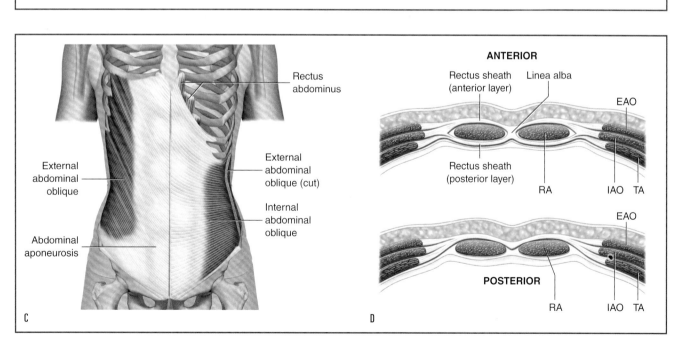

Thoracolumbar fascia. (**A**) Posterior view. (**B**) Transverse plane cross-section view. Abdominal aponeurosis. (**C**) Anterior view. (**D**) Transverse plane cross-section views. Upper figure: upper trunk. Lower figure: lower trunk. EAO, external abdominal oblique; IAO, internal abdominal oblique; SP, spinous process; TA, transversus abdominis; TP, transverse process.

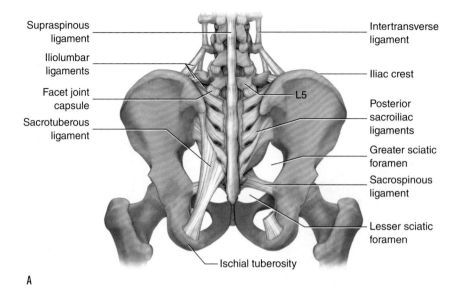

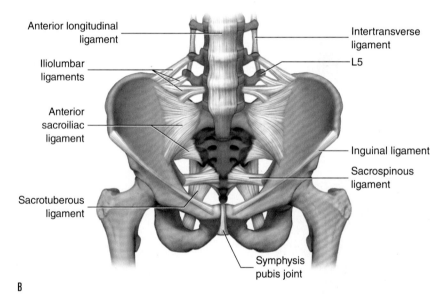

Figure 1-43 Ligaments of the pelvis. The SIJ is well stabilized posteriorly and anteriorly by ligaments. **(A)** Posterior view. **(B)** Anterior view.

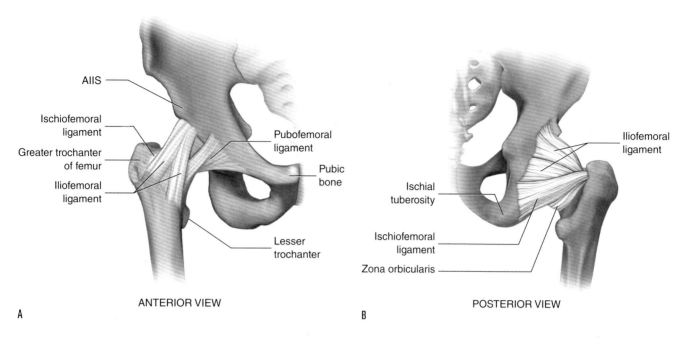

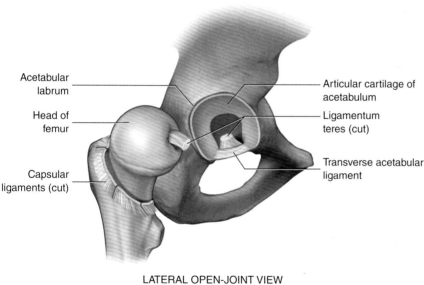

Figure 1-44 Ligaments of the hip joint. (**A**) Anterior view. (**B**) Posterior view. (**C**) Lateral open-joint view. *AIIS,* anterior inferior iliac spine. ([**C**] Modeled from Neumann DA. *Kinesiology of the Musculoskeletal System: Foundations for Physical Rehabilitation.* 2nd ed. St. Louis, MO: Mosby Elsevier; 2010.)

PRECAUTIONS

The low back and pelvic region contains a number of neurovascular structures (nerves, arteries, and veins) whose locations are important to know because they contraindicate deep pressure. These structures are located both anteriorly and posteriorly (Fig. 1-45). However, even though caution is called for in the vicinity of these structures, it should not prevent therapeutic work entirely. A good guideline when working near any neurovascular structure is to begin with light to medium pressure before transitioning to deeper pressure. Knowledge of the anatomy of the region can allow work to be performed therapeutically and safely. Chapter 3 discusses other cautions and contraindications for specific pathologic conditions.

Anterior Structures: Abdominal Aorta

The **abdominal aorta** is located within the abdominal cavity, running along the midline of the anterior surfaces of the vertebral bodies and discs (see Fig. 1-45A). Because it is

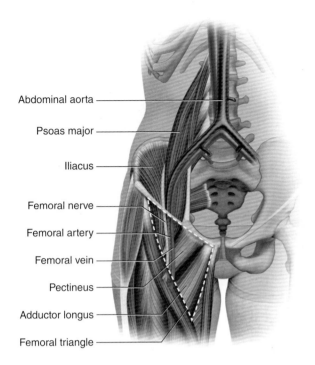

Abdominal aorta

Psoas major

Iliacus

Femoral nerve

Femoral artery

Femoral vein

Pectineus

Adductor longus

Femoral triangle

A

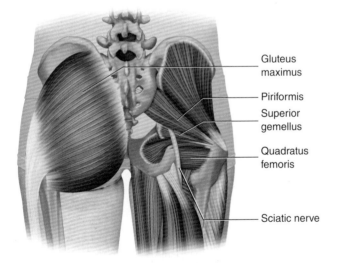

Gluteus maximus

Piriformis

Superior gemellus

Quadratus femoris

Sciatic nerve

B

Figure 1-45 Neurovascular structures of the low back and pelvis. **(A)** Anterior view showing the abdominal aorta and the femoral triangle containing the femoral nerve, artery, and vein. **(B)** Posterior view showing the sciatic nerve.

located so deeply, it is rarely accessed. However, pressure can be placed upon it if the therapist is working the belly of the psoas major within the abdomen and is working slightly too medially. For this reason, when palpating for and working the psoas major, it is important to be mindful of the location of the aorta and to make sure that no pressure is being placed upon it. It is usually easy to know when the fingers are pressing on the aorta, or any artery for that matter, because a pulse can be felt. If a pulse is felt, move laterally off the aorta.

Anterior Structures: Femoral Triangle

The **femoral triangle** is the name given to the region in the proximal anterior thigh; immediately distal to the inguinal ligament; and overlying the adductor longus, pectineus, and iliopsoas muscles. Within the femoral triangle are the **femoral nerve**, **femoral artery**, and **femoral vein** (see Fig. 1-45A). It is important to be mindful of these structures when work is being done to the proximal attachments of the hip flexor and adductor musculature. If a pulse is felt, you are on the femoral artery. It is not necessary to stop working. Instead, either slightly move your palpating fingers or try to gently displace the vessel to one side or the other and continue working in that spot. When first applying pressure in this region, be sure to begin with lighter pressure because deep pressure could compress the artery and block its blood circulation, thereby blocking palpation of its pulse as well.

If pressure is applied in this region and the client feels a sharp pain that shoots into the anterior thigh, then it is likely that the femoral nerve is being compressed. As with the femoral artery, either slightly move your palpating fingers or try to gently displace the nerve by accessing from one side or the other and continue working in that spot.

Posterior Structures: Sciatic Nerve

The **sciatic nerve** is the largest nerve in the human body; it is approximately a quarter inch in diameter. It emerges in the gluteal region between the piriformis and superior gemellus muscles (although variations are common in which part or all of the nerve emerges through or superior to the piriformis) (see Fig. 1-45B). It then runs superficial to the rest of the deep lateral rotator muscles (and deep to the gluteus maximus) in

---

1.1   THERAPIST TIP

Gluteal Work and Referral Symptoms

Pain or other referral symptoms experienced into the lower extremity when applying pressure to the gluteal region can result from pressure directly on the sciatic nerve. However, pressure to the gluteal region in the vicinity of the sciatic nerve can also refer symptoms into the lower extremity because of trigger point (TrP) referral. Therefore, it can be difficult to be certain of the cause of the referral. Referral caused by direct nerve pressure tends to feel like a shooting pain; however, this is not always the case. Consulting a TrP referral illustration may help (see Chapter 2 for illustrations of TrPs and their referral zones). If your client's pain falls within the typical TrP referral pattern, it is more likely that the pain is a TrP referral, but this is not definite. If the referral does not coincide with the typical TrP referral pattern, then you are most likely pressing directly on the sciatic nerve and should move your pressure slightly so as to remove pressure from the nerve. When in doubt, it is always wise to be cautious and change the location of your pressure.

1.2   THERAPIST TIP

Working with the Client Prone

Many clients have a difficult time spending long periods of time lying prone because this position causes the lumbar spine to be unsupported, placing stress upon the posterior musculature and ligaments. This can be true for anyone, but is especially true if the client is experiencing an acute condition of the low back. This is ironic and unfortunate because the soft tissue work necessary to help alleviate a low back problem is best done with the client prone. When confronted with this circumstance, the therapist has three choices:

- Limit the time that the client spends prone.
- Place a small roll under the client's lumbosacral area.
- Work with the client side-lying instead (and place a small pillow between the client's thighs/knees.

Also of value is to have the client stretch her low back as soon as she gets up from the prone position. The yoga Child's Pose is an excellent way to accomplish this (see accompanying figure).

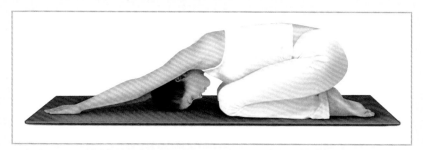

Lateral View of the Child's Pose

the gluteal region before entering the thigh. Because the sciatic nerve is deep to the gluteus maximus muscle, it is not very superficial and therefore not easily injured with soft tissue work. However, deeper work can translate to the sciatic nerve and the therapist should be mindful of this, especially when performing deep work on the quadratus femoris muscle.

Motions

Another caution should be mentioned, even though it does not involve an anatomic structure per se. When treating the client's low back, be aware that many clients do not tolerate well any extension beyond anatomic position and/or any extreme or fast rotation motions. This is especially true with elderly clients, but it may also be true for middle-aged or younger clients. The lumbar spine has limited rotation ranges of motion. Further, rotation and extension motions cause the surfaces of the facet joints to approximate each other; if they are injured or irritated in any way, and/or if there are degenerative joint changes (osteoarthritis), this can result in pain. For this reason, it is always wise to be aware of this possibility. When stretching or otherwise moving the client, it is advisable to increase these ranges of motions gradually over the span of several visits if necessary.

At the hip joint, caution must be exercised whenever the client's thigh is moved into flexion combined with adduction and medial rotation. This is especially important for clients who have had hip replacement surgery.

CHAPTER SUMMARY

This chapter presented a review of the essential anatomy and physiology of the low back and pelvis. The lumbar spine is composed of five vertebrae. Landmarks of the lumbar spine that are particularly important for stretching and joint mobilization techniques are the spinous processes and laminae. Each lumbar spinal joint level has two paired facet joints and a disc joint. The lumbar spine moves very well in all ranges of motion except rotation.

Structurally, the musculature of the low back can be divided into four quadrants: anterior right, anterior left, posterior right, and posterior left. Functionally, the muscles of the low back can be divided into six major mover groups: flexors, extensors, right and left lateral flexors, and right and left rotators.

Structurally, the muscles of the pelvis can be divided into three categories: muscles crossing the lumbosacral joint from the trunk onto the pelvis, muscles crossing the hip joint from the lower extremity onto the pelvis, and pelvic floor muscles. As with the muscles of the trunk, pelvic muscles that cross the hip joint can also be divided into four quadrants: anterior, posterior, lateral, and medial. Functionally, these muscles are usually considered from their open chain action on the thigh. However, their closed chain action on the pelvis is likely more important; certainly, it is with regard to their effect on the posture of the pelvis and therefore the lumbar spine.

CHAPTER 2

Common Musculoskeletal Pathologic Conditions

OBJECTIVES

After completing this chapter, the student should be able to:

1. Explain why it is important to understand the pathomechanics of a condition.
2. Describe the presentation, mechanism, and causes of each of the conditions covered in this chapter.
3. Describe how the gamma motor system, muscle spindles, muscle memory, and resting muscle tone work together to create hypertonic musculature.
4. Compare and contrast a globally tight muscle with a myofascial trigger point.
5. Describe the difference between the pain-spasm-pain and contraction-ischemia cycles.
6. Describe the relationship between adhesions and mobility.
7. Identify the four main ways that a muscle can become hypertonic.
8. List and describe the two major types of joint dysfunction.
9. Compare and contrast a sprain and a strain.
10. List and describe the different types of pathologic disc.
11. Describe the relationship between tight muscles and a pathologic disc.
12. Describe the relationship between tight muscles and degenerative joint disease.
13. Define scoliosis and explain how a scoliotic curve is named.
14. Describe the relationship between excessive anterior tilt and hyperlordotic lumbar spine.
15. Describe facet syndrome and explain how it is assessed.
16. Describe the causes and symptoms of spondylolisthesis.
17. Define each key term in this chapter.

KEY TERMS

adaptive shortening
adhesions
anterolisthesis
bone spurs
central canal stenosis
contraction-ischemia cycle
degenerative joint disease (DJD)
disc bulge
disc herniation
disc prolapse
disc rupture
disc thinning
facet syndrome
fascial adhesions
fibrous adhesions

gamma motor system
globally tight muscle
hyperlordosis
hyperlordotic lumbar spine
hypermobile
hypertonic
hypomobile
ischemia
joint dysfunction
locked long
locked short
lower crossed syndrome
macrotraumas
mechanism
meniscoid body
meralgia paresthetica

microtearing
microtraumas
misalignment
motion palpation
muscle memory
muscle spindle fibers
muscle spindle reflex
muscle splinting
myofascial trigger point
osteoarthritis (OA)
osteophytes
pain-spasm-pain cycle
pathomechanism
pathophysiology
piriformis syndrome
resting tone

sacral base angle
sacroiliitis
scar tissue adhesions
sciatica
scoliosis
sequestered disc
space-occupying lesions
spondylolisthesis
spondylosis
sprain
strain
stretch reflex
subluxation
swayback
trigger point (TrP)
Wolff's law

INTRODUCTION

Proper therapeutic treatment of a client's low back and pelvis depends on an accurate assessment of the client's condition(s) as well as a clear understanding of the mechanism of the pathologic condition(s) that the client is experiencing. Therefore, this chapter offers a brief description of the most common pathologic musculoskeletal conditions that affect these regions. Chapter 3 discusses the procedures used to assess these conditions.

When treating a healthy or unhealthy low back and pelvis, it is most important to understand the **mechanism**, or physiology, of how these regions function. Normal mechanics of the low back and pelvis are addressed in Chapter 1. However, when a person has a pathologic condition, the mechanics are altered. Each pathologic condition has a unique physiologic mechanism, **pathophysiology** or **pathomechanism**, that, when understood, can guide critical reasoning regarding the therapeutic tools that should be used. Rather than asking the learner to apply a memorized "cookbook" routine from one technique or another that may be ineffective or perhaps even hurt the client, this chapter will encourage learning how to choose the technique protocols that will safely and most effectively help the client.

BOX	2.1

Musculoskeletal Pathologic Conditions

The following musculoskeletal pathologic conditions are presented in this chapter:
1. Hypertonic (tight) musculature
2. Joint dysfunction
3. Sprains and strains
4. Sacroiliac joint injury
5. Pathologic disc conditions and sciatica
6. Piriformis syndrome
7. Degenerative joint disease (DJD)
8. Scoliosis
9. Anterior pelvic tilt and hyperlordotic lumbar spine
10. Facet syndrome
11. Spondylolisthesis

HYPERTONIC MUSCULATURE

Hypertonic, or tight, musculature is an important condition to discuss for two reasons:

1. It is the most common presenting complaint that a manual therapist will confront.
2. It is usually a component of every other musculoskeletal condition of the low back and pelvis.

Of further significance is the fact that tight musculature is so often ignored by conventional medical professions. There are medical specialties for every organ system of the body, but there is no "muscle doctor." Even the chiropractic profession usually relegates the importance of tight musculature to a position of lesser importance compared with joint positioning and function. Perhaps the importance of tight musculature is overlooked because it does not show on x-rays, other radiographic imaging, or in laboratory results. For this reason, manual therapists who are highly trained in muscle palpation assessment skills and soft tissue treatment techniques have the opportunity to step into this niche.

Description of Hypertonic Musculature

A **hypertonic** muscle is one that has too much tone; "hyper" denotes an excessive amount. Tone refers to tension; in other words, it is the pulling force of a muscle. The degree of tone that a muscle has varies based on the degree of its contraction. There are two types of hypertonic musculature: a **globally tight muscle** and a myofascial trigger point (TrP). The first term is used to describe an entire muscle or large portion of a muscle that is too tight; the second term is used to describe a small focal area of muscle tightness that can refer pain to a distant site.

Globally Tight Musculature

When you consciously contract a muscle, its tone is high. However, when a muscle is at rest and you are not consciously directing it to contract, other than a small amount of baseline tone to maintain the posture of the joint, it should be relaxed. This condition is called **resting tone**. A resting tone greater than the amount needed to maintain joint posture is what defines a muscle as being hypertonic. Other terms often used synonymously are spasm, cramp, and contracture, all of which essentially describe a muscle whose baseline tone is excessive or hypertonic.

Mechanism of Globally Tight Musculature

The physiologic mechanism of a globally tight muscle is determined by **muscle spindle fibers** (also known as spindle fibers or spindle cells). Muscle spindle fibers are located within the belly of a muscle and lie parallel to the regular fibers of the muscle. Similar to these regular muscle fibers, spindle fibers have the ability to contract and relax. But they also possess another feature that regular muscle fibers do not. Muscle spindles are receptor cells that have the ability to detect when they are being stretched. They are sensitive to both how quickly and how far they are stretched. The sensitivity of their setting is determined by the **gamma motor system** of the brain, which can order them to contract and tighten or allow them to be relaxed and loose. The tighter the muscle spindles are set, the more sensitive they are to stretch; the looser they are, the more tolerant they are to being stretched.

If a muscle is stretched, all of the fibers within the muscle, both regular and spindle, are lengthened. If this stretch occurs quickly or is farther than the spindle fibers can com-

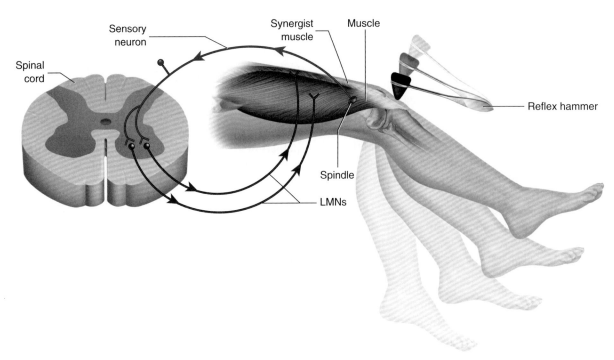

Figure 2-1 Muscle spindle reflex. A reflex hammer is used to strike and cause a quick stretch of the distal tendon of the quadriceps femoris (knee joint extensor musculature), triggering the muscle spindle reflex. A signal is sent to the spinal cord via a sensory neuron. In response, a signal is sent from the spinal cord through lower motor neurons (LMNs) to tell the muscle to contract, causing extension of the leg at the knee joint.

fortably allow, it sends a signal via a sensory neuron into the spinal cord. This sensory neuron then synapses with lower motor neurons (LMNs) that return to the muscle, ordering the regular fibers of the muscle to contract (Fig. 2-1). This is called the **muscle spindle reflex**, or **stretch reflex**, and is protective in nature. By tightening the muscle, the stretch is stopped, and the muscle is protected from being overstretched and perhaps torn.

The stretch reflex is usually only thought of as protecting a muscle from strong forces such as whiplash accidents. However, the stretch reflex is also responsible for setting resting tone of the musculature. When the gamma motor nervous system directs the spindle fibers within a muscle to contract, they shorten. Then when the person moves, as soon as that muscle is stretched even a small amount more than the length of its spindles, the stretch reflex will cause the muscle's fibers to contract to the tension level set for the spindles. In this manner, the length of a muscle's fibers, or its tone, will match the length and tone set for its spindles. The term **muscle memory** is often used to describe this baseline tone of a muscle. Muscle memory resides in the nervous system, not in the muscle itself.

Causes of Globally Tight Musculature

There are a number of causes for globally tight musculature. Four of the most common causes are as follows:

1. Overuse
2. Splinting

3. Adaptive shortening
4. Overstretching

In each case, the muscle memory tone set by the gamma motor system and the muscle's stretch reflex is increased. Although this chapter addresses each cause separately, when a client presents clinically with tight musculature, the mechanisms of the causes can and often do overlap.

Muscle Overuse

Overuse of a muscle fatigues it. Overuse also increases its level of tension. This increases the muscle's pulling force on its tendons and bony attachments, irritating these structures and causing pain. In response to this pain, the nervous system signals the muscle to contract, which creates increased tightness of the entire muscle. This is a protective mechanism meant to decrease or prevent motion that might further irritate or injure the musculature and/ or other soft tissues. Muscle tightness causing pain, which then triggers further tightness, which then triggers further pain, and so forth, is known as the **pain-spasm-pain cycle**. Prolonged contraction of a muscle can also result in a disruption of the blood circulation to the area. Initially, the prolonged contraction interrupts venous return of blood, causing a buildup of waste products. These waste products are acidic and irritate the muscle tissue, causing increased pain, which then further perpetuates the pain-spasm-pain cycle. The result is increased reflexive spasm of the muscle (Fig. 2-2).

Fascial Adhesions

When muscles are tight, another factor that must be considered is fascial adhesions. **Fascial adhesions**, also known as **scar tissue adhesions** (or **fibrous adhesions**, or more simply **adhesions**), are composed of fibrous fascia collagen fibers (see accompanying figure). These collagen fibers are the same substance that makes up tendons, ligaments, and other fibrous fascial tissues. Although adhesions are normally thought to be deposited in sites of trauma (i.e., scar tissue), they are in fact deposited continuously between the soft tissues of the body. These fibers increase the stability of the tissues by binding/connecting the tissues together. However, if adhesions build up excessively, they may bind together the two opposing surfaces of a soft tissue interface, which should slide along one another when movement is needed; this results in restricted mobility. In a client with an active lifestyle, these fibers do not get the chance to build up because as the client's body moves, adhesions that have formed are broken up and resorbed. However, a sedentary lifestyle encourages adhesions to build up progressively until mobility is greatly restricted. Although adhesions do not actually cause an increase in the baseline resting tone contraction level of a muscle, they do add to the muscle's tightness by decreasing the muscles' ability to stretch and lengthen. If a muscle cannot lengthen, then it cannot allow movements of the body performed by the antagonists to that muscle.

The mobility of ligaments, joint capsules, and all other soft tissue can be affected by adhesions as well. Manual treatment techniques such as massage, stretching, and hydrotherapy all help to break up adhesions in muscles and other soft tissues.

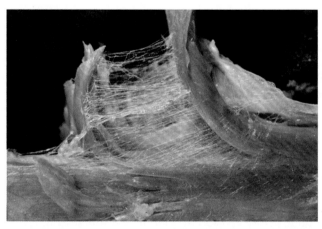

Fascial collagen fibers have a spiderweb appearance. Educator and author, Gil Hedley, uses the term *fuzz* to describe fibrous fascia. (Photo © Ronald A. Thompson. Courtesy Ron Thompson.)

Muscle overuse is often thought of in terms of an activity such as playing sports or working out at a gym. If the same muscle or muscle group is used repeatedly without rest, it will gradually fatigue and become painful. However, overuse can also result from prolonged unhealthy postures. Although less dramatic, poor posture is often a greater contributor to muscle tightness than overuse from activity.

One of the most common postures that causes tightness of low back musculature is when the trunk is flexed forward such that its weight is no longer centered over the pelvis. This happens every time that you lean forward to work down low in front of yourself, or when you bend forward to pick up something from the ground. Without muscles to counteract the force of gravity, the trunk would naturally fall forward. Low back extensor muscles, such as the erector spinae, must eccentrically contract to slow your body's descent as you flex forward, then isometrically contract if you hold the imbalanced forward-flexed posture, and then concentrically contract to extend back to anatomic position (Fig. 2-3). Because of the tremendous amount of time that many people spend in forward-flexed postures, tightness of the posterior low back musculature is very common.

If the client is pregnant or if the client is overweight with a large abdomen, the increased weight carried anteriorly can imbalance the client's center of weight anteriorly, increasing the forward flexion force upon the client's trunk. This would

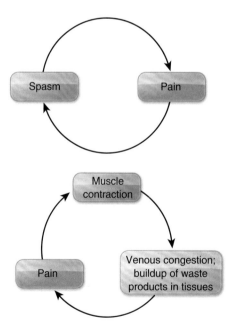

Figure 2-2 Pain-spasm-pain cycle. (**A**) A tight (spasmed) muscle pulls excessively on its attachments, causing pain. In response to the pain, the muscle's tension level increases. (**B**) When a muscle is tight, its contraction can also reduce venous blood flow, resulting in a buildup of acidic waste products in the area. This causes further pain, which perpetuates the pain-spasm-pain cycle. (Reproduced with permission from Muscolino JE. *Advanced Treatment Techniques for the Manual Therapist: Neck.* Baltimore, MD: Lippincott Williams & Wilkins; 2013.)

Figure 2-3 Prolonged postures and low back tightness. (**A**) Flexing the trunk when working down in front of the body causes the body weight of the trunk to be imbalanced. This requires isometric contraction of the posterior low back extensor muscles to hold the trunk in this posture. (**B**) Carrying a baby on a hip requires isometric muscular contraction of the elevators of the pelvis on that side.

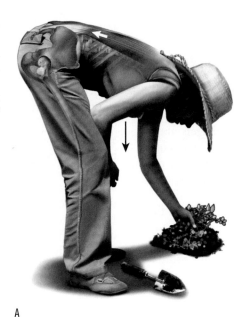

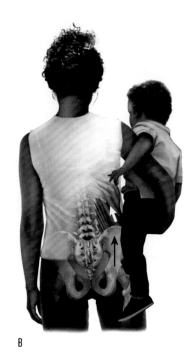

A

B

have to be counteracted by the postural isometric contraction of the low back extensor musculature. With excessive work, postural muscles of the low back will likely fatigue and tighten.

Muscle Splinting

Muscles of the low back and pelvis may tighten not only if the muscles themselves are irritated and overused but also if any other tissues of the region become irritated or injured. This is especially true of the tissues of the sacroiliac joints and the facet joint capsules and ligaments of the lumbar spine. This phenomenon is called **muscle splinting**, and it is a protective mechanism for these fragile and vulnerable tissues. By tightening, the musculature acts as a splint to the area, blocking motion and thereby allowing the tissues of the area to rest and heal. Therefore, overt traumatic injury or irritation to any tissues of the joints of the low back and pelvis can cause the muscles of the region to tighten and splint the area.

Adaptive Shortening

Adaptive shortening occurs when a muscle is held in a shortened state for a prolonged time and adapts to that shortened state by increasing its tone. Adaptive shortening is a protective mechanism. If a muscle is shortened and slackened, then when it contracts to move the body, the muscle would be unable to generate tension on its attachments until all the slack has been removed. This would not only cause an inefficient delay in movement but it could also be dangerous in a fight-or-flight scenario. For this reason, the nervous system adaptively shortens the muscle by increasing its tone to match the shortened length. The net result is that if a certain posture is held for a long time, the musculature will shorten

and adapt to that posture so it is ready to create tension and movement immediately if needed. One example of this is the posture of the hip joint when sitting. Sitting places the hip joint into flexion, shortening the hip flexor muscles that cross the joint anteriorly, attaching from the pelvis to the thigh. This chronic posture of allowing the hip joint to be flexed can result in adaptive shortening of the hip flexor musculature bilaterally. Their tightness will then tend to create an excessively anteriorly tilted pelvis because hip flexor musculature's reverse action is anterior tilt of the pelvis at the hip joint (see Anterior Pelvic Tilt and Hyperlordotic Lumbar Spine section).

Muscle Overstretching

Another common reason for the low back muscles to tighten is overstretching of the musculature. As described previously, if the low back is stretched too fast or too far, it can activate the muscle spindle's stretch reflex and cause a spasm. Even though this reflex is protective, the spasming often persists long after the initial event that triggered it, resulting in a chronic posture of tight musculature of the region.

Overstretching a muscle can be caused traumatically, as with a fall or other injury. It can also occur when doing stretches as part of a health and fitness regimen. This is especially true if stretching is done too vigorously when the muscles have not yet warmed up, as often occurs when stretching is done before an exercise routine. For this reason, it is increasingly recommended that stretching be done after exercising, when the muscle tissues are warm. Thus, even though stretching is a valuable part of a health and fitness regimen, when it is performed too aggressively, it can be detrimental to musculoskeletal health. Moderation is the key.

Overstretching also often occurs in a much more insidious and seemingly innocuous manner. Simple postures assumed and carried out during the day can be the culprit. Examples include poor ergonomics at the workplace, such as bending down to work low in front of your body instead of working up higher in front of yourself, or twisting to one side to work off to the side in front of yourself instead of working directly in front of yourself. Postures and activities outside of work can also contribute. Bending forward during hobbies or activities such as cleaning or gardening can overstretch the low back extensors of the spine. Sleep posture can be equally problematic. If the client sleeps in a position that is halfway between side-lying and being on the stomach, the lumbar spine is torqued/rotated. This posture can easily cause an overstretch of the opposing rotator musculature that is antagonistic to this position, resulting in waking during the night or the next morning with tight muscles caused by the stretch reflex.

Myofascial Trigger Points

The other type of hypertonic musculature is a **myofascial trigger point**, often referred to simply as a **trigger point (TrP)**, and known in lay terms as a muscle knot. As described previously, a TrP is a focal area of muscle tightness that can refer pain to a distant site. TrPs are often divided into active and latent TrPs. Latent TrPs require pressure to be applied to them for referral of pain to occur. Active TrPs can refer pain without pressure.

Mechanism of Myofascial Trigger Points

Unlike globally tight musculature, whose mechanism is the muscle spindle reflex under the direction of the gamma motor system of the brain, a myofascial TrP is a local phenomenon. Muscle contraction occurs via the sliding filament mechanism. During this mechanism, crossbridges of myosin and actin (filaments found within the muscle fibers) constantly form, release, and reform to create the muscle contraction. Necessary to the release of these crossbridges is supply of energy in the form of adenosine triphosphate (ATP) molecules, which are created by a supply of glucose (blood sugar) delivered in the arterial blood supply to the musculature. If this arterial blood supply is cut off (often due to compression caused by the muscle's own contraction), then the muscle tissue is deprived of nutrients, including glucose. This loss of arterial blood supply is called **ischemia**; the creation of ischemia by muscular contraction is called the **contraction-ischemia cycle** (Fig. 2-4).

When ischemia, resulting in the loss of ATP formation, occurs in a small region of muscle fibers, the crossbridges in this region cannot be released, and a TrP forms. Therefore, the mechanism for TrP formation and perpetuation is ischemia at the local level. Treatment should be aimed at relieving ischemia by manual therapy that increases local blood circulation. Deep stroking massage (usually for a duration of approximately 30 to 60 seconds) is increasingly

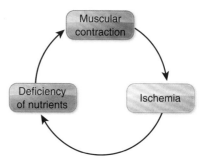

Figure 2-4 Contraction-ischemia cycle. If a muscle contraction is strong enough, it can compress arteries and reduce arterial blood flow to the local tissues. This results in ischemia, which can then cause myofascial TrPs to develop in the muscle. (Reproduced with permission from Muscolino JE. *Advanced Treatment Techniques for the Manual Therapist: Neck.* Baltimore, MD: Lippincott Williams & Wilkins; 2013.)

being recommended as the treatment of choice to work a myofascial TrP.

Causes of Myofascial Trigger Points

The four most common causes of myofascial TrPs are as follows:

1. Acute or chronic overuse of the muscle, including concentric and eccentric contraction with activity as well as isometric contraction with posture
2. Chronic stretch of the muscle
3. Prolonged immobility of the muscle
4. Trauma/injury to the muscle

Common Myofascial Trigger Points of the Low Back and Pelvis and Their Referral Zones

A TrP can form anywhere within a muscle. However, there are certain locations within muscles where TrPs tend to form more commonly than others. Further, each TrP within a muscle tends to have a characteristic referral zone. Each referral zone is usually divided into primary and secondary referral zones. A TrP most commonly refers to its primary referral zone; when more severe, it usually also refers to its secondary referral zone. Figures 2-5 to 2-22 illustrate common TrP locations and their corresponding referral zones for the muscles of the low back and pelvis. The locations of TrPs are indicated by Xs. Primary referral zones are indicated in dark red; secondary referral zones are indicated in light red.

Summary of Hypertonic Musculature

It is important to distinguish between globally tight musculature and myofascial TrPs because optimal treatment approaches differ for the two conditions. Manual and movement therapy for a globally tight muscle might be performed locally at the tight muscle, but its intended consequence is to

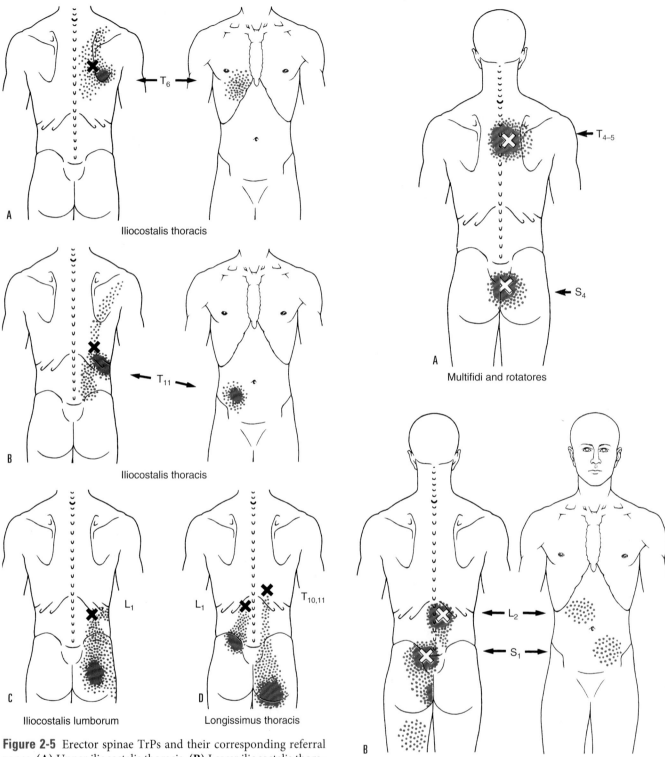

Figure 2-5 Erector spinae TrPs and their corresponding referral zones. (**A**) Upper iliocostalis thoracis. (**B**) Lower iliocostalis thoracis. (**C**) Iliocostalis lumborum. (**D**) Longissimus thoracis. *TrP*, trigger point. (Reproduced with permission from Simons DG, Travell JG, Simons LS. *Upper Half of Body*. 2nd ed. Baltimore, MD: Lippincott Williams & Wilkins; 1999. *Travell & Simons' Myofascial Pain and Dysfunction: The Trigger Point Manual*; vol 1.)

Figure 2-6 Transversospinalis multifidus and rotatores TrPs and their corresponding referral zones. (**A**) Midthoracic and sacral multifidus and rotatores. (**B**) Lumbar and upper sacral multifidus. *TrP*, trigger point. (Reproduced with permission from Simons DG, Travell JG, Simons LS. *Upper Half of Body*. 2nd ed. Baltimore, MD: Lippincott Williams & Wilkins; 1999. *Travell & Simons' Myofascial Pain and Dysfunction: The Trigger Point Manual*; vol 1.)

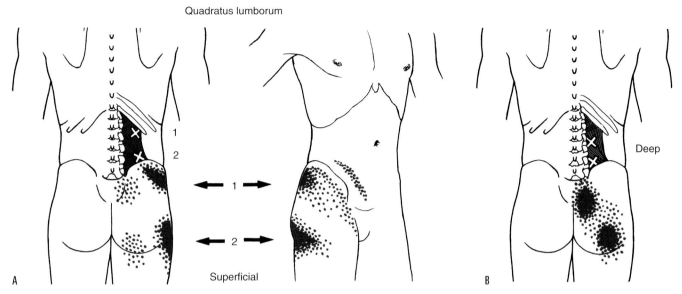

Figure 2-7 Quadratus lumborum TrPs and their corresponding referral zones. **(A)** Lateral (superficial) TrPs. **(B)** Medial (deep) TrPs. *TrP*, trigger point. (Reproduced with permission from Travell JG, Simons DG. *The Lower Extremities*. Baltimore, MD: Lippincott Williams & Wilkins; 1992. *Travell & Simons' Myofascial Pain and Dysfunction: The Trigger Point Manual*; vol 2.)

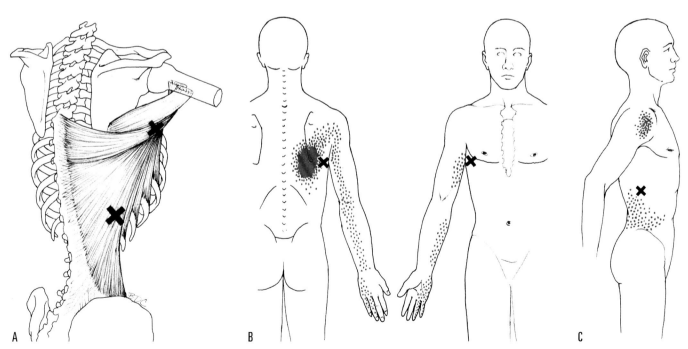

Figure 2-8 Latissimus dorsi TrPs and their corresponding referral zones. **(A)** Posterolateral view of two most common TrPs. **(B)** Upper TrP. **(C)** Lower TrP. *TrP*, trigger point. (Reproduced with permission from Simons DG, Travell JG, Simons LS. *Upper Half of Body*. 2nd ed. Baltimore, MD: Lippincott Williams & Wilkins; 1999. *Travell & Simons' Myofascial Pain and Dysfunction: The Trigger Point Manual*; vol 1.)

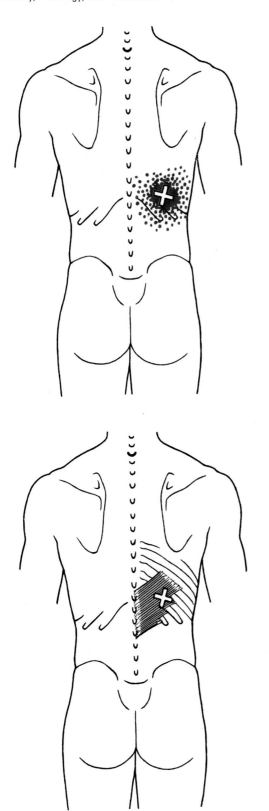

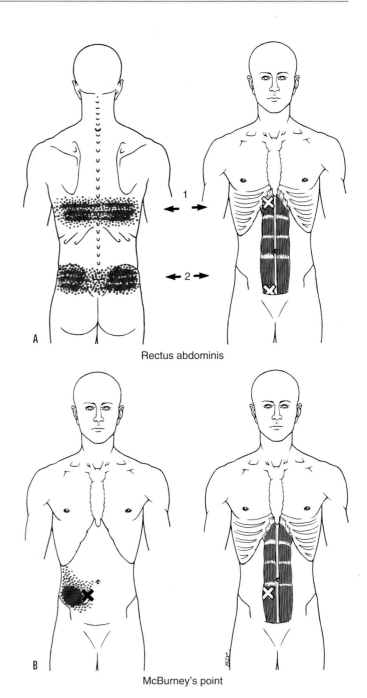

Rectus abdominis

McBurney's point

Figure 2-10 Rectus abdominis TrPs and their corresponding referral zones. **(A)** Pain can refer into the back bilaterally. **(B)** Pain from a lateral right-sided TrP can refer to the region of the appendix (over McBurney's point). *TrP*, trigger point. (Reproduced with permission from Simons DG, Travell JG, Simons LS. *Upper Half of Body.* 2nd ed. Baltimore, MD: Lippincott Williams & Wilkins; 1999. *Travell & Simons' Myofascial Pain and Dysfunction: The Trigger Point Manual*; vol 1.)

Figure 2-9 Serratus posterior inferior TrPs and their corresponding referral zones. *TrP*, trigger point. (Reproduced with permission from Simons DG, Travell JG, Simons LS. *Upper Half of Body.* 2nd ed. Baltimore, MD: Lippincott Williams & Wilkins; 1999. *Travell & Simons' Myofascial Pain and Dysfunction: The Trigger Point Manual*; vol 1.)

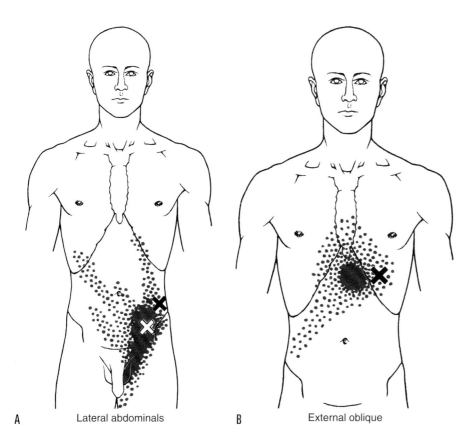

Figure 2-11 Anterolateral abdominal wall muscles: External and internal abdominal oblique and transversus abdominis TrPs and their corresponding referral zones. (**A**) Anterolateral abdominal wall TrPs. (**B**) Upper external abdominal oblique TrP. *TrP*, trigger point. (Reproduced with permission from Simons DG, Travell JG, Simons LS. *Upper Half of Body*. 2nd ed. Baltimore, MD: Lippincott Williams & Wilkins; 1999. *Travell & Simons' Myofascial Pain and Dysfunction: The Trigger Point Manual*; vol 1.)

A   Lateral abdominals   B   External oblique

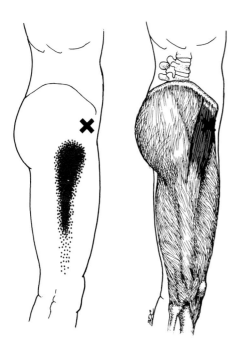

Figure 2-12 Tensor fasciae latae TrPs and their corresponding referral zones. *TrP*, trigger point. (Reproduced with permission from Travell JG, Simons DG. *The Lower Extremities*. Baltimore, MD: Lippincott Williams & Wilkins; 1992. *Travell & Simons' Myofascial Pain and Dysfunction: The Trigger Point Manual*; vol 2.)

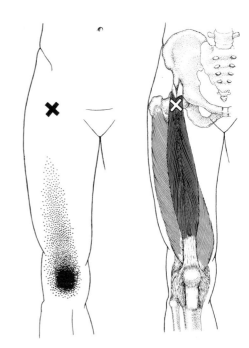

Figure 2-13 Rectus femoris TrP and its corresponding referral zones. *TrP*, trigger point. (Reproduced with permission from Travell JG, Simons DG. *The Lower Extremities*. Baltimore, MD: Lippincott Williams & Wilkins; 1992. *Travell & Simons' Myofascial Pain and Dysfunction: The Trigger Point Manual*; vol 2.)

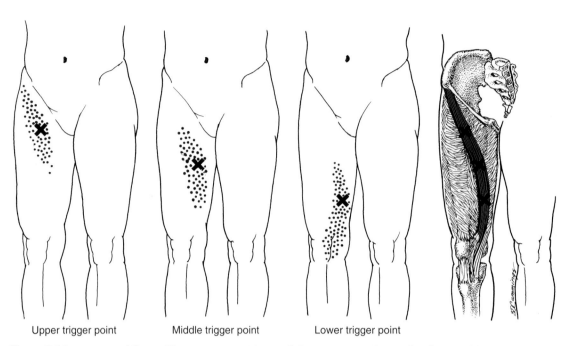

Upper trigger point   Middle trigger point   Lower trigger point

Figure 2-14 Upper, middle, and lower sartorius TrPs and their corresponding referral zones. *TrP*, trigger point. (Reproduced with permission from Travell JG, Simons DG. *The Lower Extremities*. Baltimore, MD: Lippincott Williams & Wilkins; 1992. *Travell & Simons' Myofascial Pain and Dysfunction: The Trigger Point Manual*; vol 2.)

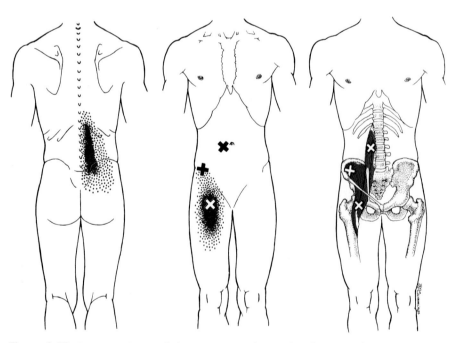

Figure 2-15 Iliopsoas TrPs and their corresponding referral zones. *TrP*, trigger point. (Reproduced with permission from Travell JG, Simons DG. *The Lower Extremities*. Baltimore, MD: Williams & Wilkins; 1992. *Travell & Simons' Myofascial Pain and Dysfunction: The Trigger Point Manual*; vol 2.)

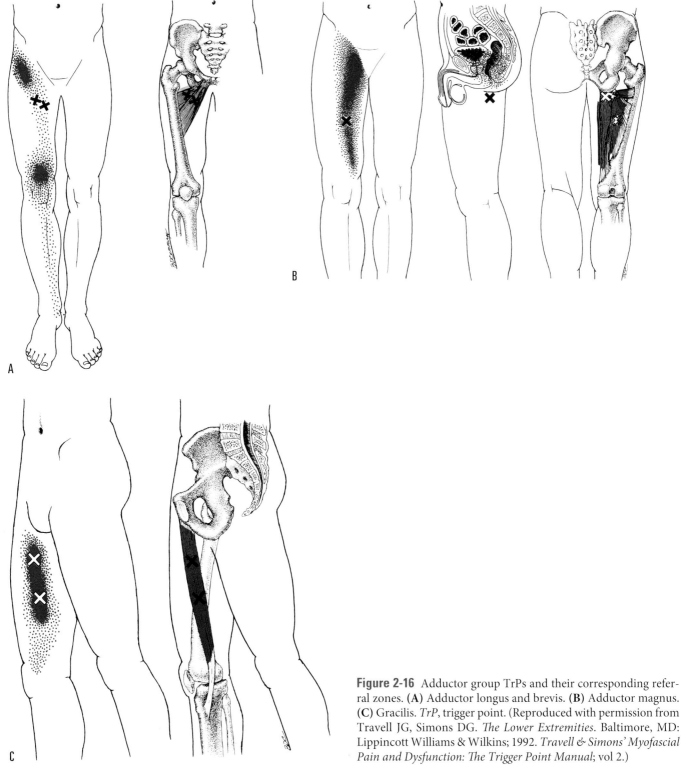

Figure 2-16 Adductor group TrPs and their corresponding referral zones. (**A**) Adductor longus and brevis. (**B**) Adductor magnus. (**C**) Gracilis. *TrP*, trigger point. (Reproduced with permission from Travell JG, Simons DG. *The Lower Extremities*. Baltimore, MD: Lippincott Williams & Wilkins; 1992. *Travell & Simons' Myofascial Pain and Dysfunction: The Trigger Point Manual*; vol 2.)

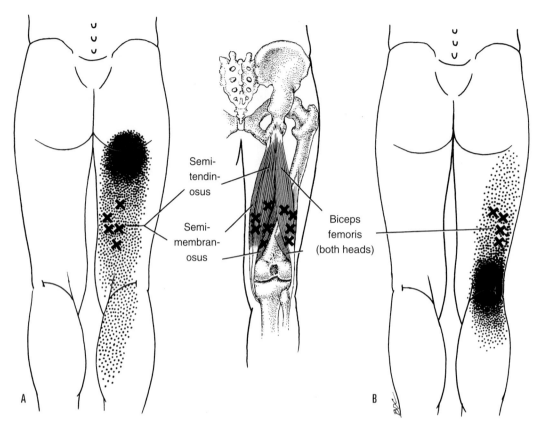

Figure 2-17 Hamstring group TrPs and their corresponding referral zones. *TrP*, trigger point. (Reproduced with permission from Travell JG, Simons DG. *The Lower Extremities*. Baltimore, MD: Lippincott Williams & Wilkins; 1992. *Travell & Simons' Myofascial Pain and Dysfunction: The Trigger Point Manual*; vol 2.)

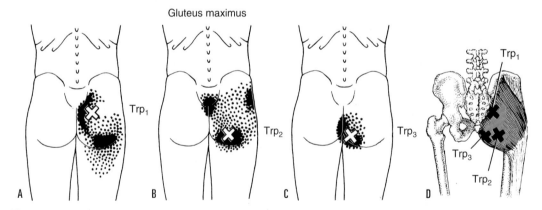

Figure 2-18 Gluteus maximus TrPs and their corresponding referral zones. **(A)** Upper TrP and its referral zone. **(B)** Lower midline TrP and its referral zone. **(C)** Lower medial TrP and its referral zone. **(D)** TrPs. *TrP*, trigger point. (Reproduced with permission from Travell JG, Simons DG. *The Lower Extremities*. Baltimore, MD: Lippincott Williams & Wilkins; 1992. *Travell & Simons' Myofascial Pain and Dysfunction: The Trigger Point Manual*; vol 2.)

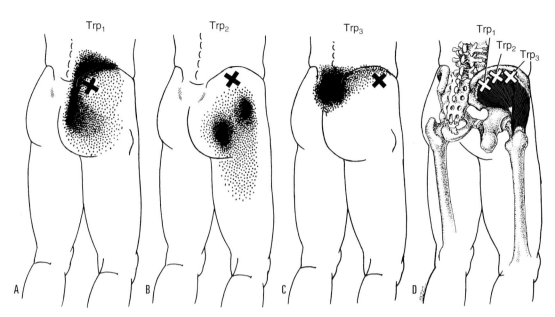

Figure 2-19 Gluteus medius TrPs and their corresponding referral zones. (**A**) Posterior TrP and its referral zone. (**B**) Midline TrP and its referral zone. (**C**) Anterior TrP and its referral zone. (**D**) TrPs. *TrP*, trigger point. (Reproduced with permission from Travell JG, Simons DG. *The Lower Extremities.* Baltimore, MD: Lippincott Williams & Wilkins; 1992. *Travell & Simons' Myofascial Pain and Dysfunction: The Trigger Point Manual*; vol 2.)

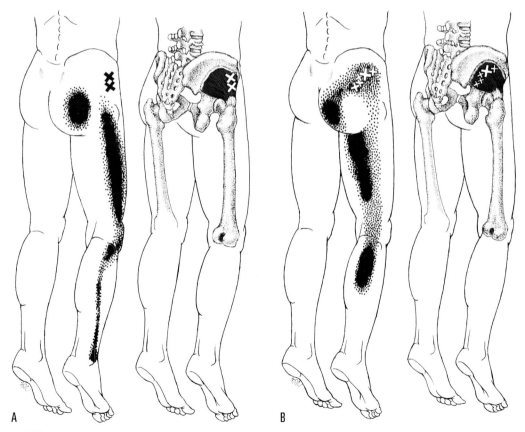

Figure 2-20 Gluteus minimus TrPs and their corresponding referral zones. (**A**) Anterior TrPs. (**B**) Posterior TrPs. *TrP*, trigger point. (Reproduced with permission from Travell JG, Simons DG. *The Lower Extremities.* Baltimore, MD: Lippincott Williams & Wilkins; 1992. *Travell & Simons' Myofascial Pain and Dysfunction: The Trigger Point Manual*; vol 2.)

Figure 2-21 Piriformis TrPs and their corresponding referral zones. *TrP*, trigger point. (Reproduced with permission from Travell JG, Simons DG. *The Lower Extremities*. Baltimore, MD: Lippincott Williams & Wilkins; 1992. *Travell & Simons' Myofascial Pain and Dysfunction: The Trigger Point Manual*; vol 2.)

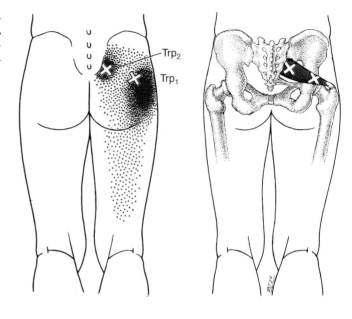

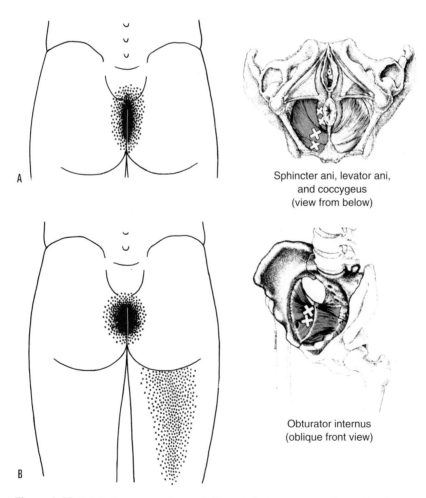

Figure 2-22 Pelvic floor musculature TrPs and their corresponding referral zones. **(A)** Coccygeus, levator ani, and sphincter ani. **(B)** Obturator internus. *TrP*, trigger point. (Reproduced with permission from Travell JG, Simons DG. *The Lower Extremities*. Baltimore, MD: Lippincott Williams & Wilkins; 1992. *Travell & Simons' Myofascial Pain and Dysfunction: The Trigger Point Manual*; vol 2.)

cause the gamma motor system of the central nervous system to change its pattern of muscle memory that determines the tone of that muscle. In contrast, treatment of a TrP is aimed directly at causing a local change in the muscle tissue itself, increasing blood supply where the TrP is located.

However, all hypertonic musculature, whether it is a globally tight muscle or a myofascial TrP, can decrease motion at the joint that is crossed by that muscle. Once joint motion has been restricted for a prolonged time, the functioning of that joint may become impaired. This condition is known as joint dysfunction and is discussed in the following section.

2.1   TREATMENT CONSIDERATIONS IN BRIEF

Hypertonic Musculature

Every technique presented in this book addresses tight musculature. Certainly, all forms of massage therapy, stretching, and hydrotherapy are effective for the treatment of hypertonic musculature. In particular, deep stroking massage is recommended for the treatment of myofascial TrPs. For more details, see Chapter 3.

JOINT DYSFUNCTION

Like hypertonic musculature, joint dysfunction is usually present as a component of most pathologic musculoskeletal conditions of the low back and pelvis. Tight muscles and joint dysfunction seem to follow a cyclical pattern. If tight muscles are present, they restrict joint motion, which leads to adhesions in the periarticular soft tissues (tissues located around the joint) and causes joint dysfunction. Similarly, if

---

2.1   THERAPIST TIP

Massage and Chiropractic

Tight musculature and joint dysfunction usually coexist in every musculoskeletal condition. For this reason, massage therapy and chiropractic (or osteopathy) ideally complement each other, and massage therapists are often employed in chiropractic offices. In chronic conditions, fibrous adhesions are also nearly always present, reinforcing the need for chiropractic manipulation and massage as well as moist heat and stretching techniques.

---

joint dysfunction is present, the lack of proper movement will either lead to adaptive shortening and tightening of the muscles, and/or the pain with attempted motion will cause splinting of the adjacent musculature. For this reason, most musculoskeletal problems involve a combination of tight musculature and joint dysfunction. The benefits of massage for the musculature are clear, as are the benefits of stretching for the musculature and joints and of joint mobilization for the joints.

BOX   2.3

Subluxation/Misalignment Versus Joint Dysfunction

The terms **subluxation** and **misalignment** are commonly used in chiropractic and osteopathic practices. Although these two terms are often used to denote joint dysfunction, they are not actually synonymous with joint dysfunction. Subluxation and misalignment, as well as saying that a bone is *out of place* refer to the static structural/postural alignment of a vertebra. If in neutral anatomic position, a vertebra is slightly rotated, laterally flexed, flexed, or extended, then it is said to be subluxated or misaligned. Joint dysfunction, on the other hand, refers to the functional motion of a vertebra at its spinal joints.

However, there often is a relationship between the static alignment of a vertebra and its functional motion. A vertebra that is misaligned is often misaligned because of asymmetry of tight musculature and/or adhesions. The same tight musculature and adhesions may certainly affect the motion of the vertebra, causing a hypomobile joint dysfunction. This relationship is not always present, however. A helpful analogy is that of a door that naturally sits slightly ajar. If you look at its static position, you would say that it is misaligned because it is ajar. However, to determine whether the door functions correctly, you would need to see if it can move through its full range of motion, opening and closing all the way. If it can do that, then it is functioning fine, even if it is "misaligned." When there is a discrepancy between structure and function, proper functioning is usually more important.

Description of Joint Dysfunction

Joint dysfunction means that the function of a joint is unhealthy. Given that joint function is to allow movement, two forms of joint dysfunction exist. A **hypomobile** joint is restricted in motion and moves too little; a **hypermobile** joint has excessive motion and moves too much.

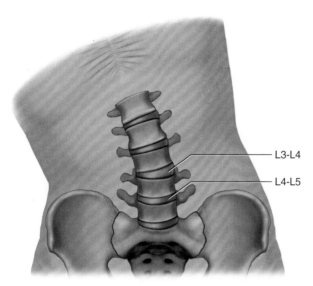

Figure 2-23 Joint hypomobility. A joint dysfunction hypomobility at one segmental level of the lumbar spine usually results in a compensatory joint dysfunction hypermobility at the adjacent level. Here, L4-L5 is hypomobile, and L3-L4 is a compensatory hypermobility.

L3-L4

L4-L5

Although both hypermobilities and hypomobilities can occur in the lumbar spine and pelvis, the more common presenting complaint, and the one that manual therapists are better able to treat, is hypomobility. Because a lumbar spinal joint can move in multiple directions, it can be hypomobile in one or more of its six cardinal ranges of motion: flexion, extension, right and left lateral flexion, and right and left rotation (for a table of average ranges of motion of the lumbar spine, see Table 1-1 in Chapter 1). For example, it is possible for a lumbar spinal joint to move perfectly well into right lateral flexion (as well as other ranges of motion) but not move well into left lateral flexion. For this reason, to accurately assess a joint hypomobility, the specific range of motion that is restricted should be determined.

However, assessing the overall gross range of motion of a specific motion of the low back (such as right lateral flexion) does not necessarily indicate the range of motion of specific segmental joint levels of the low back. In other words, a client may have a full 45-degree range of motion into right lateral flexion of the lumbar spine as a whole; however, the client may be restricted and hypomobile within a specific portion of the lumbar spine, say at the L4-L5 segmental joint level. If the client is compensating with more motion at the adjacent L3-L4 joint level, then this hypermobile L3-L4 joint will mask the hypomobile L4-L5 joint level (Fig. 2-23).

Mechanism and Causes of Joint Dysfunction

There are usually two major mechanisms that can cause a hypomobile joint. One is tight (hypertonic) muscles that

cross the joint; this is especially true of smaller, deeper intrinsic muscles of the joint, such as rotatores, interspinales, and intertransversarii of the low back. The other is taut soft tissues resulting from the buildup of fibrous adhesions; this is especially important if the adhesions build up in the joint capsules and ligaments of the joint because they directly and intimately limit the motion of the joint.

There are also two major mechanisms that cause a hypermobile joint. Certainly, an overstretching injury of the joint's soft tissues, especially the joint capsules and ligaments, will result in an unstable hypermobile joint. Another common mechanism that creates a hypermobile joint is excessive joint movement in compensation for an adjacent hypomobility. This is especially true in the spine, where multiple joints are located next to each other.

The example used in the preceding section demonstrates why it can be important to detect early a segmental hypomobility. If L4-L5 is hypomobile and L3-L4 compensates by becoming hypermobile, in time, L3-L4 level will likely be overused and become fatigued and painful. This will lead to the pain-spasm-pain cycle, which in turn will result in a tightening of the smaller intrinsic muscles around the L3-L4 joint, causing it to become hypomobile as well. As a result, demand will be placed on the next segmental level, L2-L3, to become further hypermobile to compensate for the two hypomobile segments below it. Naturally, in time, this level may be similarly overused and then become hypomobile itself. Segmental joint dysfunction hypomobilities tend to have a domino effect, spreading through the spine until sufficient hypermobile compensation is not possible and the overall gross range of motion of the spine is decreased. However, this point is often reached late in the disease process. If not detected early, delayed treatment allows tight musculature to become chronic and more fascial adhesions to form. For this reason, it is important to locate and identify segmental joint hypomobilities early when only one, or perhaps two, are present. The assessment technique for segmental joint hypomobility is called joint play assessment, or **motion palpation**, and is addressed in Chapter 3. Treatment is then aimed at introducing motion into these restricted joints.

It should be emphasized that joint dysfunction is not necessarily a problem of the entire low back and/or pelvis. Rather, it is more focused on a specific segmental joint level of the region. When joint dysfunction of a segmental joint level occurs, it is often the result of a tightening of the smaller, deeper, intrinsic postural muscles that cross just that joint or perhaps a couple of joints in that area. Examples are the rotatores, multifidus, intertransversarii, or interspinales. Similarly, taut fascial tissues, likely the result of fascial adhesions, are not necessarily present in every area of the low back. Instead, they may be present in the joint capsules and ligaments of a specific joint level or a couple of joint levels. The same process that a manual therapist often sees on a larger level is simply being played out on a smaller, more focused level.

BOX 2.4

Causes of Joint Hypomobility

In addition to tight musculature and fascial adhesions, two other mechanisms exist that can cause joint hypomobility. One is bone spur formation at the joint margins; this is part of the DJD process (DJD is covered in more detail later in this chapter). If a bone spur becomes large enough, it can block and limit joint motion at that segmental level. The other mechanism is the presence of a meniscoid body within the joint space. A **meniscoid body** is a fibrous, fatty, soft tissue that is usually present at the periphery of a joint space. The meniscoid body functions to increase the congruity of the joint by helping the two joint surfaces better fit together. However, if it displaces and moves toward the center of the joint, it can jam between the two bones and cause a blockage and restriction of motion (see accompanying figure).

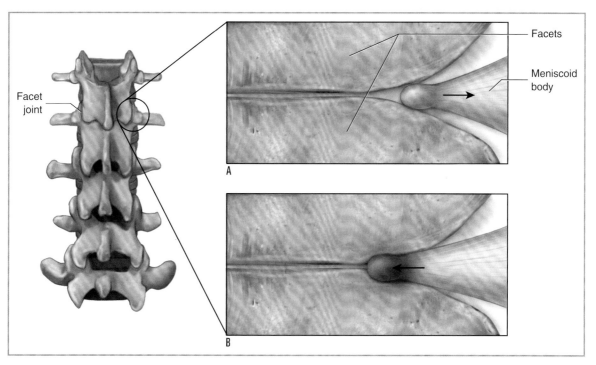

(**A**) A meniscoid body's normal and healthy relationship to the facet joint. (**B**) A meniscoid body jammed between the two facets of the joint. (Adapted with permission from Muscolino JE. *Advanced Treatment Techniques for the Manual Therapist: Neck*. Baltimore, MD: Lippincott Williams & Wilkins; 2013.)

2.2   TREATMENT CONSIDERATIONS IN BRIEF

Joint Dysfunction

Every technique presented in this book can be used to address hypomobile joint dysfunction. Massage and stretching can be used to loosen tight muscles associated with hypomobility as well as to stretch the taut soft tissues associated with it. However, the best technique to target the specific segmental hypomobilities is joint mobilization. Hydrotherapies can also be beneficial for softening and loosening these tight/taut soft tissues. Hypermobile joint dysfunction is more problematic to treat. For more details, see Chapter 3.

SPRAINS AND STRAINS

Sprains and strains are usually addressed together because they are similar in nature. Technically, when a ligament or joint capsule is torn, it is termed a **sprain**; when a muscle is torn, it is termed a **strain** (Fig. 2-24).

Description of Sprains and Strains

Sprains and strains tend to occur together because the force that is necessary to tear one tissue will likely cause tearing of the other. However, sprains and strains are not always equally present. An injury may present as a minor sprain but be a major strain or vice versa. The severity of a sprain or a strain is expressed as follows:

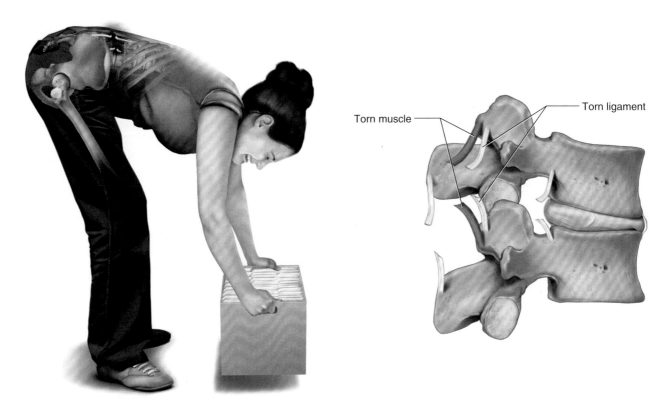

Figure 2-24 Low back strain and sprain. Attempting to lift a heavy object that is in front of the body places a strong force on the posterior tissues of the low back. If this force is excessive, a tearing of the low back extensor musculature, termed a strain, can occur. A tearing of ligament, termed a sprain, can also occur.

| 2.2 | THERAPIST TIP |

Strain

The term *strain* is often used loosely. At times, a client who is described as having a strain actually has a muscle spasm. As explained previously, when a muscle is stretched too quickly or too far, the muscle spindle's stretch reflex is initiated, which causes the muscle to contract (spasm). This reflex prevents the muscle from being torn and therefore strained. However, the resulting muscle spasm is often described as a strain (certainly, if some tearing occurred before the stretch reflex engaged, then it would truly be a strain in addition to a spasm). However, it is possible to justify the use of the term strain in this scenario from another perspective. Any strenuous use of a muscle usually results in a normal and healthy amount of **microtearing** of the muscle's fascial tissue. This fascial microtearing is necessary so that the fascia can mend and heal larger. This allows for more sarcomeres and sarcoplasm to be placed in the muscle fiber when a muscle hypertrophies after exercising. Hence, this microtearing could be interpreted as a minor strain of the muscle. The most important point is to understand the mechanism of what is occurring so that treatment is appropriate for the condition.

■ Grade I: minor tear
■ Grade II: moderate tear
■ Grade III: marked tear or complete rupture

Given that strains and sprains involve torn soft tissue, pain, inflammation, and bruising are usually present when the sprain and/or strain are in the acute stage. Muscular splinting/spasming is also present in the acute stage and often persists long-term.

Although sprains and strains are similar, functionally, they present quite differently. Sprains are worse than strains because ligaments lack a good blood supply and therefore do not heal well. For this reason, once a ligament has been stretched and torn, it usually heals stretched out and remains that way for the rest of the client's life, resulting in chronic joint hypermobility. Musculature, on the other hand, has a good blood supply, so strains usually heal well if properly treated. However, the presence of a good blood supply also causes more bleeding and bruising with strains. Strains also usually hurt more than sprains because muscle tissue has more sensory nerve endings than ligaments.

Mechanism and Causes of Sprains and Strains

The mechanism for sprains and strains is similar. An excessive pulling force causes a disruption of the fibers of the ligament or musculature (see Fig. 2-24). This pulling force can occur during a macrotrauma, such as bending over to lift a heavy object, a fall, or a car accident. It can also occur from repeated postural or movement microtraumas, such as overuse injuries that place excessive tension on ligaments and muscles over time; repeated bending is a good example of this.

The function of a ligament is to limit motion of a joint; therefore, if the ligament is torn and stretched, the joint tends to become hypermobile and less stable. This may be masked during the acute phase by muscular splinting/spasming. Strains, on the other hand, tend to result in joint hypomobility, both because of muscular spasming that occurs in the short run and often continues into the long run, as well as the formation of scar tissue adhesions that occur during the healing process. Although adhesions are necessary to repair and mend torn soft tissues, if excessive adhesions are allowed to form, the tissue will lose its mobility, resulting in decreased ranges of motion.

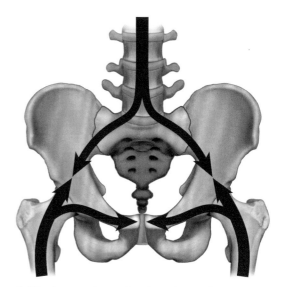

Figure 2-25 The SIJ is located in the pelvis and is subject to forces from the spine above and from the lower extremities below.

| 2.3 | TREATMENT CONSIDERATIONS IN BRIEF |

Sprains and Strains

Icing is especially useful for treating acute strains and sprains. Massage is helpful for sprains and strains when the condition is subacute and/or chronic. Stretching is helpful for subacute and chronic care of strains. For more details, see Chapter 3.

SACROILIAC JOINT INJURY

Injury to the sacroiliac joint (SIJ) is extremely common. Indeed, a large number of low back problems emanate from the SIJ.

Description of Sacroiliac Joint Injury

The SIJ is located in the pelvis, which is a transitional body part located between the lower extremities and the spine. Therefore, the SIJ is subjected to a great deal of physical stresses both from below and above (Fig. 2-25). When injured, the SIJ can be inflamed, sprained, and/or strained. Inflammation of the SIJ is termed **sacroiliitis**. If ligaments of the SIJ are overstretched or torn, it is a sprain; if muscles of the SIJ are overstretched or torn, it is a strain.

Mechanism and Causes of Sacroiliac Joint Injury

As stated, the SIJ is subjected to a great deal of physical stresses both from below and above. From below, the SIJ can be irritated from excessive motion of the lower extremities as well as impact forces from contact with the ground when walking, running, or jumping. From above, the SIJ can be irritated from excessive motion of the spine as well as weight-

bearing compression forces from the body weight above when sitting or standing and forces placed on the joint when bending over. Macrotrauma injuries such as falls and car accidents can also contribute to SIJ injuries. The sum of these physical forces can result in inflammation to the joint, in other words, sacroiliitis.

Because of the ligamentous nature of the SIJ, sprains are especially common. The SIJ has little or no musculature that crosses the joint and attaches from the sacrum to the ilium. For this reason, musculature has a limited ability to stabilize the SIJ. Although some muscles come from another bone and then attach to both the sacrum and the ilium, such as the erector spinae and the latissimus dorsi, these muscles do not cross from the sacrum to the ilium. Even the piriformis, which does cross the SIJ, does so by skipping attachment to the iliac portion of the pelvic bone, and indeed by skipping the pelvic bone entirely, to then attach to the greater trochanter of the femur; therefore, its role is involved in stabilization of the hip joint as well as the SIJ.

As a result, the SIJ must depend on its ligament complex for the vast majority of its stability. Indeed, the SIJ is extremely well supplied with ligamentous tissue (Fig. 2-26). This means that when the SIJ is injured, it is usually a sprain that occurs, not a strain. And because ligaments have a relatively poor blood supply, they do not heal well; therefore, an SIJ sprain usually results in a chronic hypermobile joint that remains unstable. A strain to SIJ musculature can occur but is far less common in occurrence and/or is usually a small component of the client's SIJ injury.

Sacroiliac Joint Muscle Splinting and Symptoms

Regardless of whether the condition is sacroiliitis, SIJ sprain, or SIJ strain, adjacent musculature commonly tightens in an attempt to splint the joint. When compensatory muscular

Figure 2-26 Ligaments of the SIJ. (**A**) Posterior view. (**B**) Anterior view.

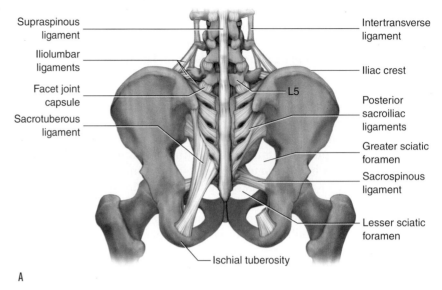

Supraspinous ligament

Iliolumbar ligaments

Facet joint capsule

Sacrotuberous ligament

Intertransverse ligament

Iliac crest

L5

Posterior sacroiliac ligaments

Greater sciatic foramen

Sacrospinous ligament

Lesser sciatic foramen

Ischial tuberosity

A

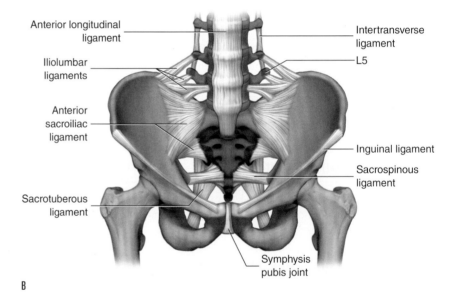

Anterior longitudinal ligament

Iliolumbar ligaments

Anterior sacroiliac ligament

Sacrotuberous ligament

Intertransverse ligament

L5

Inguinal ligament

Sacrospinous ligament

Symphysis pubis joint

B

spasming accompanies an SIJ injury, it is usually the same-side piriformis, lumbar erector spinae and transversospinalis musculature, superomedial fibers of the gluteus maximus directly next to the posterior superior iliac spine (PSIS), and the hamstrings. The same-side gluteus medius and the other deep lateral rotators are also often involved (Fig. 2-27). These same muscles on the other side may also become involved because one SIJ often becomes hypermobile to compensate for the other SIJ if the other SIJ is hypomobile or injured.

SIJ symptoms classically include pain during prolonged sitting or standing, bending, and with excessive walking. The quality of the pain is usually dull but can become sharp at times. The pain is usually located directly over the SIJ, immediately medial to the PSIS. Pain may also be located lateral to the PSIS in the superomedial fibers of the gluteus maximus or can be superior to the sacrum in the erector spinae and

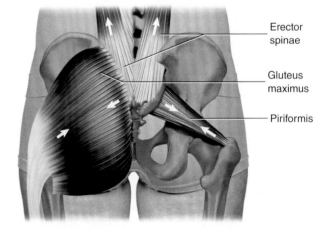

Erector spinae

Gluteus maximus

Piriformis

Figure 2-27 When the SIJ is injured, muscles in the region often splint to protect the joint.

transversospinalis musculature (overlying the lumbosacral joint). Due to the fact that injury to one SIJ often results in compensation by the other SIJ, it is common for SIJ pain to switch from one side of the body to the other.

2.4 | TREATMENT CONSIDERATIONS IN BRIEF

Sacroiliac Joint Injury and Sprain

Treatment to an irritated/injured SIJ involves moist heat, massage, and stretching to the compensatory tight muscles of the region. If the SIJ is hypomobile, then stretching and joint mobilization are especially important. If the SIJ is hypermobile, then the ultimate treatment is for the client to engage in strengthening exercise to stabilize the region. For more details, see Chapter 3.

2.3 | THERAPIST TIP

Sacroiliac Joint Injury and the Hamstrings

Hamstring musculature often tightens for stabilization and splinting when the SIJ on that side of the body is injured. The hamstrings do not attach directly into the sacrum; however, their contractile pull is transferred to the sacrum via their fascial connection into the sacrotuberous ligament, which does attach into the sacrum. The therapist should always assess the hamstrings in all clients who present with an injured SIJ.

PATHOLOGIC DISC CONDITIONS AND SCIATICA

Pathologic discs of the lumbar spine are extremely common. Although any pathologic disc is potentially serious, the degree of symptoms and functional impairment can vary tremendously. Some pathologic discs require immediate surgery, whereas others cause no problem and may be found, if at all, only incidentally when magnetic resonance imaging (MRI) or a computed tomography (CT) scan is done for another reason.

Description of Pathologic Disc Conditions

There are two major types of pathologic conditions of the intervertebral disc:

- Disc thinning
- Bulging or rupture of the fibers of the annulus fibrosus

Disc thinning involves a decrease in the height of the disc. Given that the volume of the inner nucleus pulposus determines the height of the disc, disc thinning occurs as the nucleus pulposus gradually desiccates with age. This condition usually occurs when the client is middle-aged or older. The danger of disc thinning is that as the two adjacent vertebrae approach each other, there is a decrease in size of the intervertebral foramina at that level through which the spinal nerves pass (Fig. 2-28). Because greater disc thickness allows for greater range of motion of that intervertebral joint, disc thinning can also result in decreased range of motion.

Thus, if disc thinning becomes marked in degree, spinal nerve compression is possible. Because a spinal nerve carries both sensory and motor neurons, altered sensation can occur wherever the sensory neurons of that spinal nerve originated

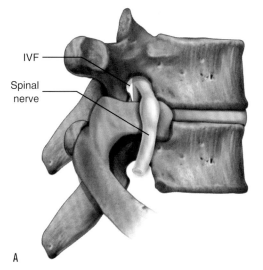
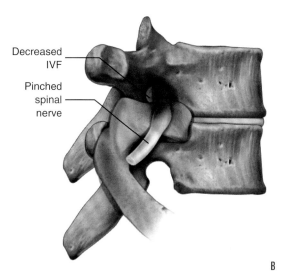

Figure 2-28 Disc height and the size of the intervertebral foramen. (**A**) The disc is healthy and there is a normal-sized intervertebral foramen (IVF) through which the spinal nerve travels. (**B**) The disc has thinned, resulting in an IVF that is decreased in size and impingement of the spinal nerve. (Reproduced with permission from Muscolino JE. *Advanced Treatment Techniques for the Manual Therapist: Neck*. Baltimore, MD: Lippincott Williams & Wilkins; 2013.)

and/or altered motor function can occur wherever the motor neurons of that spinal nerve end. Sensory symptoms can include tingling, numbness, or pain; motor symptoms can include twitching, weakness, or flaccid paralysis of the musculature. Because the lumbar and sacral spinal nerves innervate the lower extremity, these symptoms occur in the pelvic (gluteal) region, thigh, leg, and/or foot. However, for most clients, disc thinning does not usually progress to the point that nerve compression with lower extremity referral occurs.

The other major type of pathologic disc condition is a weakening of the outer annulus fibrosus that leads to a bulging or rupture of its fibers. This condition has three major types/gradations of severity:

- Disc bulge
- Disc rupture
- Sequestered disc

The mildest form is a **disc bulge**. In this condition, the annular fibers weaken and allow the nucleus pulposus to push against the annulus, causing it to bulge outward (Fig. 2-29A). A disc bulge is considered the mildest form because the annular fibers are still intact. A **disc rupture** is considered the next degree of severity because the annular fibers have weakened to the point that the pressure of the nucleus pulposus causes them to rupture. In this case, the nucleus pulposus can actually extrude through the annulus and enter into the intervertebral foramen or spinal canal. A disc rupture is also known as a **disc herniation** or **disc prolapse** (Fig. 2-29B). The third and most severe form of this pathologic disc condition is the sequestered disc. A **sequestered disc** is a disc rupture in which a portion of the nucleus pulposus that extrudes through the annular fibers separates from the inner core of nucleus pulposus (the term "sequester" literally means to set apart or separate) (Fig. 2-29C). It cannot rejoin the disc and is left to float within the intervertebral foramen or spinal canal.

The danger with disc bulges, herniations, and sequestrations is that the disc can push outward and compress the spinal nerve within the intervertebral foraminal space or the spinal cord within the central spinal canal at that level. Therefore, they are considered to be **space-occupying lesions**. (*Note*: DJD, covered later in this chapter, is another common example of a space-occupying lesion that can compress spinal nerves). With a bulging disc, the bulging annular fibers can compress the neural structures; with a ruptured or sequestered disc, the nucleus pulposus can create the compression.

If a pathologic disc compresses nerve roots of the sciatic nerve, a condition called **sciatica** can occur. The sciatic nerve is the largest nerve in the human body. It measures approximately a quarter inch in diameter and is composed of L3, L4, L5, S1, and S2 nerve roots. Symptoms of sciatica can be sensory and/or motor because both sensory and motor neurons are located in the sciatic nerve. Pain and/or motor weakness of sciatica can occur in the posterior thigh, or leg, or anywhere in the foot (Fig. 2-30).

The actual determinant of the severity of these conditions is the degree of nerve compression that occurs. For this reason, a large disc bulge can be much more problematic than a small disc rupture. Sequestered discs are usually the worst because the extruded fragment of nucleus pulposus remains in the intervertebral foramen or spinal canal and can continue to compress the spinal nerve or spinal cord, respectively.

Mechanism of Pathologic Disc Conditions

Annular bulges and ruptures occur as a result of forces that stress and weaken the annular fibers. These can be **microtraumas** or **macrotraumas**. Microtraumas are small physical stresses. One example is the everyday compression that results from supporting the weight of the trunk, neck, head, and upper extremities. Another example is holding a prolonged posture that stresses the disc, such as maintaining a bent-over posture of the trunk to work down in front of the body. Postures in which the trunk is held forward in flexion are especially prevalent and contribute to disc problems. The po-

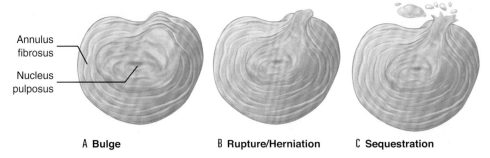

Annulus fibrosus

Nucleus pulposus

A Bulge　　　**B Rupture/Herniation**　　　**C Sequestration**

Figure 2-29 Three forms of pathologic disc conditions. (**A**) Disc bulge. The annulus fibrosus weakens and bulges, but the nucleus pulposus remains within the annular fibers. (**B**) Disc rupture/herniation. The annular fibers have ruptured/herniated, and the nucleus pulposus material extrudes through the annulus but remains attached to the core of nuclear material. (**C**) Sequestered disc. A sequestered disc is a disc rupture/herniation in which a piece of the nucleus pulposus that has extruded through the annulus separates from the core of inner nuclear material. (Reproduced with permission from Muscolino JE. *Advanced Treatment Techniques for the Manual Therapist: Neck.* Baltimore, MD: Lippincott Williams & Wilkins; 2013.)

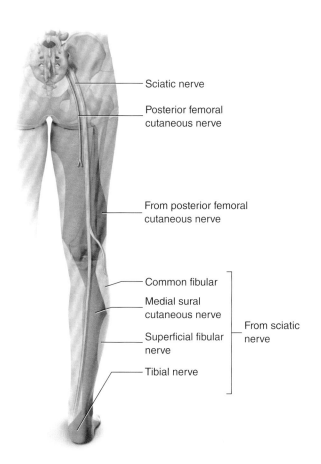

Figure 2-30 The sciatic nerve provides sensory innervation into the lower extremity.

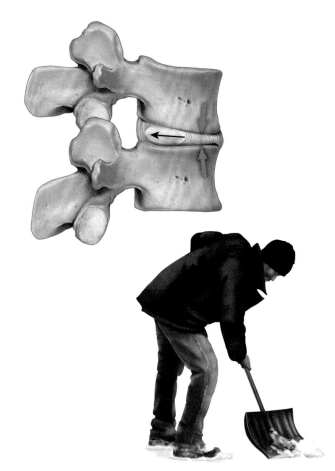

Figure 2-31 Nucleus pressure against the posterior annular fibers. Flexion of a vertebral joint creates a compression force at the anterior disc that pushes the nucleus pulposus posteriorly against taut posterior annular fibers. Repeated flexion postures can lead to excessive wear against the posterior annulus. (Adapted with permission from Muscolino JE. *Advanced Treatment Techniques for the Manual Therapist: Neck*. Baltimore, MD: Lippincott Williams & Wilkins; 2013.)

sition of flexion pulls taut the posterior annular fibers while at the same time pushing the nucleus pulposus posteriorly against these taut fibers. Continual flexion postures cause eventual weakness and fraying of the posterior fibers of the annulus (Fig. 2-31). These microtraumas accrue over time and gradually weaken the annulus until the nucleus either causes it to bulge or ruptures through it.

Macrotraumas such as severe traumatic sports injuries or falls may also cause discs to bulge or rupture. Often, a weakened disc from repeated postural microtraumas coupled with a somewhat traumatic event will cause the integrity of the fibers of the annulus fibrosus to fail, resulting in a bulge or rupture of its fibers.

Most often, the annulus weakens and/or ruptures posterolaterally regardless of whether the pathologic disc occurs as a result of microtrauma or macrotrauma. The prevalence of flexion postures contributes to this problem because flexion causes the nucleus pulposus to push backward against the posterior annular fibers, gradually weakening them. However, because the posterior longitudinal ligament of the spine reinforces the annulus midline posteriorly (posteromedially), the effect of the physical stress of constant and recurring flexion postures usually manifests posterolaterally. Because the intervertebral foramina are located posterolaterally, most

disc conditions result in compression of a spinal nerve in the intervertebral foramen on one side. If a disc were to bulge or rupture in the midline posteriorly, it would compress directly on the spinal cord in the central spinal canal.

The symptoms of a lumbar disc bulge or rupture may refer to the lower extremity, occur in the low back alone, or both. Because most disc bulges/ruptures occur posterolaterally, compressing the spinal nerve in the intervertebral foramen, the result is unilateral sensory or motor symptoms that occur in the lower extremity on that side. Occasionally, a disc bulge or rupture may occur in the midline posteriorly. In such an instance, depending on which neurons of the cord are compressed, symptoms may be felt in the lower extremity unilaterally or bilaterally (Fig. 2-32).

Symptoms may also be local if the small nerves in the disc area are compressed. When this occurs, pain occurs directly from this compression. Low back muscles may then protectively splint to stop movement that may further harm the

Tight Muscles and Disc Problems

Perhaps the least appreciated but common microtrauma that contributes to spinal disc problems is tight muscles. When spinal muscles become tight, their attachments pull toward the center, drawing the vertebrae crossed by these muscles toward each other. This results in an increased compression on the discs (see accompanying figure). Clients commonly have chronically tight low back muscles, which can contribute significantly to an eventual pathologic disc.

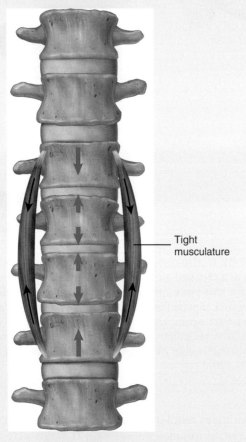

Tight musculature

(Reproduced with permission from Muscolino JE. *Advanced Treatment Techniques for the Manual Therapist: Neck.* Baltimore, MD: Lippincott Williams & Wilkins; 2013.)

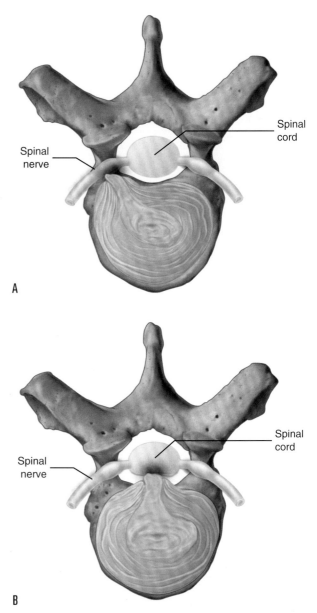

Spinal cord

Spinal nerve

A

Spinal cord

Spinal nerve

B

Figure 2-32 Disc herniation. **(A)** A posterolateral disc herniation presses on the spinal nerve as it passes through the intervertebral foramen. **(B)** A midline posterior herniation compresses the spinal cord in the spinal canal. (Reproduced with permission from Muscolino JE. *Advanced Treatment Techniques for the Manual Therapist: Neck.* Baltimore, MD: Lippincott Williams & Wilkins; 2013.)

Central Canal Stenosis

Another space-occupying condition that can cause referral into the lower extremity is **central canal stenosis**. As its name implies, the space within the central spinal canal where the spinal cord is located becomes stenotic (narrowed/closed). This condition usually occurs in the elderly as ligaments hypertrophy (thicken) and bone spurs from DJD develop, pushing into the central spinal canal and compressing the spinal cord. This condition usually continues to progress and can become very debilitating. Extension of the lumbar spine usually increases lower extremity pain/symptoms because extension narrows the diameter of the spinal canal; flexion usually relieves lower extremity pain/referral because flexion increases the diameter of the lumbar spinal canal.

disc. Unfortunately, the severity of the muscle spasming it-self may cause pain, and the muscle splinting can increase the compression force on the discs, further aggravating the condition by increasing the size of the bulge or rupture. Note that when a disc condition is acute, inflammation can contribute to the neural compression, with the swelling itself producing symptoms. As the episode passes from the acute stage to the subacute and chronic stages, symptoms often decrease because swelling has diminished.

Although local low back pain or spasming may occur, lumbar pathologic discs often show no local symptoms at all and present with only lower extremity referral symptoms. Pain, tingling, numbness, or weaknesses that are referred in the lower extremity should be a red flag that a disc problem may exist. However, this does not mean that all lower extremity referral symptoms come from a lumbar disc bulge or rupture. Other conditions such as piriformis syndrome (see next section) or meralgia paresthetica (Box 2.6) may also

---

BOX 2.6

Meralgia Paresthetica

The sciatic nerve is not the only nerve that can be compressed and cause referral into the lower extremity. The lateral femoral cutaneous nerve, which exits from the pelvis into the anterolateral thigh between the pelvic bone and the inguinal ligament, can also be compressed. When this occurs, the resulting condition is called **meralgia paresthetica**.

Because the lateral femoral cutaneous nerve is solely sensory, this condition results only in altered sensation,

usually tingling or pain, into the anterolateral thigh (see accompanying figures). The most common causes of meralgia paresthetica are wearing low-rise jeans or a belt too tightly, being overweight with increased weight carried in the anterior abdominal region, and tightness of various hip flexor muscles, including the iliopsoas, sartorius, and/or tensor fasciae latae. With the increased rates of obesity in the United States, the incidence of meralgia paresthetica will likely increase in the future.

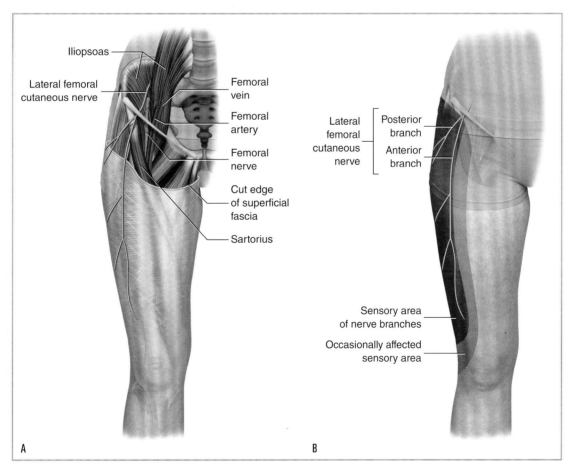

Meralgia paresthetica. (**A**) Meralgia paresthetica is caused by compression of the lateral femoral cutaneous nerve. (**B**) Area of sensory symptoms in the anterolateral thigh.

refer symptoms to the lower extremity. Although a reasonably accurate assessment can be made with the appropriate orthopedic assessment procedures (see Chapter 3), if a lumbar disc condition is suspected, the client should be referred immediately to a physician for a definitive diagnosis.

| 2.5 | TREATMENT CONSIDERATIONS IN BRIEF |

Pathologic Disc

Massage can be extremely beneficial to help decrease muscular spasms associated with a pathologic disc. Stretching is also helpful, but caution is advised if the client's trunk is extended or laterally flexed to the side of a pathologic disc. It is contraindicated to place the client in any position that causes or increases referral of symptoms into the lower extremity. Icing may help decrease some of the inflammation that accompanies a pathologic disc. For more details, see Chapter 3.

PIRIFORMIS SYNDROME

Piriformis syndrome is a condition in which the piriformis muscle compresses the sciatic nerve, causing symptoms of sciatica into the lower extremity (see previous section).

Description of Piriformis Syndrome

Normally, the sciatic nerve exits from the internal pelvis into the buttocks between the piriformis muscle and the superior gemellus muscle. However, approximately 10% to 20% of the time, part or all of the sciatic nerve either exits through the piriformis, or above it, between the piriformis and the gluteus medius (Fig. 2-33). Regardless of the relationship of the piriformis and sciatic nerve, if the muscle is tight enough, the nerve may be compressed, resulting in sciatica. This condition is often said to cause "pseudo sciatica"; however, this term does not make sense and shows a bias toward bony or disc impingement on the nerve. If compression of the sciatic nerve occurs and symptoms of sciatica are experienced, then regardless of the cause, it can be correctly termed sciatica.

Mechanism and Causes of Piriformis Syndrome

The piriformis muscle can become tight due to overuse. The piriformis acts as a lateral rotator of the thigh at the hip joint as well as a contralateral rotator of the pelvis at the hip joint (contralateral rotation of the pelvis occurs when planting and cutting [planting the foot and pivoting to change directions] during sports). The piriformis is also functionally important toward stabilizing the sacrum at the sacroiliac joint and stabilizing the hip joint.

| 2.6 | TREATMENT CONSIDERATIONS IN BRIEF |

Piriformis Syndrome

Because piriformis syndrome is a condition of muscular origin, it makes sense that it will respond well to soft tissue manipulation. Moist heat, massage, and stretching are all very beneficial. For more details, see Chapter 3.

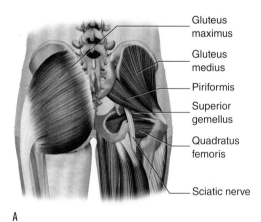
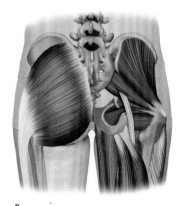
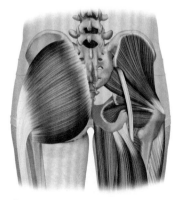

Gluteus maximus
Gluteus medius
Piriformis
Superior gemellus
Quadratus femoris
Sciatic nerve

A   B   C

Figure 2-33 Relationship of the sciatic nerve to the piriformis. **(A)** The usual relationship is for the sciatic nerve to emerge from the internal pelvis into the gluteal region between the piriformis and the superior gemellus. **(B, C)** Sometimes, part or all of the sciatic nerve exits through the piriformis or above the piriformis, between it and the gluteus medius.

DEGENERATIVE JOINT DISEASE

Degenerative joint disease (DJD) is a disease in which the joint surfaces of bones deteriorate. DJD is a normal response to the physical forces that are placed on the joints as you age. However, if the degree of progression is either more than is typical for the client's age or impairs function, it is considered a pathologic disease process. DJD is also known as **osteoarthritis (OA)**; when this condition occurs in the spine, it may also be called **spondylosis**. Most older middle-aged and elderly clients who state that they have "arthritis" have DJD.

2.5   THERAPIST TIP

The Terms *Degenerative Joint Disease* and *Osteoarthritis*

Arthritis literally means "joint inflammation" ("arthr" means joint; "itis" means inflammation). The term *degenerative joint disease* is gradually replacing the term *osteoarthritis* because inflammation is rarely involved in this condition, making the suffix "itis" inappropriate. Inflammation is usually present only when the condition has progressed and is more severe.

Description of Degenerative Joint Disease

The beginning stage of DJD involves breakdown of the articular cartilage that covers the joint surfaces of the two bones of the joint. As the condition progresses, calcium is deposited within the bone that underlies the articular cartilage (subchondral bone). In the later stage of DJD, calcium deposition begins to occur on the outer surfaces of the bones of the joints, and **bone spurs** (also known as **osteophytes**) protrude at the joint margins (Fig. 2-34). DJD can affect both the disc and facet joints of the spine. These bone spurs are easily seen on radiography, making radiographic analysis (x-ray) the best and easiest means to assess DJD.

Because DJD occurs as a result of accumulated physical stresses, radiographs of most middle-aged people will reveal at least some lumbar spinal DJD. Most of the time, the presence of DJD is an incidental finding, and the condition causes no symptoms. However, if the condition progresses to the point of functional impairment, a decrease of motion can occur at the joint where the DJD is present. This is a result of the presence of bone spurs that block full range of motion of the affected joint. Furthermore, if the calcium deposition creates bone spurs that are large enough to encroach on the spinal nerve in the intervertebral foramen or on the spinal cord within the spinal canal, the calcium deposition can cause compression of nervous tissue, resulting in referral into the lower extremities. When the calcium deposits of DJD cause compression of a spinal nerve or the spinal cord, DJD is similar in mechanism to a bulging or ruptured disc in that it is a space-occupying lesion that compresses nerve tissue.

Mechanism and Causes of Degenerative Joint Disease

The mechanism of DJD is a simple wear and tear response of the cartilage and bony surfaces of a joint resulting from the physical stress that is placed on the bones at the joint. If the degree of physical stress is more than the joint can absorb, the articular cartilage begins to degrade, and in so doing, more stress is transmitted to the subchondral bone. Excessive stress on the subchondral bone then causes calcium to be deposited along the margins of the bones of the joint, a physical process known as **Wolff's law**. Wolff's law states that calcium is deposited in response to the physical stress that is placed on a bone. This process is meant to strengthen bone by increasing its calcium mass; however, if the stresses placed on the bone are excessive, ex-

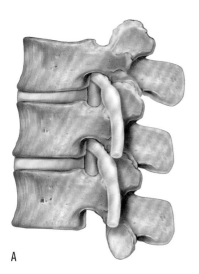
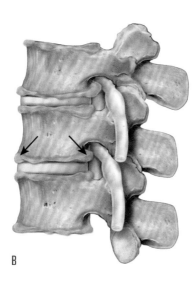

A   B

Figure 2-34 DJD and bone spur formation. (**A**) Healthy spine. (**B**) Bone spurs along the joint margins. (Reproduced with permission from Muscolino JE. *Advanced Treatment Techniques for the Manual Therapist: Neck.* Baltimore, MD: Lippincott Williams & Wilkins; 2013.)

cessive calcium deposition occurs, resulting in bone spurs, as described previously. Movement and weight bearing are everyday microtrauma stresses that affect joints. Tight musculature, especially chronically tight postural muscles, can also be viewed as repeated microtrauma that adds compression forces to the joints that the tight muscles cross. Certainly, more powerful macrotraumas, such as falls and other traumatic injuries, can also greatly contribute to the progression of DJD.

2.6	**THERAPIST TIP**

Is Degenerative Joint Disease the Cause of the Client's Pain?

DJD must be fairly marked in its progression to actually compress spinal nerves or the spinal cord and cause symptoms. However, physicians often wrongly blame DJD for a client's pain when the pain is actually caused by tight muscles and other taut or irritated periarticular soft tissues located around the joint. Tight muscles are probably the most common aggravated periarticular soft tissue. When the physician orders and views radiographs (x-rays) of the client's low back, if any DJD is present, as is usually the case in most middle-aged and older adults, it is often blamed for the client's pain. But the muscles and other soft tissues are not visible on radiographs, and these tissues often are the real culprit. When this is the case, the manual therapist can provide an important service by relaxing, softening, and loosening the muscles and other soft tissues of the low back and pelvis. Further, because tight muscles and other soft tissues can add to the physical stress on joints, improving the health of the soft tissues can also decrease the progression of the client's DJD and possibly even help to keep it from causing nerve compression.

2.7	**TREATMENT CONSIDERATIONS IN BRIEF**

Degenerative Joint Disease

Massage can be extremely beneficial in helping to decrease the muscular spasms that often coexist with and increase the physical stresses that foster DJD. Stretching is also helpful for the taut soft tissues that likely exist. However, if the DJD is advanced to the point that it is causing neural compression, then the client should not be laterally flexed to the side of a bone spur or placed in any position that causes or increases referral of symptoms into the lower extremity. If neural compression and/or nerve irritation is present, icing may help to decrease some of the accompanying inflammation. For more details, see Chapter 3.

SCOLIOSIS

Scoliosis is, by definition, a lateral flexion deformity of the spine. Although the spine should have curves in the sagittal plane, in the frontal plane, it should ideally be straight. Any curve that is present in the frontal plane is a scoliosis.

Description of Scoliosis

The shape of a scoliotic curve is usually described as being a C-curve, an S-curve, or a double S-curve (Fig. 2-35). Further, like most conditions, a scoliosis can be mild in presentation or more severe. The severity of a scoliotic curve can be measured by drawing a line along the superior surface of the body of the uppermost vertebra of the scoliotic curve and another line along the inferior surface of the body of the lowermost vertebra of the scoliotic curve, and then measuring the angle that is created by their intersection (Fig. 2-36). It is also important to note that although scoliosis is defined by its frontal plane lateral flexion, transverse plane rotation is also present. In the lumbar spine, facet joint lateral flexion couples with contralateral rotation; this results in the spinous processes rotating into the concavity of the curve (see Fig. 2-35). This coupled rotation can have repercussions during the postural assessment exam because if the therapist uses visualization of the spinous processes to assess the degree of scoliosis, when the spinous processes rotate into the concavity, the degree of scoliosis appears to be less (Fig. 2-37). For this reason, when possible, it is best to view an x-ray to determine the degree of a client's scoliosis.

Mechanism and Causes of Scoliosis

The curvature of the lumbar spine is largely determined by the posture of the pelvis. The 5th lumbar vertebra sits on the base of the sacrum of the pelvis; therefore, if the sacrum

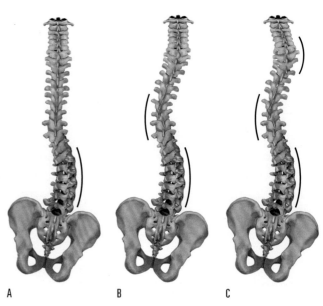

A   B   C

Figure 2-35 Scoliotic curves. (**A**) C-curve. (**B**) S-curve. (**C**) Double S-curve.

changes its posture, the lumbar spine must accordingly change its posture. If the sacrum tilts in the frontal plane, then like the Leaning Tower of Pisa, the spine will lean to that side. This would result in the head being unlevel, and therefore the eyes and inner ears being unlevel, throwing off our sense of balance and making it difficult to see. To compensate, the spine bends in the frontal plane to bring the head back to level, thereby creating a scoliotic curve (Fig. 2-38). A number of factors can unlevel the sacrum. A tight quadratus lumborum could pull the pelvis and sacrum up on one side; similarly, tight hip abductors (e.g., gluteus medius) could pull the pelvis and sacrum down on one side. An anatomically short femur or tibia can create a lower extremity that is shorter on one side than the other, dropping the pelvis/sacrum on that side. Excessive pronation of the foot, resulting in a dropped arch, can also result in a shorter lower extremity on that side.

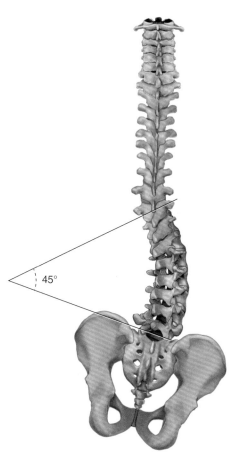

Figure 2-36 A scoliotic curve can be measured by drawing a line along the superior margin of the body of the upper vertebra of the curve, another line along the inferior margin of the body of the lower vertebra of the curve, and then measuring the angle formed by their intersection.

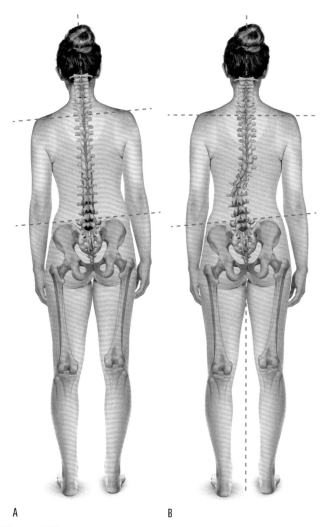

A   B

Figure 2-38 Scoliosis as a compensation for unlevel sacral posture. (**A**) If the sacrum is unlevel in the frontal plane, the spine would slant to the side where the sacrum is low. This results in the head, and therefore the eyes and inner ears being unlevel. (**B**) As a compensation, a scoliotic curve of the spine brings the eyes and inner ears to be level.

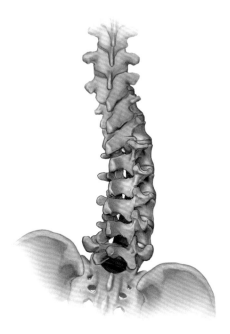

Figure 2-37 In the lumbar spine, the spinous processes rotate into the concavity of a scoliosis, making the scoliosis less evident during visual examination.

Sometimes, the cause of a scoliotic curve is unknown. Idiopathic scoliosis, which usually occurs in adolescent girls and is often quite severe, has no known cause (idiopathic literally means "of unknown origin").

Regardless of the cause, it is important to treat scoliosis because it can continue to progress throughout a person's life, often increasing between one-half and one degree per year.

2.7 THERAPIST TIP

Scoliosis and Tight Muscles

Muscles are usually tight on both sides of a scoliotic curve. The muscles are lengthened and tight on the convex side (often termed "**locked long**") and shortened and tight on the concave side (often termed "**locked short**"). Although it is important to work both sides, it is especially important to work the shortened concave-side muscles with massage and stretching and to work the lengthened convex-side muscles with massage and strengthening exercise.

2.8 TREATMENT CONSIDERATIONS IN BRIEF

Scoliosis

Moist heat, massage, and stretching can be very beneficial for clients with scoliosis. When stretching, it is important that the client focus the stretch so that the lateral flexion component of the stretch is opposite to the concavity of the curve. In other words, if the concavity is oriented to the right, the stretch should be into left lateral flexion. For more details, see Chapter 3.

ANTERIOR PELVIC TILT AND HYPERLORDOTIC LUMBAR SPINE

The healthy lumbar spine should have a lordotic curve (also known as a lordosis). However, it is very common for the degree of lumbar extension, described as lordosis, to be excessive.

Description of Anterior Pelvic Tilt and Hyperlordotic Lumbar Spine

When the lumbar lordosis is excessive, it is described as a **hyperlordotic lumbar spine** (**hyperlordosis**), and commonly called a **swayback**. The problem with this condition is that it places excessive pressure on the facet joints of the spine and the posterior margins of the discs (Fig. 2-39). This can lead to irritation, injury, and pain. This can be easily felt by simply tilting the pelvis anteriorly and arching the back; this usually

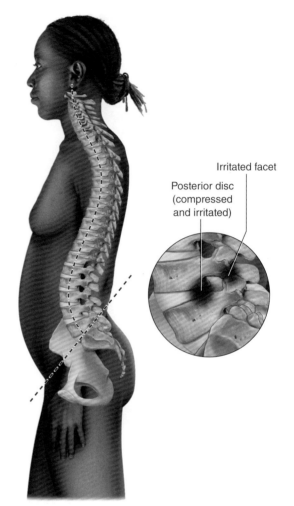

Figure 2-39 A hyperlordotic lumbar spine places greater weight-bearing force on the facet joints and the posterior discs.

causes immediate low back discomfort or pain. More seriously, because lumbar extension/lordosis decreases the size of the intervertebral foramina as well as the central spinal canal, this condition can predispose the client to nerve compression. Increased compression to the facets and posterior disc margins can also further the progression of DJD (see section on Degenerative Joint Disease earlier in this chapter), causing increased bone spurs, which can also further aggravate nerve compression.

2.8 THERAPIST TIP

The Terms *Lordosis* and *Lordotic*

Because many people use the terms *lordosis* and *lordotic* to denote an excessive and unhealthy lordotic curve/lordosis, it is important to understand whether a person is referencing to a normal lordosis or an excessive lordosis when using these terms. An excessive lordosis is most accurately termed a hyperlordosis/hyperlordotic curve.

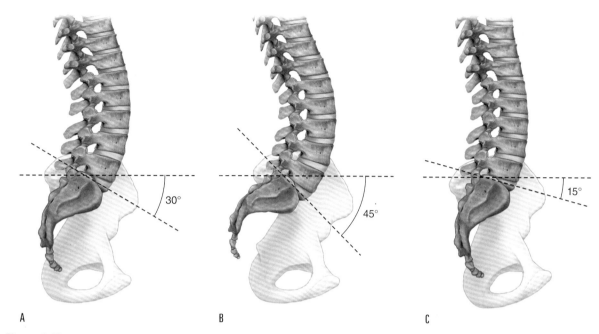

Figure 2-40 Sacral base angle and lumbar lordosis. The sacral base angle is formed by measuring the intersection of a line drawn along the base of the sacrum and a horizontal line. (**A**) Normal sacral base angle of 30 degrees and a healthy lumbar lordosis. (**B**) An increased sacral base angle results in increased lumbar lordosis. (**C**) A decreased sacral base angle results in decreased lumbar lordosis.

Mechanism and Causes of Anterior Pelvic Tilt and Lumbar Hyperlordosis

The cause of a hyperlordotic lumbar spine is almost always an increased anterior tilt posture of the pelvis. The lumbar spine sits on the sacrum of the pelvis. If the sacrum tilts anteriorly within the sagittal plane, the lumbar spine must compensate by increasing its extension/lordosis to maintain the head upright so that you can see forward and have your ears level for balance. The degree of a person's pelvic tilt is measured by the **sacral base angle**. The sacral base angle is formed by drawing two lines, one horizontal and another along the base of the sacrum, and then measuring the angle formed between them. A sacral base angle of approximately 30 degrees is usually stated as being ideal. A greater sacral base angle results in a hyperlordotic lumbar spine, and a lesser sacral base angle results in a hypolordotic lumbar spine (Fig. 2-40). Therefore, the root of a lumbar hyperlordosis usually rests in the sagittal plane posture of the pelvis. Treatment must be directed toward remedying the increased anterior pelvic tilt.

Muscles of Pelvic Tilt

The tilt posture of the pelvis in the sagittal plane is determined by the forces placed on it. Most commonly, these forces result from muscle pulls. Within the sagittal plane, the hip flexor muscle group and the low back extensor muscle group do anterior tilt of the pelvis, and the hip extensor muscle group (gluteals and hamstrings) and the anterior abdominal wall muscle group do posterior tilt of the pelvis (see Chapter 1 for more details on the musculature of pelvic tilt). It is very common for hip flexor and low back extensor anterior tilters to be excessively tight and for the anterior abdominal wall and gluteal region posterior tilters to be excessively weak. It is often stated that the anterior tilters are facilitated and the posterior tilters are inhibited in tone. When viewing this pattern from the side, you see that a cross ("X") is formed, with one arm of the cross representing the facilitated anterior tilters and the other arm representing the inhibited posterior tilters. Because of this crossed pat-

---

2.9 | TREATMENT CONSIDERATIONS IN BRIEF

Anterior Pelvic Tilt and Hyperlordotic Lumbar Spine

Soft tissue work for clients with increased anterior tilt of the pelvis and the compensatory hyperlordosis of the lumbar spine that follows is extremely valuable. The primary goal for the manual therapist is to loosen anterior tilters of the pelvis (hip flexors and low back extensors) and to have the client strengthen posterior tilters of the pelvis (anterior abdominal wall and gluteal muscles in the buttocks). For more details, see Chapter 3.

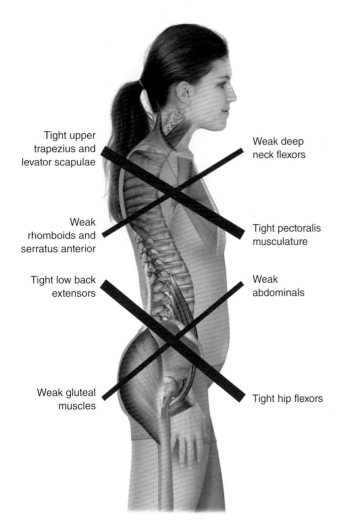

Figure 2-41 Lower crossed syndrome.

Tight upper trapezius and levator scapulae

Weak deep neck flexors

Weak rhomboids and serratus anterior

Tight pectoralis musculature

Tight low back extensors

Weak abdominals

Weak gluteal muscles

Tight hip flexors

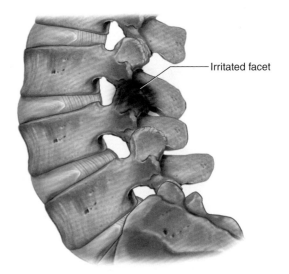

Irritated facet

Figure 2-42 Facet syndrome is caused by excessive physical stress on the facets.

tern, this condition is often described as the **lower crossed syndrome** (there is an upper crossed syndrome in the upper body as well) (Fig. 2-41).

Excessive anterior tilt can also be caused or increased by excessive weight carried anteriorly in the abdominal region. Further, if an excessive pelvic anterior tilt and lumbar hyperlordotic posture become chronic, ligament laxity/tautness will occur as well as fascial adhesions that resist normalization of this condition.

FACET SYNDROME

As described in its name, facet syndrome is a condition of the facet joints of the spine.

Description of Facet Syndrome

Disc joints and facet joints each have their own functional role within the spine. As a rule, disc joints bear weight and facet joints guide motion. When excessive compression force is placed upon the lumbar facet joints, they can become irritated and painful. The resulting condition is termed **facet syndrome**.

Mechanism and Causes of Facet Syndrome

Facet syndrome can occur for a number of reasons. Common among them is excessive time spent in a posture of extension or motions into extension because extension transfers weight bearing from the anteriorly located discs to the posteriorly located facets (Fig. 2-42). Having an increased anterior pelvic tilt with a compensatory hyperlordotic lumbar spine (see previous section) is a major predisposing factor

---

2.9   THERAPIST TIP

Pelvic Posture and Swayback

A hyperlordotic lumbar spine (swayback) is a postural syndrome that is ultimately related to an increased anterior tilt of the pelvis. For this reason, assessment of the sagittal plane anterior and posterior tilt muscle groups of the pelvis is essential in all clients who present with this condition.

2.10   THERAPIST TIP

Assessing Facet Syndrome

Facet syndrome is extremely simple to assess. Have the client move his or her lumbar spine into extension. If there is no pain, he or she does not have facet syndrome. If he or she has facet syndrome, this motion will reproduce low back pain (of course, it should be kept in mind that pain resulting from lumbar extension can also be caused by other conditions).

for this condition. Facet syndrome is extremely easy to assess because lumbar extension range of motion will reproduce the client's pain. Although facet syndrome is an irritation/inflammation of the articular surfaces of the lumbar facets, it is usually accompanied by spasming/hypertonicity of the paraspinal musculature. This muscle tightening can then add to the client's pain.

2.10 | TREATMENT CONSIDERATIONS IN BRIEF

Facet Syndrome

Moist heat, massage, and stretching can all be very beneficial for clients with facet syndrome. The primary focus for the manual therapist is to counsel the client on decreasing the causes of the condition, usually excessive postures and motions into extension. Also important is to relax the concomitant muscle spasming that usually accompanies the facet joint irritation. For more details, see Chapter 3.

SPONDYLOLISTHESIS

Spondylolisthesis is a condition of the spine in which one vertebra slips on the vertebra below it. This condition usually occurs in the lumbar spine. *Note:* Spondylolisthesis should not be confused with spondylosis; spondylosis is another term for DJD (OA) of the spine.

Description of Spondylolisthesis

As stated, spondylolisthesis is a slippage of one vertebra on the vertebra below it. This slippage is usually anterior in direction and can therefore also be described as an **anterolisthesis** (Fig. 2-43). Lateral slippage (laterolisthesis) and posterior slippage (posterolisthesis) may occur but are far less common. Indeed, when the term *spondylolisthesis* is used, unless otherwise specified, it is usually assumed that an anterolisthesis is present.

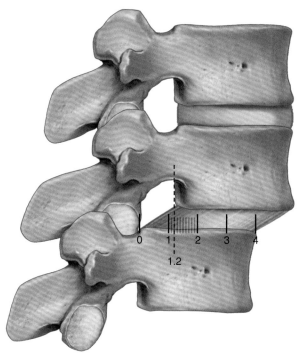

Figure 2-44 A spondylolisthesis can be measured by dividing the superior margin of the body of the vertebra below into four equal sections and then subdividing each of these four sections by 10. The spondylolisthesis seen here is grade 1.2.

Mechanism and Causes of Spondylolisthesis

Most often, a spondylolisthesis is due to a break in the pars interarticularis of the vertebra (see Fig. 1-3), allowing the body of the superior vertebra to slip anteriorly along the body of the vertebra below. This break could be congenital or it could be acquired via trauma. The degree of spondylolisthesis can be measured by how far the superior vertebral body slips on the inferior vertebral body. Generally, the grading is done on a scale of 1 to 4; the grading may be further defined by subdividing each grade by 10 (Fig. 2-44).

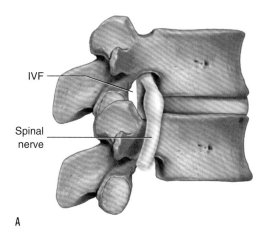
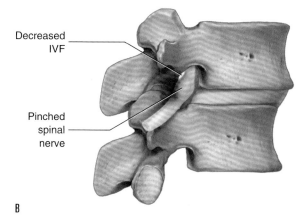

Figure 2-43 Spondylolisthesis. **(A)** Healthy posture of L4 on L5. **(B)** Spondylolisthesis of L4 on L5. Right lateral views.

The symptomology of spondylolisthesis can be due to tension on the soft tissues that are tractioned by the slippage. It is also common for spasming of the adjacent musculature to occur in an attempt to splint the region; this muscle spasming can increase the client's pain. More seriously, if the vertebra slips sufficiently, the intervertebral foramina can be narrowed, resulting in compression of the exiting spinal nerve(s) at that level (see Fig. 2-43). When this occurs, referral into the lower extremity can occur. Spondylolistheses (plural of spondylolisthesis) tend to be very unstable. The posture of the vertebra may be healthy for an extended period of time, and then a particular motion or posture of the body may cause it to slip, thereby exacerbating the condition.

2.11   **THERAPIST TIP**

Spondylolisthesis

If a client has a lumbar spondylolisthesis (anterolisthesis), it can be helpful to place a roll under his or her lumbosacral region to help support the spine when he or she is lying prone. This prevents the spondylolisthesis vertebra from slipping anteriorly. In fact, placing a roll under the lumbosacral region can be beneficial for most all clients lying prone, not just those with spondylolisthesis or other low back problems.

2.11   **TREATMENT CONSIDERATIONS IN BRIEF**

Spondylolisthesis

Soft tissue work into the tight musculature that usually accompanies a spondylolisthesis can be very helpful. But ultimately, the best treatment for this condition is for the client to strengthen his or her core musculature to stabilize the region. For more details, see Chapter 3 and Chapter 12 (available online at thePoint.lww.com).

CHAPTER SUMMARY

Clinical manual therapy requires a knowledge base of normal anatomy and physiology of the human body. It also requires an understanding of the altered physiology, in other words, pathophysiology, that occurs with each musculoskeletal condition with which the client might present. In addition, it requires the ability to accurately assess these conditions. Chapter 1 reviewed the anatomy and physiology of the low back and pelvis, this chapter presented the most common musculoskeletal conditions of the low back and pelvis that a manual therapist will encounter in practice, and Chapter 3 discusses the assessment of these conditions. Competent clinical orthopedic practice rests on a clear understanding of these three cornerstones of knowledge and understanding: anatomy and physiology, pathophysiology, and assessment.

Assessment and Treatment Strategy

OBJECTIVES

After completing this chapter, the student should be able to:

1. Explain why it is important to understand the mechanics of a healthy low back and pelvis and the pathomechanics of a pathologic condition when doing assessment.
2. Explain the difference between a diagnosis and an assessment.
3. Describe the purpose and role of the health history in assessment.
4. Describe the principle by which assessment tests work.
5. Explain what is meant by a positive result and a negative result for an assessment procedure.
6. Describe the difference between a sign and a symptom and give an example of each.
7. Describe the purpose of postural assessment and give an example of a postural deviation.
8. Perform and describe the roles in assessment of active range of motion (ROM), passive ROM, and manual resistance.
9. Describe the role of palpation in assessment.
10. Describe joint play assessment.
11. List the special assessment tests for a lumbar disc and the special assessment tests for the sacroiliac joint.
12. Describe and perform each of the special assessment tests presented in this chapter.
13. Describe the mechanism underlying each of the special assessment tests presented in this chapter.
14. State and be able to perform the assessment procedures for each of the conditions presented in this chapter.
15. Define each key term in this chapter.

KEY TERMS

active range of motion (active ROM)
active straight leg raise (active SLR)
ASIS compression test
assessment
assessment procedure
assessment test
bad posture
cough test
diagnosis
end-feel
full SLR test

Gaenslen's test
good posture
health history
iliac crest compression test
intrathecal pressure
joint play assessment
manual resistance (MR) assessment
motion palpation
Nachlas' test
negative test result
palpation
passive range of motion

passive straight leg raise (passive SLR)
physical assessment examination
piriformis stretch test
positive test result
postural assessment
posture
PSIS compression test
range of motion (ROM) assessment
report of findings
sacroiliac joint medley of tests

sign
slump test
special assessment tests
symptom
thigh thrust test
treatment plan
treatment strategy
Valsalva maneuver/test
Yeoman's test

INTRODUCTION

To provide proper therapeutic treatment to a client's low back and pelvis, it is necessary to perform an accurate assessment of the client's condition and gain a clear understanding of the mechanism behind the pathologic condition. This chapter covers the assessment procedures that should be performed before treatment can be decided upon. The review of anatomy and physiology in Chapter 1 and the discussion of pathologic conditions in Chapter 2 form the foundation for this chapter. Therefore, both chapters should be read before starting this chapter.

Assessment usually consists of two main parts:

- **Health history.** When meeting with a new client, or when seeing a repeat client who has a new condition, begin the assessment by obtaining the health history, which is a written and/or verbal history of the client's health. The intention behind the health history and the examination is to gain a thorough understanding of the client's specific condition(s) so that proper treatment can be applied.
- **Physical assessment examination.** This examination usually involves several components:
  - Postural assessment
  - Range of motion (ROM) assessment
  - Palpation assessment
  - Joint play/mobilization assessment
  - Special assessment

These assessments are recommended to all therapists when assessing a client's condition, although they need not be done in the order shown here. *Note*: Before performing joint play/mobilization, be sure to check with local and state licensure/certification regulations for compliance with scope of practice.

After gathering all the information from the health history and physical assessment examination, the assessment is made, and the appropriate treatment strategy is determined. The next step is to complete a **report of findings**, in which the client is informed of what was found in the assessment and what treatment is recommended. With the client's consent, treatment can begin.

3.1 | **THERAPIST TIP**

Diagnosis and Assessment

Although it is a fine line, there is a distinction between diagnosis and assessment. With a **diagnosis**, a physician definitively determines the condition that a patient has and informs the patient of the findings. **Assessment**, on the other hand, is carried out not for the purpose of informing the client of the condition but to help the therapist determine which treatment techniques are safe and effective to perform and which treatment techniques to avoid. Of course, if there is any doubt as to the safety and efficacy of treatment, referral of the client to a physician for a definitive diagnosis is strongly recommended.

HEALTH HISTORY

Think of the health history as a conversation between the therapist and the client. The health history may begin by having the client complete a written questionnaire about the present condition as well as his or her past health history. The conversation continues with a verbal history in which the client answers additional questions regarding his or her health.

The health history is usually done before the physical assessment exam because it helps reveal the problem regions that need to be assessed during the physical exam. If the history is thorough enough, the signs and symptoms discussed during the conversation will often indicate the client's condition or conditions, allowing the examination to be more focused and efficient. During the history, there is no one required order to the questions asked, however, it may be helpful to the individual therapist to develop and follow a consistent order when conducting health histories. Such consistency not only helps keep thoughts organized but also increases efficiency when returning later to review a client's information. However, it is also important to be flexible with questions. The client's answer to one question will often determine the follow-up questions. Although it is impossible to state every question that should be asked during a health history, some of the key questions are listed in Box 3.1.

BOX 3.1

Health History Questions

1. What are your height and weight?
2. Are you right-hand or left-hand dominant?
3. What is the problem area?
4. When did symptoms first begin?
5. What precipitated the problem? Was there a trauma or did it begin insidiously?
6. Have you had this problem before?
7. Have you had any other problems with your low back or pelvis before?
8. If there is pain, is the quality of the pain sharp or dull?
9. On a scale of 0 to 10, where 0 is no pain at all and 10 is the worst pain you can imagine having, what number would you assign your pain level?
10. Are there shooting pains or other referral of symptoms down into the lower extremities (buttock, thigh, leg, or foot)?
11. Are the symptoms (pain or other symptoms) related to the time of day? If so, is it worse first thing in the morning or at the end of the day?
12. Are the symptoms related to certain postures or activities?
13. Does the pain increase with prolonged standing or prolonged sitting?
14. Are there other precipitating factors that cause the symptoms?
15. What increases the symptoms? What decreases the symptoms?
16. Overall, since the problem began, is the severity getting better, worse, or staying the same?
17. Have you had this condition treated yet? If so, by whom? What was their assessment/diagnosis? What was their treatment? What was your progress with this treatment? May I have written permission to contact the therapist/physician about your treatment?
18. What do you think is the cause of your condition?

In addition to questions that are specific to the client's presenting complaint, it is also valuable to gather information about the client's general health.

1. Do you have any other health conditions, musculoskeletal, or otherwise?
2. What is your history of broken bones/fractures, car accidents, and other physical traumas?
3. Are you on any medications? Do you take them regularly, or are they only for a temporary condition?
4. How much do you exercise?
5. What postures (at work and home) do you assume most often?
6. In what position(s) do you sleep?
7. Do you smoke? Do you drink alcohol? If so, how much, and how often?
8. What is your stress level?
9. Is there a family history of musculoskeletal problems?
10. Is there anything else that you would like to add that I have not asked about?

PHYSICAL ASSESSMENT EXAMINATION

As discussed in Chapter 2, what is most important when assessing and treating the low back and pelvis is to understand the mechanisms of lumbar, pelvic, and hip joint function. When a person has a pathologic condition, the mechanics of these regions are altered. This alteration usually results in a tissue or tissues whose integrity has been compromised. Knowing this can help guide the therapist's assessment of the client's condition. The essence of an **assessment test (assessment procedure)** is to further stress the compromised tissue with the intention of reproducing or creating signs or symptoms of the problem. If the therapist understands the mechanics that underlie pathologic conditions, it is possible to use critical thinking to reason out not only which tissues are stressed but also how to further stress those tissues. In this manner, almost every assessment test can be thought through logically and understood without rote memorization.

3.2 THERAPIST TIP

Signs and Symptoms

When an assessment test yields signs and/or symptoms, it is important to distinguish between the two. A **symptom**, by definition, is subjective in nature and can be experienced only by the client. For example, pain is a symptom. No one can tell the client that he or she does or does not have pain; only the client can report having pain and what level it is. In contrast, a **sign**, by definition, is objective—that is, the therapist can verify and report it. The degree of the sign can also often be measured. For example, when a client is performing joint range of motion (ROM), the therapist can objectively determine whether the client's motion is decreased and even measure it in degrees. The client history and exam should include both the objective signs found and the subjective symptoms that the client reports.

If an assessment test reproduces signs and/or symptoms of the condition, it is a **positive test result**, and the therapist knows that tissue is unhealthy. For example, if Nachlas' test (a special assessment test for the sacroiliac joint [SIJ]) results in pain in the SIJ, the test result is considered to be positive for a pathologic condition of the SIJ. If no signs or symptoms are reproduced, then it is a **negative test result**. A negative test result may indicate one of two things: either the client does not have the condition or the degree of the condition is mild and below the threshold to yield a positive finding. Every assessment procedure has a certain sensitivity to detecting the presence of the condition for which it is designed.

It is important to note that if the test creates signs and symptoms, but not the signs or symptoms of the condition for which the test is designed, then the assessment test result is still considered to be negative. In the case of Nachlas' test, knee pain that occurs during the procedure does not indicate injury to the SIJ, even though knee pain is a symptom reported by the client. Knee pain during the assessment test is likely due to the knee joint compression that occurs during the test and is not relevant to assessment of the SIJ.

When assessing the client's low back and pelvis, it is important to perform all pertinent assessment procedures. Even if one test result is positive and indicates that the client has a certain condition, the other assessment procedures should still be done because a client may have more than one condition.

The following are the components of a thorough physical assessment examination of the client's low back and pelvis:

1. Postural assessment
2. ROM and manual resistance (MR)
3. Palpation
4. Joint play/mobilization
5. Special assessment tests

The next section addresses each physical assessment in more detail.

Postural Assessment

Postural assessment is usually the first physical assessment procedure that is performed. The term **posture** means position; therefore, in postural assessment, the client's static position is evaluated. Before evaluating a client's posture, it is important to understand what is meant by good posture and poor posture. **Good posture** is defined as a balanced posture that is symmetrical and does not place excessive stress on the tissues of the body (Fig. 3-1A). **Bad posture**, in contrast, is asymmetrical and/or imbalanced and places excessive physical stress on the tissues of the body (Fig. 3-1B). When evaluating a client's posture, look for asymmetries and deviations, as these will indicate increased stress forces on the tissues of the body. When a client has a postural deviation, it is important to determine why it is occurring and what tissues are stressed as a result of the posture.

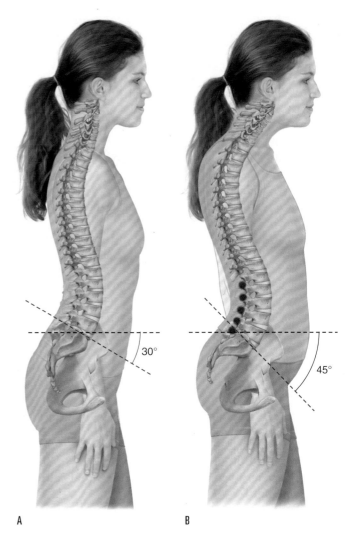

A   B

Figure 3-1 Good and bad low back posture. (**A**) The client's posture is considered good because the sagittal plane tilt of the pelvis and the lumbar lordotic curve are within normal limits. (**B**) The posture could be called bad because the pelvis is excessively anteriorly tilted and the lumbar lordosis is increased. This places increased weight-bearing stress on the facet joints of the lumbar spine and creates shortening of some muscles and lengthening of others.

A client may assume an infinite number of postures during the day. Unfortunately, therapists usually perform only standing postural assessment, often using a plumb line. (A plumb line is a string that has a weight attached to it ["plumb" comes from the Latin word for *lead*] so that the string hangs perfectly vertical, allowing the therapist to check for symmetry relative to the vertical line.) Although standing posture may be important to evaluate, it is not the only posture that should be assessed. In fact, depending on the client's profession, hobbies, and activities, it may not even be pertinent to the client's condition. It is important to assess all postures that the client assumes. For clients with low back and pelvis problems, sitting posture is especially important, such as when sitting at a desk or driving a car. For this reason, it is important to inquire about what types of seated postures the client engages in and how many hours of the day the client spends in each. Given that most people spend 6 to 8 hours a day sleeping, it is also important to find out what position or posture the client usually sleeps in (this is usually done during the health history).

A few examples will illustrate the critical reasoning skills involved in a client's postural assessment in which a postural deviation is found.

- **Example 1:** A common postural deviation occurs when one iliac crest is higher than the other. This is often caused by increased tension of some of the muscles in the region, for example, hip joint abductors (e.g., gluteus medius) on the low iliac crest side and/or elevators of the pelvis (e.g., quadratus lumborum) on the high iliac crest side. The therapist would need to know to specifically evaluate for these tight muscles during the palpation and ROM assessments. If these muscles are tight, treatment might target these muscles and include home advice for the client regarding stretching and/or hydrotherapy. A high iliac crest may also result in a compensatory scoliosis; therefore, the therapist should know to assess for this condition. Other recommendations to help alleviate unlevel iliac crest height might include avoiding certain postures or modifying postures, and activities that cause or perpetuate this condition.
- **Example 2:** If the client's posture shows that the pelvis is excessively anteriorly tilted, it would be reasonable to suspect that the hip flexor muscles and/or low back extensor muscles are tight because these are muscles that pull the pelvis into anterior tilt. The therapist would then focus on assessing these muscles; if they are revealed to be tight, the therapist would direct treatment and home advice toward their care.

Given the focus and scope of this book, only postural deviations of the low back and pelvis have been mentioned. However, postural deviations often involve the entire body, with a problem in one area causing secondary consequences and compensations in other regions. For example, a dropped arch in the foot may lead to an iliac crest height that is low on one side with a compensatory scoliosis that may reach to the cervical spine. For this reason, postural assessment should always address the client's entire body from the feet to the head. After the therapist has taken a look at a full body assessment of the client's posture, then appropriate treatment can be performed.

Range of Motion and Manual Resistance Assessment

Range of motion (ROM) assessment is usually performed directly after postural assessment. There are two types:

- **Active ROM**
- **Passive ROM**

Active ROM is performed by asking the client to actively contract the muscles of the low back, pelvis, and hip joint to move through the cardinal plane ROMs (Fig. 3-2A). Passive

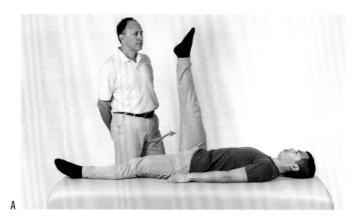

A

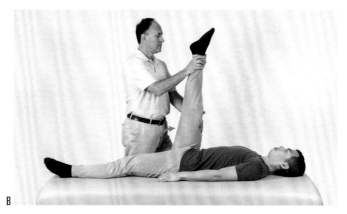

B

Figure 3-2 Active and passive ROM. **(A)** The client is actively moving the right thigh into flexion. **(B)** The client's right thigh is being passively moved into flexion by the therapist.

ROM is performed by passively moving the client through these cardinal plane ROMs (Fig. 3-2B). *Note*: Oblique plane ROMs can and often should also be assessed. The six cardinal plane ROMs for the lumbar spine and hip joint are as follows:

- Sagittal plane: flexion and extension
- Frontal plane: right lateral flexion and left lateral flexion for the lumbar spine; abduction and adduction for the hip joint
- Transverse plane: right rotation and left rotation for the lumbar spine; lateral rotation and medial rotation for the hip joint

When performing ROM assessment, two important factors should be considered:

- The presence of pain at any point during the ROM
- The actual amount of the ROM measured in degrees

The discussion that follows illustrates how critical reasoning is used when performing ROM assessment.

If pain is present with active ROM, the assessment is considered positive. The presence of pain indicates that three possible circumstances exist:

1. The "mover" muscles that are contracting to create the motion are strained, causing the client to experience pain when contracting them.

2. The ligaments/joint capsules of the joint(s) being moved are sprained, causing the client to feel pain when these structures are moved.
3. The (antagonist) muscles on the other side of the joint from the direction of motion performed are strained and/or spasmed, causing the client to feel pain when these muscles are stretched.

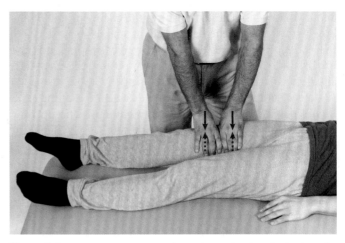

Figure 3-3   The therapist is providing MR to the client's thigh as the client attempts to move the thigh into flexion.

3.3 THERAPIST TIP

Unhealthy Joint Surfaces

In addition to strain of mover musculature, sprain of ligaments and joint capsules, and strain/spasm of antagonist musculature, a fourth condition can cause pain with active or passive ROM: an unhealthy joint surface at the joint being moved. For example, if there is degenerative joint disease (DJD) (osteoarthritis) of a joint surface, then motion at that joint may result in compression of that joint surface with resultant pain.

Therefore, pain with active ROM can result from a strain of the mover musculature, a sprain of the joint(s), and/or a strain or spasm of the antagonist muscles. One or any combination of these conditions can exist. Conversely, if no pain is present, then the client does not have any of these conditions.

If the client has pain with one or more active ROMs, then it is necessary to repeat these motions passively. If the client also experiences pain with passive motion, then the client has either a sprain, because ligaments and joint capsules are still being moved, or a strain or spasm of the antagonist muscles, because they are still being stretched. During passive ROM, mover muscles are no longer contracting, so pain with passive ROM does not indicate a strain of the mover musculature of that motion.

The process of elimination leads to the conclusion that if active motion causes pain and passive motion does not, then the client must have a strain of the mover musculature. If the client experiences pain with both active and passive motion, then the client at least has a sprain and/or a problem with the antagonist muscles.

To now determine whether the client also has a strain of the mover musculature, a third assessment procedure must be performed: **manual resistance (MR) assessment**. The client attempts to perform the ROM that caused pain while the therapist provides resistance to prevent the client from actually moving the joint(s). This causes the client's mover musculature to contract isometrically (Fig. 3-3). Both the therapist and the client should exert a moderately strong force that is enough to challenge the mover muscles and determine if they are healthy. Pain with resisted motion indicates a strain of the mover musculature because the

mover muscles are working in this scenario. Given that the ligaments/joint capsules and the antagonist muscles are not moved with an isometric contraction, pain with resisted motion does not indicate a ligament sprain or strain/spasm of the antagonist muscles.

The challenge is discerning pain that occurs from a sprain (resulting from ligaments/joint capsules being moved) from pain that occurs from a strain/spasm of the antagonist muscles (resulting from the antagonist muscles being moved/stretched). Each of these conditions can cause pain with both active and passive ROM, and neither condition causes pain with resisted motion. The best way to differentiate between them is to ask the client where the pain is occurring, if pain is present. Pain that is located in soft tissue on the other side of the joint where the antagonist muscles are located indicates strain/spasm of the antagonist muscles. If the pain is located deep in the joint, it indicates a sprain of the ligamentous and joint capsule tissues of the joint. Another approach is to have the client isometrically contract the antagonist muscles against your resistance. This will stress the antagonist muscles but not the ligaments/joint capsules (because the joint did not move).

In addition to the presence of pain, the other factor to consider when performing ROM assessment is the actual ROM—that is, the joint's degree of movement in each direction. In effect, ROM assessment is an assessment of the ability of the tissues to stretch when being moved. The amount of movement that the client exhibits can be compared to the standard ideal ROMs that are listed in Chapter 1. This comparison helps determine if the client's motion is normal and healthy or if the joints are hypermobile or hypomobile. If the client's ROM is greater than the standard ROM, the joint is hypermobile, usually indicating lax ligaments and joint capsules. If the client's ROM is less than standard, the joint is hypomobile, indicating overly contracting muscles (muscle spasming), excessively taut ligaments/joint capsule, fibrous adhesions within the soft tissues, and/or joint dysfunction.

Evaluating Range of Motion

It is important to keep an open mind when comparing a client's ROMs with the standard ROMs presented in the table in Chapter 1. The standard values are an average across the population, so a difference of the client's motion by a few degrees is not necessarily important. In addition, younger clients usually have greater ROMs than do older clients.

In addition to evaluating the absolute measure (in degrees) of motion at the joint, it is also important to compare the motion of the client's lumbar spine to the right with its motion to the left. This should be done for lateral flexions in the frontal plane and rotations in the transverse plane. If motion to one side is decreased, then assuming that the other side is healthy, the therapist knows what normal ROM for the client is and can determine what the treatment goal is when working to restore motion to the hypomobile side. Similarly, motions of the thighs at the right and left hip joints can be compared; this can be done for all three cardinal plane motions. *Note*: The client's other side is not always healthy; this can usually be determined by evaluating the client's history.

Active ROM, passive ROM, and MR are extremely valuable techniques when assessing a client's low back and pelvis. These procedures assess strains, sprains, and spasmed muscles, all of which are common musculoskeletal conditions that lead clients to consult manual and movement therapists.

Palpation

Perhaps no assessment procedure is more important to the manual therapist and integral to musculoskeletal assessment than palpation. **Palpation** involves the physical assessment of the client's bony and soft tissues through touch, usually with the pads of the fingers.

Palpation of bony landmarks can be important for determining the underlying skeletal structure that could otherwise be seen only on radiographic imaging (x-ray). In the low back/pelvis region, it is important to feel for the iliac crests, anterior superior iliac spines (ASISs), and posterior superior iliac spines (PSISs) to assess the posture of the client's pelvis (Fig. 3-4A). It is also important to palpate the spinous processes of the lumbar spine to assess the degree of the client's lordosis (Fig. 3-4B). Through chronic postures and physical traumas, the normal lordotic curve may be increased, decreased, or even, at times, reversed. Because a lordotic curve is concave posteriorly, it can be challenging to palpate all five lumbar spinous processes. If all the spinous processes of the lumbar spine can be easily felt, this indicates a decreased lumbar curve.

After assessing the bony posture of the lumbar spine and pelvis, soft tissue palpation can be performed. Once a soft

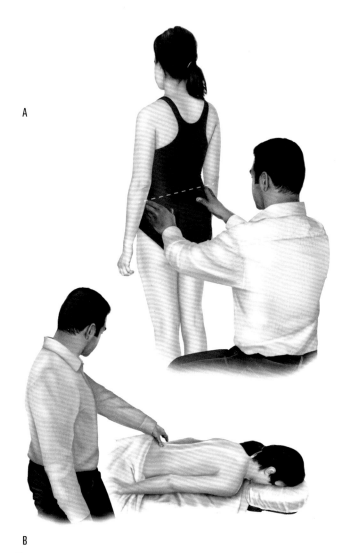

A

B

Figure 3-4 Standing palpation of the iliac crests. **(A)** The iliac crest on the right side is higher than the iliac crest on the left side, indicating an asymmetry of the pelvis in the frontal plane. **(B)** Palpation of the lumbar spinous processes.

tissue has been located, the quality of the tissue is assessed. If the tissue being assessed is a muscle, the qualities to look for are whether it is hard or soft. Tight (overly contracted) muscles feel hard; loose, relaxed muscles are soft. If the muscle is hard, is the entire muscle hard? Or are there perhaps small knots of tightness or taut bands within the muscle? Small knots may be myofascial trigger points, whereas taut bands are usually a result of bundles of muscle fibers that are either overly contracted and bunched up or overly stretched and pulled taut. Taut bands are usually strummable, similar to twanging a guitar string.

Whether muscle tissue, other soft tissues, or bone is being assessed, palpation can provide a great deal of useful information. Palpating for swelling and increased temperature may reveal tissue inflammation; palpating for thickness and increased density within a soft tissue may reveal the buildup of fibrous adhesions within the tissues. It is also important to palpate the end-feel of a joint's ROM. The **end-feel** of the low back's joint motion occurs at the end of passive ROM and should have a small, healthy bounce or spring to it. An end-feel that is hard and unyielding, as if a concrete wall has been reached, usually indicates DJD (arthritic) bone spurs, or perhaps markedly spasmed muscles or adhesions in the soft tissues.

The health history and ROM examination, which are usually done before palpation, often give the therapist some advance guidance about where to focus attention when palpating. Palpation often serves to confirm or eliminate the clinical impression that the therapist began to form during the earlier phases of the assessment procedures.

Joint Play/Mobilization Assessment

Joint play assessment is essentially a focused and specific form of passive ROM assessment. Instead of moving or stretching the entire low back or pelvis in a certain direction, the motion is directed at one segmental joint level. This is important because it helps narrow down the area where the problem ex-

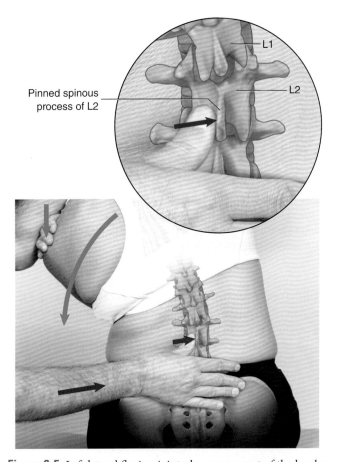

Figure 3-5 Left lateral flexion joint play assessment of the lumbar spine. The pelvis and lower lumbar spine are stabilized by body weight and the therapist's thumb while the rest of the body, and therefore the vertebra immediately superior, is moved into left lateral flexion relative to it. Joint play allows for specific assessment of the soft tissues of only that segmental level of the spine. In this figure, the L1-L2 joint is being assessed.

ists. For example, if the therapist passively moves the client's entire low back into right lateral flexion and the motion is decreased, the only information that procedure reveals is that decreased motion, or hypomobility, exists in that direction. It does not reveal whether every joint of the lumbar spine is hypomobile in that direction, or whether the hypomobility is present at just one or a few of the segmental joint levels. Joint play assessment makes it possible to discern this.

In fact, it is entirely possible for there to be a hypomobile joint level within the lumbar spine in right lateral flexion passive ROM while the entire lumbar spine has a normal degree of motion. If one segmental level is hypomobile and produces insufficient movement, another adjacent joint level might become hypermobile to compensate. This makes it possible for the gross ROM of the entire lumbar spine to be normal while lumbar hypomobilities and hypermobilities are present. Therefore, the only way to determine the health of a specific segmental joint level is to employ joint play assessment.

Joint play assessment is performed similarly to the joint mobilization technique (for a detailed explanation of how to perform joint mobilization, see Chapter 10). The therapist pins (fixes/stabilizes) one lumbar vertebra, usually by positioning the client such that body weight creates the stabilization force or by pinning the vertebra with a thumb pad, while moving the vertebra immediately above (along with the rest of the spine above that point) relative to the lower vertebra (Fig. 3-5). This procedure isolates the motion to the segmental joint level that is located between these two vertebrae, thereby allowing the therapist to assess specifically that joint level's end-feel motion. By performing joint play assessment at each level of the low back, it is possible to assess specific hypomobilities and hypermobilities throughout the lumbar spine and target treatment to those levels. This technique can also be used to assess the segmental motion of one SIJ of the pelvis relative to the other. This is accomplished in a similar manner: one pelvic bone is stabilized and the other pelvic bone or sacrum is moved relative to it (see Chapter 10). Joint play assessment is also known as **motion palpation**.

3.5	THERAPIST TIP

Joint Play Assessment

Joint play assessment, like joint mobilization technique, is performed by bringing the client's joint to the end of its passive ROM and then gently applying a small, even, steady force for less than a second that further stretches the joint in the desired direction. It cannot be emphasized too strongly that the force applied to assess joint play must be gentle, even, steady, and for less than 1 second. Joint play assessment and joint mobilization technique should never involve any type of fast or sudden thrust. A fast thrust within the realm of joint play is defined as a chiropractic or osteopathic adjustment and cannot be legally performed by most manual therapists.

Before employing joint play/mobilization, be certain it is within the scope of practice of your profession. If there is any doubt about the ethical or legal application of joint play/mobilization within your profession, please check with your local, state, or provincial licensing body; your certifying body; and/or your professional organization.

Special Assessment Tests

Although most sprains, strains, and spasms can be assessed accurately with the procedures already introduced, several conditions of the lumbar spine and pelvis require knowledge of specific procedures known as **special assessment tests**. Each special assessment test yields valuable information about the possible existence of a specific condition or type of condition. The most frequently used special assessment tests for the low back and pelvis are listed in Box 3.2.

BOX 3.2

Special Assessment Tests

- Space-occupying lesion tests
  - Straight leg raise (SLR)
  - Cough test
  - Valsalva maneuver
  - Slump test
  - Piriformis stretch test
- Test for injured tissue
  - Passive SLR
  - Active SLR
  - MR
  - Nachlas' test
  - Yeoman's test
  - SIJ medley

Common uses of the special tests in Box 3.2 include the following:
- SLR tests, cough test, Valsalva maneuver, slump test, and piriformis stretch test are used to assess a space-occupying lesion of the lumbar spine and buttocks. The lesions these tests are most often used to assess are pathologic (bulging or herniated) lumbar discs and lumbar spine bone spurs from DJD (osteoarthritis), but these four tests may also be used to assess swelling or a tumor in the lumbar spine, or piriformis syndrome in the buttock.
- Piriformis stretch test is used to assess a tight piriformis that might be compressing the sciatic nerve in the buttock.
- Active and passive SLR tests can also be used to assess for sacroiliac and lumbar strains and sprains as well as sacroiliitis.
- Nachlas', Yeoman's, and SIJ medley tests are used to assess injury to the SIJ.

Space-Occupying Lesion Tests

Following are assessment tests that are used to assess conditions caused by space-occupying lesions.

Straight Leg Raise Tests

Both **active SLR** and **passive SLR** tests are designed to pull long and taut the sciatic nerve on the posterior side of the body. If a space-occupying lesion in the lumbar spine such as a pathologic disc or bone spur is encroaching into the central canal or the intervertebral foramen, a nerve root that contributes to the sciatic nerve will be pulled against the encroachment and compressed. This compression can refer symptoms into the lower extremity.

Active SLR test is performed by asking the client to actively raise the thigh into flexion at the hip joint while keeping the knee joint fully extended. Passive SLR test is performed in a similar manner except that the client is passive as the therapist moves the client's lower extremity. In each case, it is important that the knee joint remains fully extended (hence the name *straight* leg raise) (Fig. 3-6A). If flexion is introduced into the knee joint, tension on the sciatic nerve will be lost, and it will be slackened and no longer compressed against the disc or bone spur. Compression of the sciatic nerve against the space-occupying lesion can cause sensory symptoms such as pain or tingling to refer down into the lower extremity (buttock, thigh, leg, and/or foot). SLR test for a space-occupying condition is considered to be positive if lower extremity referral symptoms are experienced. It is important to note that local low back pain alone does not constitute a positive SLR test for a space-occupying lesion (local pain can occur with SLR if the client has a sacroiliac or lumbar sprain or strain, or sacroiliitis); lower extremity referral symptoms must occur for a space-occupying lesion to be assessed. It should be pointed out that compression of the sciatic nerve due to a tight piriformis (piriformis syndrome) may also yield a positive with SLR. SLR test to assess a space-occupying condition can be performed actively or

---

3.6 THERAPIST TIP

Straight Leg Raise

SLR assessment requires the client to be able to flex the thigh at the hip joint while maintaining the knee joint in full extension. This posture is extremely difficult for a client who has very tight hamstrings because hip joint flexion and knee joint extension stretch these muscles. If the client's hamstrings are so tight that the client cannot bring the thigh very far up into flexion, then the SLR test is not valid because sufficient tension could not be placed on the sciatic nerve to assess a space-occupying lesion. It is also important to make sure the client does not compensate for tight hamstrings by posteriorly tilting the pelvis; doing so would diminish the tension on the sciatic nerve, thereby lessening the efficacy of the SLR assessment test.

Figure 3-6 SLR tests. **(A)** Active SLR. **(B)** Passive SLR. **(C)** Full SLR test. SLR tests tense and pull long the sciatic nerve. If a space-occupying lesion is present, such as a bulging disc as seen here, compression of the associated nerve can occur, causing sensory symptoms into the lower extremity on that side.

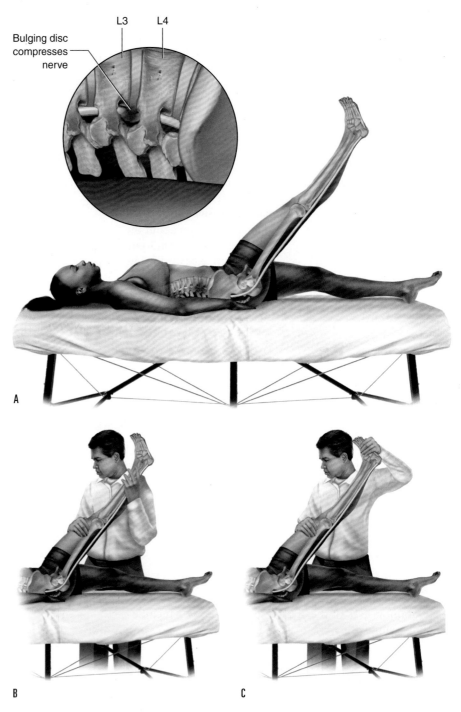

passively because the same mechanism of pulling long the sciatic nerve occurs in either case; however, it is most often performed passively.

SLR test can be augmented to become **full SLR test** by adding in adduction of the thigh at the hip joint, dorsiflexion of the foot at the ankle joint, and eversion of the foot at the subtalar joint (Fig. 3-6B). The idea behind full SLR test is that these added joint postures increase the tension on the sciatic nerve. Thigh adduction stretches the entire sciatic nerve around the ischial tuberosity as it crosses the hip joint. Dorsiflexion and eversion of the foot increase the stretch ten-

sion on the tibial nerve portion of the sciatic nerve because the tibial nerve enters the foot by crossing the ankle joint region posteriorly and medially.

Cough Test and Valsalva Maneuver

Both the **cough test** and **Valsalva maneuver/test** are designed to increase **intrathecal pressure**, or pressure on the spinal nerves in the intervertebral foraminal spaces. The mechanics are the same as with the SLR tests: Increased compression on these neural structures can cause referral of symptoms into the lower extremity in a client with a space-occupying

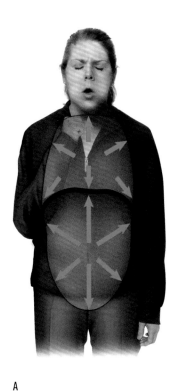 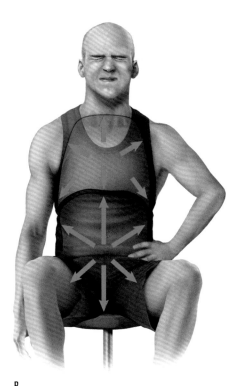

A   B

Figure 3-7 Cough test and Valsalva maneuver. **(A)** In the cough test, the client is asked to cough forcefully. **(B)** In the Valsalva maneuver, the client is asked to inhale a deep breath and hold it and then bear down as if moving the bowels. ([**A**] Reproduced with permission from Muscolino JE. *Advanced Treatment Techniques for the Manual Therapist: Neck.* Baltimore, MD: Lippincott Williams & Wilkins; 2013. [**B**] Adapted with permission from Muscolino JE. *Advanced Treatment Techniques for the Manual Therapist: Neck.* Baltimore, MD: Lippincott Williams & Wilkins; 2013.)

lesion. However, whereas the SLR test only increases compression to the lumbar spine (and perhaps the lower thoracic spine), the cough test and Valsalva maneuver cause increased compression to be experienced throughout the entire spine. Therefore, they will also assess a pathologic disc and advanced DJD of the cervical spine (if the client experiences referral symptoms into the upper extremity).

The cough test is performed by asking the seated (or standing) client to forcefully cough (Fig. 3-7A). The Valsalva maneuver is performed by asking the seated client to take in a deep breath, hold it in, and bear down as if moving the bowels (Fig. 3-7B). To preserve client modesty and avoid possible embarrassment, avoid eye contact with the client when the Valsalva maneuver is being performed. In each case, as

3.7   THERAPIST TIP

Valsalva Maneuver

Performing the Valsalva maneuver also results in a temporary decrease in blood flow to the heart and brain, possibly causing the client to become dizzy and perhaps even faint. Completing the maneuver also causes a sudden increase in blood flow to the heart. This can cause an increased strain on the heart and may be risky for clients who have a weak heart (as from congestive heart failure or other advanced cardiac disease). Therefore, it is safer to perform the Valsalva maneuver with the client seated.

with the SLR tests, local pain in the low back is not a positive sign. A positive sign is the presence of referral symptoms into the lower extremity (or upper extremity for a cervical spine space-occupying lesion).

Slump Test

 View the video "Slump Test" online on thePoint.lww.com

The **slump test** places tension on the entire spinal cord and peripheral nerves of the upper and lower extremities. Although this test is most effective at assessing a pathologic condition of the lumbar spine and sciatica, it can also be useful for assessing a space-occupying lesion in the cervical spine and thoracic outlet syndrome. (For a detailed description of cervical spine conditions and thoracic outlet syndrome, see Muscolino JE. *Advanced Treatment Techniques for the Manual Therapist: Neck.* Baltimore, MD: Lippincott Williams & Wilkins; 2013.)

The slump test works by increasing tension on the spinal cord and spinal nerves by means of a pulling force. If a space-occupying lesion is already compressing the nervous system structures, then pulling on the nerves by means of the test will likely tether the spinal nerves against this space-occupying lesion. Referral of sensory symptoms into the lower extremity is considered a positive result for a space-occupying lesion of the lumbar spine. (If sensory symptoms refer into the upper extremity, the result is positive for a space-occupying lesion of the cervical spine or thoracic outlet syndrome.)

As with the other special tests, local low back (or neck) pain does not constitute a positive test result.

The slump test is performed in several sequential steps, each one adding to the tension placed on the spinal cord and nerves. The motions may be performed actively or passively.

1. Begin with the client seated, hands clasped behind the back (Fig. 3-8A). (Clasping the hands behind the back places tension on the brachial plexus and begins the assessment for thoracic outlet syndrome.)
2. Next, ask the client to slump the thoracic and lumbar spine (Fig. 3-8B).
3. Now ask the client to flex the neck and head (Fig. 3-8C).
4. You can then add to neck/head flexion by pressing the client's head and neck further into flexion (Fig. 3-8D). These flexion motions of the spine stretch the spinal cord and also add to the tension on the brachial plexus.
5. The client's knee joint is then fully extended (Fig. 3-8E).
6. Finally, the foot can be dorsiflexed (Fig. 3-8F). These motions of the lower extremity add more stretch to the spinal cord and also stretch the sciatic nerve in the lower extremity, thereby assessing a space-occupying lesion of the lumbar spine (as well as piriformis syndrome).

Figure 3-8G illustrates the sum tension of these steps on the neural structures. Because the slump test places so much tension on the spinal cord and nerves, it is common for a healthy client to feel some pain and discomfort during the procedure. Thus, for the test result to be considered positive, the client should either experience a reproduction of the lower or upper extremity symptoms that they have been experiencing or a high level of pain/discomfort during the procedure.

Piriformis Stretch Test

The **piriformis stretch test** is used to assess piriformis syndrome, that is, compression of the sciatic nerve by the piriformis. As its name implies, the piriformis muscle is stretched, thereby increasing its tautness and its compression on the sciatic nerve. Stretching a muscle is done by simply moving the client's body into the opposite of its joint actions. Two excellent stretches for the piriformis are shown in Figure 3-9. In Figure 3-9A, the client's thigh is flexed and then horizontally adducted (horizontally flexed) because the piriformis is a horizontal abductor (horizontal extensor) when the thigh is first flexed. In Figure 3-9B, the client's thigh is flexed and laterally rotated because the piriformis is a medial rotator when the thigh is first flexed. If the client experiences a pulling (stretching) sensation or pain in the buttock, it is likely due to a tight piriformis but does not indicate compression of the sciatic nerve, therefore the test is not considered to be positive. For the piriformis stretch test to be considered positive, the client must experience referral of symptoms distally into the lower extremity (thigh, leg, and/or foot).

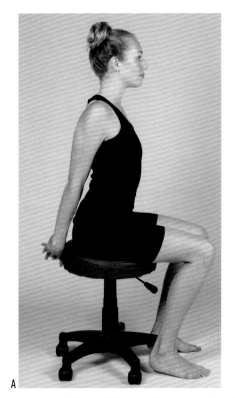
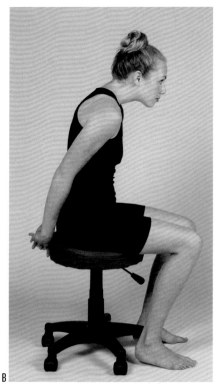
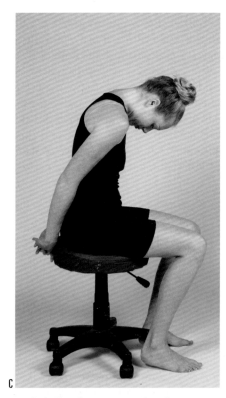

Figure 3-8 The slump test. The slump test is performed in several sequential steps. (**A**) The client is seated and clasps the hands behind the back. (**B**) The client slumps the thoracic and lumbar spine forward into flexion. (**C**) The client flexes the neck and head. *(continued)*

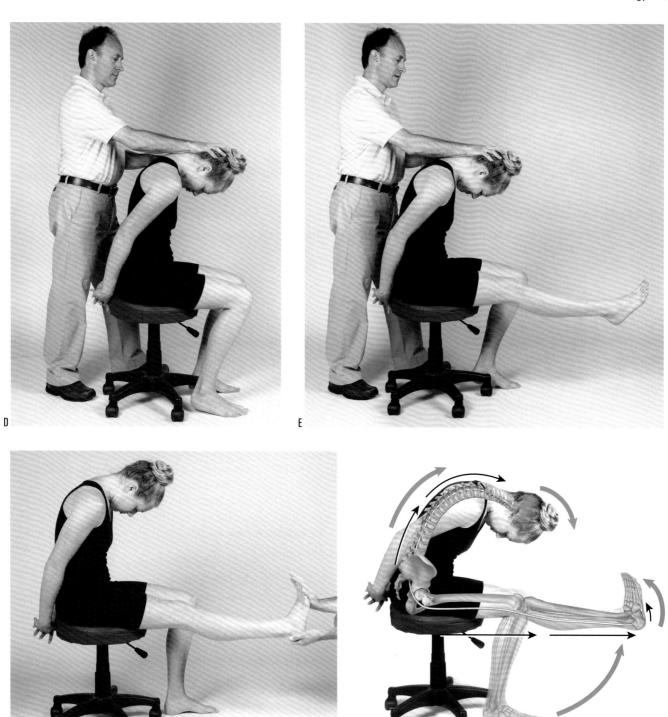

Figure 3-8 *(continued)* (**D**) The therapist adds to the neck/head flexion. (**E**) The client's knee joint is extended. (**F**) The client's foot is dorsiflexed. (**G**) This figure shows the biomechanics of the slump test, highlighting the stretch/tension that is placed on the spinal cord and nerves. (Reproduced with permission from Muscolino JE. *Advanced Treatment Techniques for the Manual Therapist: Neck.* Baltimore, MD: Lippincott Williams & Wilkins; 2013.)

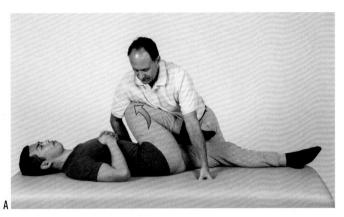
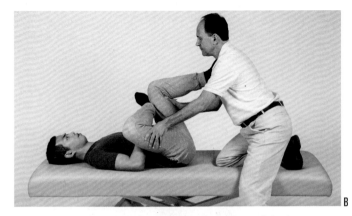

Figure 3-9 Stretches for the piriformis. **(A)** Horizontal adduction of the flexed thigh. **(B)** Lateral rotation of the flexed thigh.

Note: The relationship between the piriformis muscle and sciatic nerve can vary. Usually, the sciatic nerve exits the pelvis inferior to the piriformis. However, some or all of the nerve may exit through or above the piriformis. Regardless of the relative relationship between these two structures, a tight piriformis can potentially compress the sciatic nerve and cause piriformis syndrome.

Tests for Injured Tissue

Following are assessment tests that are used to assess conditions caused by injury to soft tissues at a joint such as sprain, strain, and irritation/inflammation. *Note*: Even though SLR tests are forms of active and passive ROM tests and have therefore already been discussed under the "Range of Motion and Manual Resistance Assessment" section, they and MR are discussed again here in their context to other assessment tests for injured tissue.

Passive Straight Leg Raise

Passive SLR test is performed as described earlier in this chapter in the section on special orthopedic assessment tests for space-occupying lesions. The difference is that now the intended assessment is for sprains and irritation/inflammation of the SIJ and lumbar spinal joints; the test is considered to be positive if local pain is felt in the SIJ region or lumbar spine (referral pain down the lower extremity is not the criterion for a positive test now). Passive SLR test is performed by the therapist raising the client's thigh into flexion at the hip joint while keeping the client's knee joint fully extended. It is important that the knee joint remains fully extended (hence the name *straight* leg raise) (Fig. 3-10A). Because the client is not engaging musculature of the region to create this motion, the client is passive. Flexing the thigh at the hip joint and keeping the knee joint fully extended places a stretch on the hamstrings. This pulls them taut, creating a tension/pulling force on the pelvic bone on that side. Therefore, as the client's thigh is lifted into flexion, that side pelvic bone will be pulled into posterior tilt. Because the other pelvic bone is stabilized on the table and not moving, motion will occur between the pelvic bones at the SIJs. If either side SIJ is sprained/inflamed, pain will be felt locally at the SIJ (Therapist Tip 3.8).

Most commonly, an SIJ sprain/inflammation will be felt when the thigh is at approximately 30 degrees of flexion. As the thigh is lifted higher than 30 degrees, the sacrum will posteriorly tilt with the pelvic bone, and as the sacrum reaches the end of its posterior tilt ROM at the lumbosacral joint relative to the L5 vertebra, it will begin to pull L5 into flexion. Once L5 is pulled into flexion to the end of its flexion ROM, L4 will flex. This motion will continue up to the lumbar spine as the thigh is moved farther and farther into flexion. If any of these lumbar spinal joints are sprained/inflamed, pain will be felt locally at that level. Generally, the higher the thigh is raised when pain occurs, the higher the region of the spine that is assessed.

Active Straight Leg Raise Test

Active SLR test is performed in a similar manner to passive SLR test except that the client is asked to actively raise the thigh into flexion at the hip joint by engaging the hip flexor muscles (Fig. 3-10B). This will also cause pelvic and lumbar musculature to engage to stabilize the pelvis and spine as the thigh is lifted. (*Note*: It will also cause the psoas major to contract as a mover of the thigh. When contracting, the psoas major will exert tension on its spinal attachments as well as the thigh, causing compression and anterior shear of the lumbar spine, which could add to the local low back pain of active SLR.) The joints are being moved in an identical manner as when the test was performed passively; therefore, active SLR test will assess sprains and irritations/inflammations of the sacroiliac and lumbar spinal joints just as passive SLR test did. However, because the client is actively contracting the musculature of the region, active SLR test will also assess strains of musculature. Active SLR test is considered to be an excellent screening test for the region because it will be positive with both sprains (and inflammations) of the joint ligaments and capsules, and strains of the musculature of the joint.

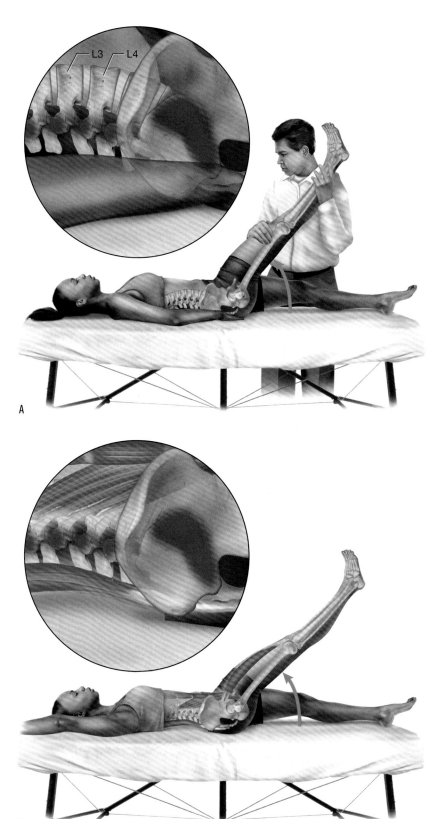

A

B

Figure 3-10 SLR tests to assess sprains and strains. **(A)** Passive SLR moves the sacroiliac and lumbar spinal joints and therefore assesses for a sprain of these joints. **(B)** Active SLR moves the joint tissues, and it requires musculature to engage; therefore, it assesses both sprains and strains.

Straight Leg Raise and Sacroiliac Joint Assessment

When performing the SLR test to assess for sprains/inflammations and/or strains of the SIJ, although it is typical to assess the same-side SIJ as the thigh being raised, the SIJ on the opposite side of the body of the thigh being raised is also sometimes assessed. The mechanism for the SLR test is as follows: If the right thigh is flexed, then the right pelvic bone will move into posterior tilt. Because the left pelvic bone is stabilized on the table, it will not move. Therefore, motion occurs between the two pelvic bones. If the right SIJ is mobile, the right pelvic bone will move relative to the sacrum at the right SIJ. Therefore, motion is introduced into the right SIJ and if it is injured, pain would occur locally at that joint; therefore, the right SIJ is assessed. However, if the right SIJ is hypomobile and does not move, then when the right thigh is raised and the right pelvic bone posteriorly tilts, the sacrum will be "locked" to the right pelvic bone, and they will move as a unit relative to the left pelvic bone. This motion will occur at the left SIJ. When this occurs, if the left SIJ is injured, then pain would be felt at that joint and that joint is assessed. Further, even if the right SIJ is mobile and allows motion, as the thigh is lifted higher, there will be a point where the end of ROM of the right SIJ will be reached and motion will start to occur at the left SIJ, assessing the left-sided SIJ. For these reasons, regardless of which thigh is lifted into flexion, either SIJ could be assessed. Even though performing SLR test on one side could assess either SIJ, it is usual and customary to perform this test on both sides of the client's body.

Straight Leg Raise Test and Antagonist Musculature

It is usually stated that passive SLR test assesses only sprains, and that active SLR test assesses both sprains and strains. However, this is a bit of an oversimplification. Both passive and active SLR tests also assess for strains and spasms of the antagonistic musculature of the joint(s) because both tests require them to stretch to allow the joint to move (whether the joint moved passively or actively).

Manual Resistance Test

MR is another test that is used to assess strains of musculature. As its name implies, MR test is performed by the therapist using his or her hands to add resistance to the client's attempted joint motion. The MR must be strong enough to stop the client from actually moving the joint. Therefore, the contraction is isometric (see Fig. 3-3). If the client's musculature engages but no joint motion occurs, then the musculature will be stressed and assessed, but the joint ligaments and capsule will not. Therefore, MR test assesses for strain of the mover muscles of the joint, but not sprains of the joint.

Nachlas' and Yeoman's Tests

 View the video "Nachlas Orthopedic Assessment Test for the Sacroiliac Joint" online on thePoint.lww.com

Nachlas' test and **Yeoman's test** both assess injury to the SIJ, primarily sprain and irritation/inflammation. These two tests are similar in that each one introduces a motion/torque into the SIJ of the prone client; if the joint is injured, this motion will stress the tissues and cause pain. Nachlas' test is performed by passively flexing the client's knee joint by bringing the client's heel toward the same-side buttock (Fig. 3-11A). This causes a stretch of the quadriceps femoris muscles. Specifically, when the rectus femoris of the quadriceps is stretched, it is pulled taut, causing a pulling force to be placed on its attachments. This pulls on the anterior inferior iliac spine (AIIS), causing anterior tilt of the pelvic bone on that side. Because that pelvic bone moves and the other pelvic bone does not because it is stabilized against the table, motion is introduced into the SIJs. Usually, Nachlas' test primarily assesses the same-side SIJ, but as explained in Therapist Tip 3.8, the opposite-side SIJ can be assessed as well.

Yeoman's test works on a similar principle. It is performed by the therapist using one hand to lift the client's thigh into extension, with the client's knee joint partially flexed (Fig. 3-11B). The client's rectus femoris, as well as all hip flexor musculature, is stretched, causing a force of anterior tilt on the client's same-side pelvic bone. Because the other pelvic bone is stabilized against the table, the force is introduced into the SIJs. The therapist uses the other hand to press down on the client's PSIS to both stabilize the pelvic bone on that side from lifting off the table and to increase the anterior tilt motion of that side pelvic bone.

Nachlas' test causes only a mild stress to the SIJs, so it usually only shows positive if the SIJ injury is moderate or marked in degree. Yeoman's test is more forceful and will show positive with a mild SIJ injury as well. One limitation to the Nachlas' test is that because it requires maximal flexion of the client's knee joint, it cannot be performed if the client has a unhealthy knee joint on that side that cannot tolerate full flexion.

Sacroiliac Joint Medley of Tests

The **sacroiliac joint medley of tests** is a series of five assessment tests to determine if the SIJ is the causative agent of the client's pain. It assesses if the SIJ is sprained and/or irritated/inflamed. If three or more of the five tests reproduce the client's pain, the medley of tests is considered to be positive. The five tests are the PSIS compression test, iliac crest compression test, ASIS compression test, thigh thrust test, and Gaenslen's test. Each test is considered to be positive if the client experiences pain at the SIJ.

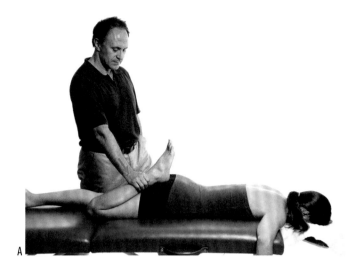

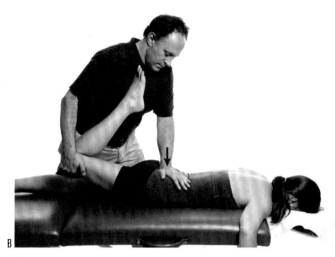

Figure 3-11 Nachlas' and Yeoman's tests for the SIJ. (**A**) Nachlas' test is performed by bringing the client's heel to the same-side buttock. (**B**) Yeoman's test is performed by lifting the client's thigh into extension with the knee joint flexed while stabilizing the same-side pelvic bone from lifting into the air and adding to the anterior tilt of the pelvic bone on that side of the body. (Reproduced with permission from Muscolino JE. Orthopedic assessment of the sacroiliac joint. *MTJ.* Fall 2010: 91–95.)

PSIS compression test is performed with the client prone. The therapist places his hands on the client's PSISs. Each PSIS is placed in the groove between the thenar and hypothenar eminences of the therapist's hand (the intereminential groove), and the therapist then adds a compression force downward (Fig. 3-12A). Both SIJs are tested simultaneously with this test.

Iliac crest compression test is performed with the client side-lying. The therapist places his hands on the client's iliac crest and adds a compression force downward (Fig. 3-12B). This test primarily assesses the SIJ that is away from the table, although some compression force is transferred to the other SIJ, so it may elicit pain there as well. The test is usually performed again with the client on the other side.

ASIS compression test, thigh thrust test, and Gaenslen's test are performed with the client supine. For the **ASIS com-**

pression test, the therapist places his hands on the client's ASISs. As with the PSIS compression test, each ASIS is placed in the intereminential groove of the therapist's hand. The therapist then adds a compression force downward and somewhat laterally (Fig. 3-12C). Both SIJs are tested simultaneously with this test.

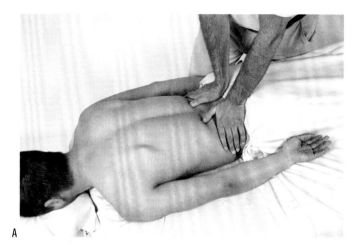

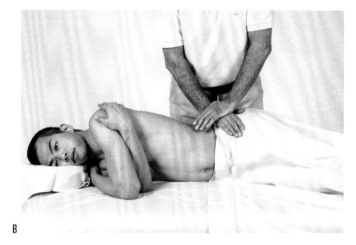

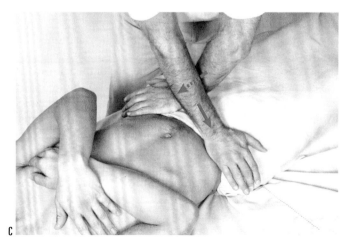

Figure 3-12 SIJ medley of tests. If three or more of these five tests are positive, the SIJ is considered to be the causative agent of the client's low back/pelvic pain. (**A**) PSIS compression test. (**B**) Iliac crest compression test. (**C**) ASIS compression test. *(continued)*

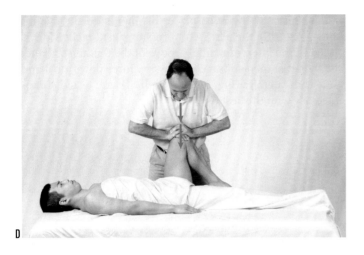

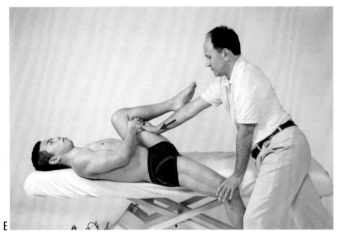

Figure 3-12 *(continued)* **(D)** Thigh thrust test. **(E)** Gaenslen's test.

Thigh thrust test is performed by placing a downward compression force on the client's knee with the client's thigh flexed to 90 degrees (Fig. 3-12D). This test assesses only the side where the pressure is applied, so it is repeated on the other side of the body.

For **Gaenslen's test**, the client needs to be positioned far to the side of the table where the therapist is standing. One thigh is dropped into extension off the side of the table while the client hugs the other thigh into the chest. The therapist adds downward pressure on the thigh that is off the table, bringing it farther into extension. This stretches the client's hip flexors, causing the same-side pelvic bone to anteriorly tilt. Having the client hug the other thigh into the chest posteriorly tilts and stabilizes the other pelvic bone. The therapist can add to this stabilization of the other side of the pelvis by pressing against the client's posterior thigh (Fig. 3-12E). The mechanism for Gaenslen's test is that torque is added into the SIJs by having one pelvic bone anteriorly tilted while the other is posteriorly tilted. Both SIJs are assessed with this test, but the dropped-thigh side is primarily tested. For this reason, Gaenslen's test is usually repeated on the other side of the body.

TREATMENT STRATEGY

Once the health history and physical assessment examination have been performed, a **treatment strategy** can be developed. This involves creating a **treatment plan** for the client. Three principle components of a treatment plan must be determined:

1. Treatment techniques that will be used during the sessions
2. Frequency of sessions
3. Self-care advice that will be given to the client

Treatment Techniques

The pathomechanics of the condition will determine the objectives of care, which in turn will determine the treatment techniques to be used. Most conditions of the low back and pelvis involve tight/taut soft tissues (hypertonic musculature and fascial adhesions), so loosening these tissues is usually the primary focus of treatment. Most conditions that have been present for some time also involve joint dysfunction hypomobilities, so joint mobilization should be another focus. It is essential to address both of these aspects of the condition if the client's musculoskeletal health is to improve.

The treatment techniques presented in this book are designed to address tight muscles and other taut soft tissues as well as joint dysfunction hypomobilities. These techniques tend to be most effective if performed after the client's tissues have been warmed up. Choosing which technique to use is often a matter of both the therapist's and the client's personal preferences. The most effective approach is usually to combine multiple techniques within the treatment plan. (Before employing any new technique in your practice, be sure that it is within the scope of practice of your profession.)

Frequency of Sessions

Once the techniques have been chosen, the next step is to decide the optimal frequency of care. Again, this depends on the circumstance. If a client is basically healthy and simply wants to maintain good health, the frequency might vary from once a week to once a month, depending on the client's lifestyle and health. However, if a client has a musculoskeletal condition that needs to be remedied, physical rehabilitation requires a frequency of two to three times per week. This is common in physical therapy, chiropractic, strength training, and sport training, and the same holds true for manual therapy.

Each treatment session must build on the previous one if the client is to improve. Performing a treatment physically changes both the state of the tissues and the neural patterns for muscle contraction. As time passes after the session, these changes are gradually lost as the body reverts back to the pattern of its pathologic condition. If too much time elapses between visits, then the client continually regresses back to his or her dysfunctional pattern before the successive treat-

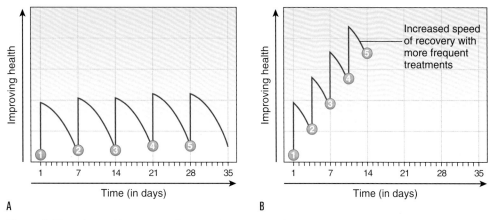

Figure 3-13 Effects of frequency of care. (**A**) Treatment frequency of once per week. (**B**) Treatment frequency of twice per week. Note the increased speed of recovery of the client's condition when treatments are more frequent. Numbered treatments are indicated in blue circles. (Reproduced with permission from Muscolino JE. Treatment planning and client education. *MTJ.* Winter 2010: 91–95.)

ment occurs. Therefore, for care to be effective and efficient, treatments should be spaced no more than 2 to 3 days apart until the desired improvement has been achieved (Fig. 3-13). Although this may seem like a strong commitment to ask of a client, it is the most time-efficient and cost-efficient approach.

Self-Care Advice

It can be very helpful to involve the client in his or her own treatment plan. Regarding self-care advice, it is extremely valuable to offer the client suggestions about postures, hydrotherapy (hot and cold), stretching, and strengthening (if your scope of practice permits). After all, even if a client sees the therapist three times a week for an hour at each session, the client is still on his or her own for the other 165 hours of the week. If the client is engaging in unhealthy postures and activities at home and work, this can easily overwhelm the

| 3.10 | THERAPIST TIP |

Giving Self-Care Advice

It is best to avoid overrecommending when giving self-care advice to clients. Whereas many clients will do one, two, or, perhaps, three recommended stretches, if the therapist gives them four, they will probably become overwhelmed and do nothing. Whether the threshold for being overwhelmed is 4 or 10, in general, the best rule regarding self-care advice is to give the client as much as he or she will do, and no more. The exact amount will vary according to the client's level of self-discipline and enthusiasm. Once the client is comfortable with the stretches or other self-care advice that is recommended, more can gradually be added in future sessions.

therapist's ability to assist. If instead the client uses that time to further the objectives of the treatment plan, then recovery will proceed more quickly. For more on self-care advice, see Chapter 11 (available online at thePoint.lww.com).

ASSESSMENT AND TREATMENT OF SPECIFIC CONDITIONS

Chapter 2 discussed the musculoskeletal conditions of the low back and pelvis that a manual therapist is most likely to encounter. This chapter has introduced and explained how to perform orthopedic assessment tests that are available to the manual therapist to assess these musculoskeletal conditions. Part 2 of this book explains how to perform the advanced treatment techniques that can be used to treat these conditions. The following is a brief overview that links the condition with its corresponding assessment procedure and its corresponding treatment.

Hypertonic Musculature

Tight muscles are assessed by measuring the client's passive ROMs. If an ROM is restricted, then the antagonistic muscles (generally located on the other side of the joint) to that motion are most likely tight. Tight musculature is not the only tissue that can restrict joint motion. Whenever an active or passive ROM is restricted, any taut tissues on the other side of the joint may contribute to the restriction in motion, including ligaments and joint capsules.

Whether they are a result of increased active muscle tone or adhesions, the treatment options available to the manual therapist to help loosen tight musculature and other soft tissues are many, ranging from soft tissue manipulation, to hydrotherapy, and to stretching techniques and joint mobilization.

Joint Dysfunction

Joint dysfunction is assessed with joint play assessment, also known as motion palpation.

If a specific segmental vertebral level is found to be hypomobile, then the only effective treatment option is to perform joint mobilization technique. If a client has a hypermobility, a manual therapist can do little to nothing to directly help because every treatment tool that a manual therapist employs is aimed at increasing, not decreasing, mobility. However, if the joint hypermobility exists as a compensation for an adjacent hypomobility, then the hypermobility may be alleviated if the adjacent hypomobility is mobilized. *Note*: Strengthening musculature around a hypermobile joint is helpful. If strength training is within your scope of practice/license, then it should be employed.

Lumbar Sprains and Strains

Assessing a sprain or a strain of the low back can be done by using active ROM and passive ROM (specifically active and passive SLR tests) as well as MR. The acronym commonly used to describe the care routine for an acute sprain or strain is RICE (rest, ice, compression, and elevation). RICE care should continue as long as inflammation is present in the tissues. This may be days, weeks, or even months or more—do not follow a cookbook rule for when to apply ice application. If inflammation is present, icing is appropriate.

Care for a chronic sprain is usually geared toward the tight muscles that usually occur as a compensation for the excessive motion. These tight muscles often cause pain and are in need of treatment. In addition, the best long-term approach that a client can take with a sprain is to strengthen the musculature of the region. Stronger musculature can compensate for the loss of stability of the stretched ligaments and help prevent painful muscle spasms.

Care for a chronic strain is geared toward loosening the muscles if they have become hypertonic and also eliminating or decreasing the formation of further adhesions. For this reason, once adhesions have mended the strained (torn) muscle tissue, and the tissue's integrity has returned, it is important to begin soft tissue manipulation and stretching to minimize tightness and prevent the formation of further adhesions. If there is any doubt about whether tissue integrity has returned, consent from a physician should be obtained.

Sacroiliac Joint Injury

Injury (sprain, strain, or irritation/inflammation) to the SIJ can be assessed with active SLR test, passive SLR test, Nachlas' test, Yeoman's test, and the sacroiliac medley of tests. If either SLR test is used, injury to the SIJ will usually cause pain at approximately 30 degrees of thigh flexion. Nachlas' test will usually only show positive if the injury is moderate or marked in degree; Yeoman's test is more sensitive and will usually detect a mild SIJ injury. For the SIJ medley of tests to

be considered positive, at least three of the five tests should elicit pain in the SIJ.

Care for a SIJ injury depends on what type of injury is present. SIJ sprains and strains should be treated similarly to lumbar sprains and strains (see preceding section). If no sprain or strain is present and the SIJ is simply irritated/swollen, then icing and rest are appropriate. Prolonged sitting, particularly prolonged driving, is especially stressful to the SIJs and should be eliminated or decreased.

Pathologic Disc and Sciatica

Assessing a pathologic lumbar disc condition (a disc bulge or rupture) and the resultant pressure on the sciatic nerve (sciatica) can only be done definitively by magnetic resonance imaging (MRI) or computed tomography (CT) scan. However, the SLR test, cough test, Valsalva maneuver, and slump test may also be used. Although these assessment procedures are not as accurate as an MRI, they are usually effective at accurately assessing a pathologic disc that is moderate or marked in severity. If a lumbar disc bulge or rupture is moderate or severe in presentation, it will likely produce a positive test result for most or all assessment procedures. However, a mild case may produce a negative result for many of the tests and a positive result for others. If there is any question about whether a client has a pathologic disc bulge or rupture, it is advisable to refer the client to a physician for a definitive diagnosis.

Treating a client with a lumbar disc problem contraindicates doing anything that would increase pressure on the disc, thereby increasing the size of the bulge or rupture. Strong compression over the spine should be avoided, and all movements of the client's lumbar spine should be done with caution. As a rule, anything that increases the referral symptoms of the disc lesion is contraindicated. There are opposing viewpoints on what type of motions are safe and effective for a client with a lumbar disc injury. Some authorities recommend flexion motions and avoiding extension (or avoiding extension with lateral flexion if the disc injury is posterolateral); others recommend that the client perform extension motions and avoid flexion. The argument for flexion is that it opens up the vertebral and intervertebral foramina. The argument for extension is that it removes tension on the posterior annular fibers and pushes the nucleus pulposus anteriorly away from the posterior annular fibers. See Chapter 11 (available online at thePoint.lww.com) for both flexion and extension exercises for the lumbar spine.

The primary focus of manual therapy is to loosen the tight muscles that surround the disc because they can increase compression on the disc, furthering the problem. As a general rule, Western-based Swedish strokes are usually fine as long as the pressure is not so great that the vertebral joints are actually moved, thereby placing stress on the discs. Because of the movement involved in stretching and joint mobilization, these treatment techniques should be avoided or done prudently at or near the level of the disc lesion. Lumbar spine traction/distraction, if performed prudently, is indicated and can be beneficial for relieving disc pressure.

Piriformis Syndrome

Piriformis syndrome is best assessed with the piriformis stretch test as well as palpation of the piriformis muscle. However, any of the assessment tests for pathologic discs or other space-occupying lesions may also show positive for piriformis syndrome. These tests include SLR, cough test, Valsalva maneuver, and slump test.

Treatment for piriformis syndrome is aimed at relaxing and loosening the piriformis muscle. Heat, soft tissue manipulation, and stretching are all effective means to accomplish this. If the piriformis is tight as a compensation to stabilize the sacrum when there is an underlying SIJ injury, resolving the SIJ condition is necessary if any lasting relief of the piriformis is to occur.

Degenerative Joint Disease

Physicians assess DJD by radiograph or other radiologic examination such as MRI or CT scan. Manually, DJD of the lumbar spine and SIJs is difficult to assess through palpation because the bone spurs of DJD are located deep within the client's tissues. Advanced DJD will impede motion of the affected joints so passive ROM will be decreased and will often have a hard palpatory end-feel to the motions.

There is nothing that a manual therapist can do to directly affect the bone spurs of DJD itself. However, manual therapy can play an extremely important role indirectly. The principal cause of DJD is physical stress to the joint, and one of the components of the physical stress is the compression force caused by tight muscles that cross the joint. If manual therapy relaxes tight musculature, less physical stress will be placed on the joint, and that can lead to a decrease or cessation in the rate at which the condition progresses. Therefore, even though manual therapy cannot reverse the condition, it can decrease its progression.

If the DJD is advanced and the client has a bone spur that is pushing on adjacent tissue, causing inflammation, another treatment option is the use of cryotherapy (the application of ice). If the bone spur is pressing on a spinal nerve, any positioning/stretching/joint mobilization that increases that nerve compression should be avoided.

Scoliosis

If scoliosis is severe enough, it can be assessed through visual and palpatory examination. However, for a definitive diagnosis, radiographic examination via an x-ray should be ordered by a physician.

Treatment of scoliosis by a manual therapist has two objectives: one is to work on the spinal joints and the other is to work the spinal musculature. Joint mobilization can be performed to increase motion of hypomobilities found within the scoliotic spine. Each vertebra within a scoliotic curve is laterally flexed and rotated. As a result, the vertebral segment will usually have decreased ROM in the opposite lateral flexion direction and also in the opposite rotation direction. The manual therapist can perform joint mobilization to decrease these hypomobilities. If the scoliosis is severe and/or very chronic, it is unlikely that joint mobilization will greatly reduce the degree of scoliosis, but it is often very effective at decreasing or stopping the progression of the condition.

Perhaps even more important is the role of the manual therapist in treating the associated spinal musculature. Asymmetric muscular pull can contribute to a scoliotic curvature by pulling the vertebrae in one direction. Therefore, the role of the manual therapist is to reduce muscular hypertonicities that can contribute to the problem. This can be done via heat, soft tissue manipulation, and stretching. If strengthening is within the therapist's scope of practice, it should also be done. Although it is beneficial to relax and stretch as well as strengthen all musculature of a scoliotic curve, as a general rule, musculature in the concavity of the curve needs to be loosened, and musculature on the convex side of the curve needs to be strengthened.

Anterior Pelvic Tilt and Hyperlordotic Lumbar Spine

Anterior pelvic tilt and hyperlordotic lumbar curvature can be assessed via visual examination. A more definitive diagnosis of the degree of the condition can be obtained via a physician-ordered radiograph.

Treatment of this condition is aimed at loosening the anteriorly placed hip flexor musculature as well as the posteriorly placed low back extensor musculature. This can be accomplished by using heat, soft tissue manipulation, and stretching. If strengthening is within the therapist's scope of practice, strengthening of the posterior hip extensor musculature and the anterior abdominal wall musculature should also be done. Although self-care is important in all conditions, it is especially important with dysfunctional postural patterns such as excessive anterior tilt. The client should be counseled regarding proper posture and stretches for the hip flexors and low back extensor muscles.

Facet Syndrome

Facet syndrome is assessed by asking the client to perform extension of the lumbar spine; pain located at the spinal joints indicates facet syndrome.

Because facet syndrome is often caused by excessive anterior pelvic tilt with resultant increased lumbar lordosis, treatment should be directed at improving the client's posture. This can be best accomplished by applying moist heat, soft tissue manipulation, and stretching to the musculature of anterior tilt, in other words, the hip flexors and low back extensors. And if strengthening is within the therapist's scope of practice, then strengthening of the posterior tilt musculature, hip extensors, and trunk flexors (anterior abdominal wall) should also be done. Self-care stretches that posteriorly tilt the client's pelvis and flex the client's lumbar spine should also be recommended (see Chapter 11, available online at thePoint.lww.com). Because facet syndrome is often accompanied by muscular spasming, it is important to relax this musculature as well.

Spondylolisthesis

Spondylolisthesis is diagnosed by a physician from lateral view radiographs. A break in the pars interarticularis and/or a slippage of one vertebra on the vertebra below indicates spondylolisthesis. By far, the most common type of spondylolisthesis involves an anterior slippage of the upper vertebra and is termed an *anterolisthesis*. Less common, the upper vertebra slips posteriorly and is termed a *posterolisthesis*, or slips laterally and is termed a *laterolisthesis*.

Manual therapy treatment of a spondylolisthesis cannot change the break in the pars interarticularis. Instead, treatment is aimed at reducing any associated muscle spasm and increasing the stability of the lumbar spine through core stabilization strengthening, if this is within the therapist's scope of practice. Muscle spasm is best reduced via moist heat, soft tissue manipulation, and stretching. Core stabilization strengthening should be directed toward the anterior abdominal wall musculature as well as the low back extensor muscles (see Chapter 12, available online at thePoint.lww.com).

Because an excessive lumbar lordotic curve, often caused by excessive anterior tilt of the pelvis, exacerbates the slippage of an anterolisthesis, remedying this postural condition through hands-on care and self-care advice (see the previous section on "Anterior Pelvic Tilt and Hyperlordotic Lumbar Spine") is an important component of the care of this condition.

CHAPTER SUMMARY

There is an adage in the world of medicine that treatment should never be administered without a diagnosis. Similarly, in the world of clinical orthopedic manual therapy, treatment should only be performed if an assessment is first made. This chapter covers the orthopedic assessment tests that manual therapists can perform to assess their clients' lower back and pelvic conditions. Of course, there are limits to the ability of these tests to fully and accurately assess every condition. If after performing these assessment tests, there is still doubt about the client's condition, referral should be made to a physician for an accurate and thorough diagnosis/assessment. Once the therapist is armed with an accurate assessment, and therefore a fundamental understanding of the pathomechanics of the client's condition, safe and effective treatment can be determined and carried out.

PART TWO

Treatment Techniques

CHAPTER **4**

Body Mechanics for Deep Tissue Work to the Low Back and Posterior Pelvis

CHAPTER OUTLINE

OBJECTIVES

After completing this chapter, the student should be able to:

1. Describe the mechanism for producing deep tissue pressure.
2. Discuss the roles of internally and externally generated forces when doing deep tissue work.
3. Describe in steps an overview of the usual protocol for performing deep tissue work to the low back and pelvis.
4. Explain why the therapist's position and the client's placement on the table are important.
5. Describe the roles of the treatment contact hand and the bracing/support hand.
6. Describe the importance of the positioning of the feet when doing deep tissue work.
7. Explain the importance of stacking the upper extremity joints when doing deep tissue work.
8. Explain why it is important to align your core with the stroke and use your core and/or lower extremities when performing deep tissue work.
9. Explain why it is important to communicate with the client when doing deep tissue work.
10. Describe the possible role of ice when doing deep tissue work.
11. Describe the usual breathing protocol for the client during deep tissue work.
12. Explain how to transition from sustained compression to short deep stroking massage and long, deep strokes with proper body mechanics.
13. Define each key term in this chapter and explain its relationship to deep tissue work to the low back and pelvis.
14. Perform deep tissue work to the client's low back and pelvis using the five routines presented in this chapter.

KEY TERMS

brace hand	external generation of force	slide	treatment contacts
contact hand	inclined back	stacked joints	trigger point (TrP)
deep pressure	internal generation of force	stooped back	vertical back
deep stroking massage	ischemic compression	support hand	
deep tissue work	knife-edge	sustained compression	
drag	myofascial TrP	target musculature	

INTRODUCTION

Western-based massage technique is a type of bodywork that involves the introduction of force (pressure) by physically pressing into the soft tissues of the client's body, usually the muscular and fascial tissues. The purposes of introducing pressure to physically work on the client's tissues are many. They

---

Body Mechanics for Deep Tissue Work Routines

The following body mechanics for deep tissue work routines are presented in this chapter:
1. Medial low back—paraspinal musculature
2. Lateral low back—quadratus lumborum
3. Middle and upper back—paraspinal musculature
4. Posterior pelvis—gluteal region
5. Lateral pelvis—abductor musculature

| 4.1 | THERAPIST TIP |

Strokes and Techniques

This chapter is not about recommending any one massage stroke (e.g., compression or effleurage) or proprietary technique over another. Every stroke and every technique has merit. Similarly, no one stroke or technique is the magic bullet. If it were, everyone would be doing that stroke or technique, and no others would exist. Learning to be a clinical orthopedic manual therapist involves learning how to choose which strokes to use for which client based on the needs of the client who is lying on the table at that point in time. Strictly adhering to cookbook techniques is not recommended. The thrust of this book is to employ critical thinking based on a fundamental understanding of the anatomy, physiology, and kinesiology of the body as well as an assessment and understanding of the pathomechanics of the client's condition presented in Part 1 of this book. Once that is accomplished, the goal is to then effectively and appropriately apply the advanced techniques that are presented here in Part 2 of this book.

Note: For the most part, this text uses the terms *deep pressure* and *deep tissue work* synonymously, but a distinction can be made. Deep tissue work implies that deeper tissues are the target structures being worked. Deep pressure does not; it can be employed for deeper or superficial tissues. However, because deep tissues usually require deeper pressure to reach them, this text uses these terms somewhat interchangeably.

Note: In the Technique and Self-Care chapters of this book (Chapters 4 to 12), green arrows indicate movement, red arrows indicate stabilization, and black arrows indicate a position that is statically held.

---

include producing changes in local fluid circulation, affecting neural proprioceptive feedback loops, and physically breaking patterns of fascial adhesions. The pressure that is applied can range from very light to very deep. Not everyone wants or needs to have **deep pressure/deep tissue work** performed; certainly, there are times when light work is preferable. However, when deep tissue work is desired or needed, it is important for you to be able to generate this deep pressure with the least amount of effort and physical stress to your body. In essence, this chapter is about learning how to employ proper body mechanics so that you work smart instead of working hard. The body mechanics that are demonstrated in this chapter can be applied to all manual therapy strokes and techniques.

MECHANISM

Because biomechanical principles follow the basic laws of physics, efficient biomechanics for performing deep tissue work techniques for the musculature of the low back and pelvis are identical to the biomechanical principles and guidelines for doing deep tissue work for any part of the body. Creating pressure is a matter of generating force into the client's tissues. Force can be generated in two ways: externally or internally. The **external generation of force** comes from the force of gravity by using your body weight. The **internal generation of force** comes from the contraction of your muscles.

Externally, the force of gravity acts on the mass of your body to create body weight. You can take advantage of your body weight to generate pressure into the client's tissues by simply dropping down and leaning into the client. Pressure derived this way is effectively free because it takes no effort on your part. For this reason, it should be used whenever possible. Because your core is the largest, most massive part of your body, you need to position it over the client and behind your contact whenever possible.

After you have generated as much force as possible via gravity and body weight, any additional force that you generate must come internally from the contraction of your muscles. This requires effort on your part, so it can be tiring. To minimize fatigue and wear and tear on your body, it is important to always use the largest muscles possible. This is especially important when it comes to deep tissue work. These larger muscles primarily are located proximally in the body.

| 4.2 | THERAPIST TIP |

Choosing the Right Table

 View the video "Body Mechanics and Electric Lift Table" online on thePoint.lww.com

Choosing the right table can be critically important to good body mechanics. The two most important parameters of a table when considering body mechanics are its width and

continued

height. When considering the width of a table, two compet-
ing concepts are client comfort and therapist body mechanics. The wider a table is, the more comfortable it is for the
larger client. However, a wider table places the client farther
from the therapist and forces the therapist to work much
harder to position the core over the client's body. This often
results in the therapist having to lean over and compromise
his body mechanics. In effect, having a wide table provides
comfort for the occasional large client, but the therapist
must struggle with all the rest of the clients. Possible compromises include tables that have sidepieces that can make
the table wider for the larger client but be removed when
working with smaller clients **(Fig. A)**. Other tables have a
scoop in the middle that narrows the table width around
the low back and pelvis of the client **(Fig. B)**. This allows
the therapist to place his core closer to the client for efficient
body mechanics. Another feature that some tables have is
additional face cradle holes that allow for the face cradle to
be moved to one side, thereby allowing the client to lie closer
to the side of the table **(Fig. C)**. This prevents you from having to lean over, thereby reducing stress to your back. It also
allows you to get your core in closer to the client, permitting
more efficient use of your body weight and the engagement
of larger muscles. If your table has these holes, it is wise to
take advantage of them for better body mechanics.

Even more important than table width is table height.
As a rule, when generating deep pressure, you want the table
to be as low as possible so that you can more easily position
your body above the client to take advantage of gravity and
body weight. It is likely that the most common error when
trying to employ efficient body mechanics is that the therapist positions the table too high. This likely happens because
many therapists begin their massage education in school with
classes that teach light pressure work. Therefore, it is easy to
work with the table high. Often, the therapist becomes accustomed to keeping the table at this height even though
deeper pressure techniques are later learned and employed.
With the table too high for the techniques now being used,
the therapist struggles to achieve pressure, believing that he is
too weak when the real culprit is a table that is too high. Even
though most tables are adjustable in height, it is important to
choose a table that can go low enough so that the top of the
table is well below the bottom of your knee joint.

For any therapist who has a stationary practice in one
location, it is an extremely wise decision to buy an electric
lift table. This allows easy adjustment of the table height
with the touch of a pedal. Adjusting the table height is
not only important between clients of different sizes but
it is also important when working on the same client if the
client changes position, such as when changing from supine

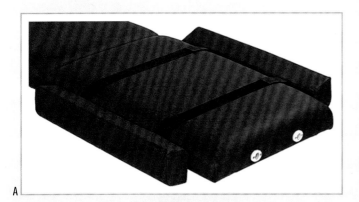

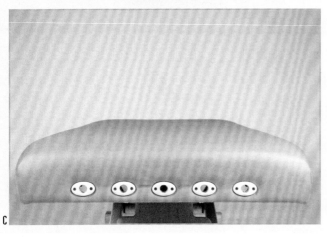

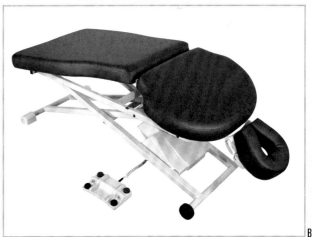

A

B

C

continued

| 4.2 | **THERAPIST TIP** *(continued)* |

or prone to side-lying. It is also important when changing contacts that are used to work on the client. For example, work with thumb or finger pads requires a far lower table than work with the elbow or forearm. Further, there are many stretches for the low back and pelvis that require the table to be very low and others that require the table to be high. It is logistically impossible to change the table height between each of these stretches. The purchase of an electric lift table is an investment in the quality of your practice as well as an investment in your success!

OVERVIEW OF TECHNIQUE

The *science* of performing deep tissue work to the low back and pelvis follows the laws of physics and, whenever possible, involves the use of body weight and the contraction of larger muscles instead of smaller ones. The *art* of performing deep tissue work lies in exactly how these guidelines are carried out and applied. The following is an overview of deep tissue work to the medial low back region of the client. In this example, the **target musculature**, the musculature being worked, is composed of the paraspinal muscles that lie directly lateral to spinous processes in the lumbar region.

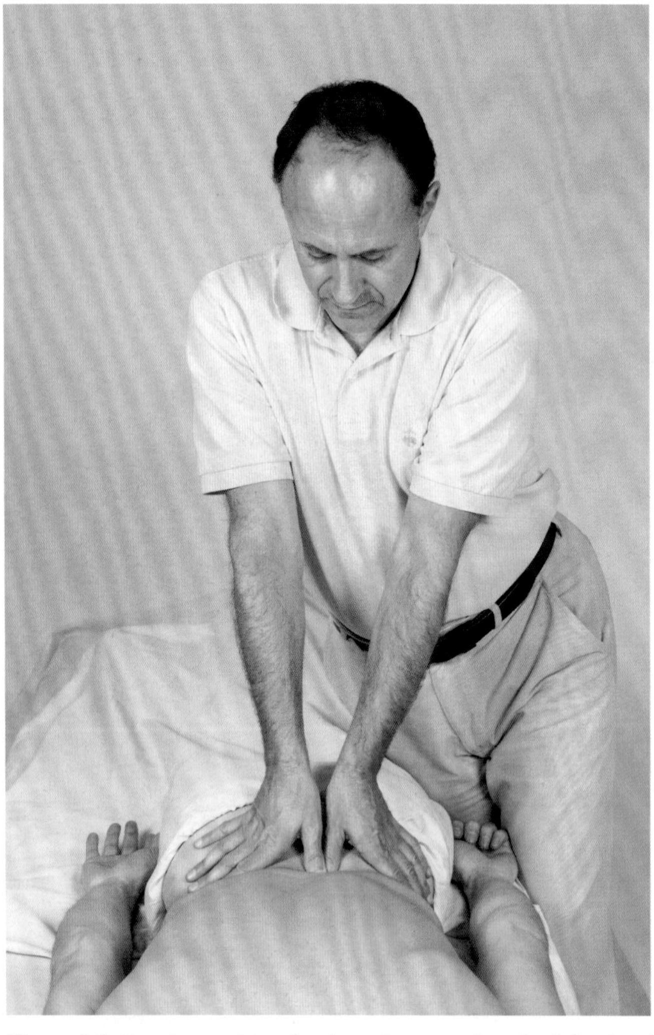

Starting Position:
- The client is prone. You are standing at the side of the table, close to the client.
- Your left hand is the **contact hand**, and it is placed on the left side of the client's low back.
- Your right hand is the **brace hand** or **support hand**, and it is placed over the contact hand.
- Note that your elbows are tucked in front of your body so that you can use your core body weight behind your contact when pressing into the client (Fig. 4-1).

Step 1: Place Contact on the Client's Musculature:
- The contact hand is the one that actually contacts the client.
- A wide choice of contacts can be used when working the client's low back (see Choosing the Treatment Contact section).
- In Figure 4-2, the thumb pad of the left hand is being shown as the contact and is placed directly lateral to the midline on the left side of the client's body over the lumbar region.

Step 2: Brace/Support the Contact:
- Place the thumb pad of your right hand over the thumb pad contact of the left hand to brace/support it. Proper

Figure 4-1 Starting position for deep tissue work to the left side of the low back.

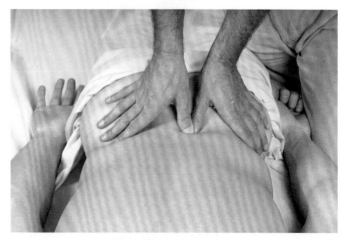

Figure 4-2 Thumb pad contact with the other thumb as the brace.

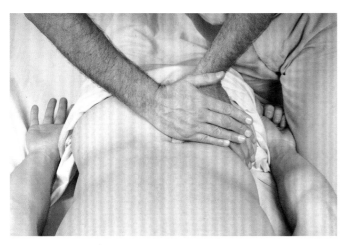

Figure 4-3 The thumb pad contact with the ulnar side of the other hand as the brace.

location of the brace is to place the right thumb pad on the dorsal surface of the distal phalanx of the thumb, in other words, on the thumb nail (Fig. 4-2).

■ An alternative brace/support contact is shown in Figure 4-3.

Step 3: Apply Pressure:
■ Now perform the deep tissue work by pressing into the client's musculature with the thumb pad of your left hand.
■ This pressure is supplemented by pressure from the right hand that braces the left (contact) hand. In effect, both hands function as treatment hands to generate pressure into the client.
■ It is important to slowly sink into the client's tissues and to apply the pressure as close as possible to perpendicular to the contour of the client's body that you are working.
■ The movement for this pressure should originate from your core body weight (Fig. 4-4).

PERFORMING THE TECHNIQUE

4.1 Positioning the Client

Generating deep pressure with body weight works best when you are directly over the client. This is facilitated by having the client as close to the edge of the table as possible. When working with the client supine, it is easy to ask the client to lie toward one side of the table or the other. But when the client is prone, because of the location of the face cradle, the client usually has to lie at the center of the table. If your table allows for the placement of the face cradle to be changed to be more to the side of the table, then it is helpful to position the client closer to the side so that it is easier to lean over and use your body weight (Fig. 4-5).

4.2 Adjusting Where You Stand

When working the back with the client prone, it is important for the therapist to stand as close as possible to the region of the client that is being worked. This allows the therapist to better position the trunk/core of the body over the client, allowing for optimal use of body weight. When working the pelvis or lumbar region, the therapist should stand directly to the side of the pelvis or lumbar spine of the client (Fig. 4-6A). If the lower thoracic region is worked, then the therapist should adjust the standing position to be at the side of the table next to the lower thoracic spine of the client (Fig. 4-6B).

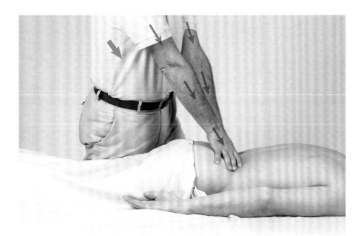

Figure 4-4 Generation of force from the core. When applying pressure into the client, as much of the force as possible should originate from the core body weight.

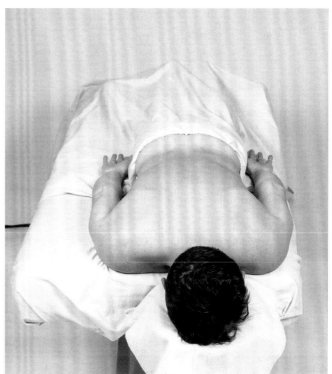

Figure 4-5 If the table allows for the prone client to lie close to the side of the table, it allows for the therapist to more easily position body weight over the client.

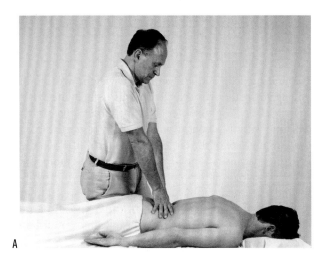

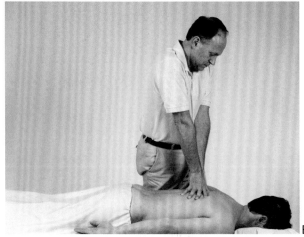

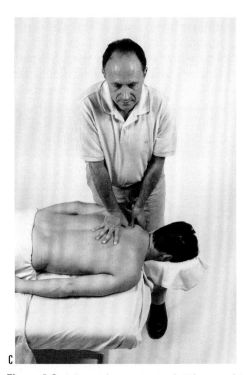

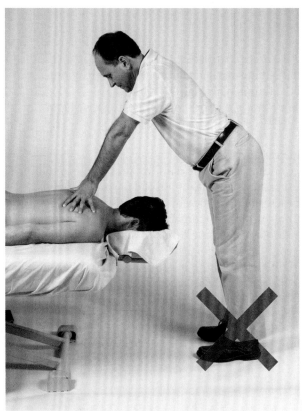

Figure 4-6 Adjust where you stand. When working the lumbosacral region (**A**) or the lower thoracic region (**B**), the therapist stands at the side of the table, adjacent to the region being worked. When working the upper and middle thoracic region, the therapist stands at the head of the table, between the face cradle and the top of the table (**C**). Standing above the face cradle leads to poor body mechanics (**D**).

To work the upper and middle thoracic region, you need to choose which side of the client you want to work and stand on that side of the table, between the face cradle and the top of the table. This allows you to place your core directly over the client's upper thoracic region on that side of the body (Fig. 4-6C). A common error is for the therapist to stand above the face cradle at the head end of the table. Standing here only distances you from the client, causing you to lean over the client to reach the low back; this compromises body mechanics and does not allow for the efficient use of body

weight (Fig. 4-6D). Optimally positioning your core requires you to optimally position where you stand.

4.3 Positioning the Feet

View the video "Foot Position and Body Mechanics" online on thePoint.lww.com

Positioning the feet is extremely important because it determines where the core of the body is oriented. If the stroke

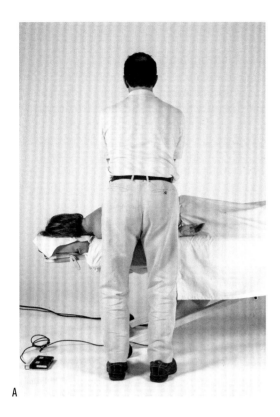

A

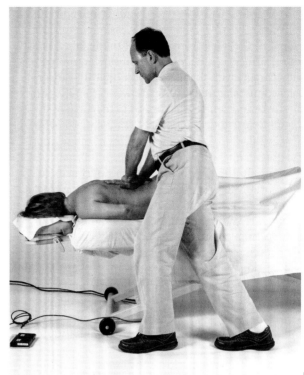

B

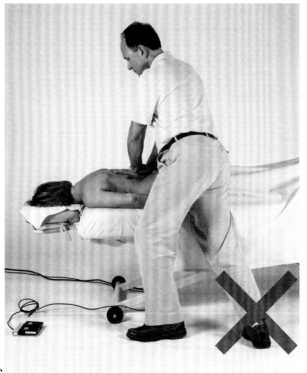

C

Figure 4-7 Positioning the feet. (**A**) When working across the client's body, the feet should be pointed across the client's body. (**B**) When working longitudinally up the client's body, the feet should be in a sagittal plane stance, pointed up the client's body. Note that the stance is not too wide, and the rear foot is oriented in the sagittal plane. (**C**) The rear foot should not be oriented perpendicular to the front foot.

is being done across the client's back or pelvis, then the feet should be oriented transversely across the table (Fig. 4-7A). If the stroke is being done up along the client's pelvis and back, then the feet should be oriented longitudinally up along the length of the table (Fig. 4-7B). In effect, the feet should point in the direction of the stroke that is being performed. It is also

important to place the feet in a sagittal plane stance, with one foot forward and the other foot in back (as seen in Fig. 4-7B). This provides a stable base when working and also allows for a transfer of weight from the rear foot to the front foot if a stroke is being performed. Also, make sure that the feet are not too far apart. A wide stance may feel more stable but creates a static position that makes it difficult to transfer weight from one foot to the other. With a narrower stance, it is easier to shift the center of weight of the body from one foot to the other as a stroke is done. Further, it is better to orient the foot in back approximately parallel with the front foot so that the powerful sagittal plane musculature of the rear lower extremity is in line with the stroke and can be used to add to the force of the stroke. Placing the rear foot transversely is a common error and should be avoided because it does not orient the sagittal plane musculature in line with the stroke (Fig. 4-7C).

When working up the client's back from inferior to superior, it is important to orient the core of the body so that it is in line with the stroke, in other words, facing the head end of the table. It is also important to position the trunk as close to being over the client's body as possible. This can be especially challenging if the table is wide. Without climbing on the table, there are two ways to facilitate this.

One way is to begin by standing next to the table, facing the head end (Fig. 4-8A). Now take the outer foot (the one that is farther from the table) and place it behind the inner foot (the one that is closer to the table). This will naturally lean the thighs against the table and place the pelvis over the table so that your trunk is closer to the middle of the table and facing the head of the table in line with your stroke (Fig. 4-8B). If any adjustment of the orientation of the core of your body is necessary, this adjustment should be done by rotating the pelvis at the hip joints and not by rotating the spinal joints. *Note:* This position should be avoided if you have genu valgum of the knee joint in front.

The other way is to begin by again standing next to the table, facing the head end (see Fig. 4-8A). This time, place the outer foot in front of the inner foot (Fig. 4-8C). Now adduct the thigh of the inner foot by moving your inner foot away from the table, allowing your thigh to rest against the side of the table (be sure that there are no hard or sharp projections where you are leaning against the side of the table). This will place your trunk over the table, oriented toward the head of the table, in line with your stroke. As with the previous method just described, if any adjustment of the orientation of the trunk is necessary, this adjustment should be done by rotating the pelvis at the hip joints and not by rotating the spinal joints.

4.4 Choosing the Treatment Contact

When working on the low back of the prone client, there are many **treatment contacts** that can be used to contact the client. From small to large, these contacts range from finger or thumb pad; to palm or ulnar side of the hand, also known as the "**knife-edge**" contact; to fist; and to elbow or forearm (Fig. 4-9). The advantage of smaller contacts is that they allow for more precision both when assessing the client's soft tissues and when working the tissues. The disadvantage is that smaller contacts are less able to deliver deep pressure and are more prone to injury when deeper pressure is being employed. Larger contacts are less precise for assessment and treatment but can better deliver deeper pressure without injury.

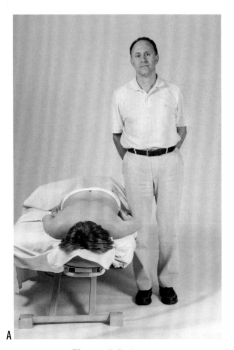 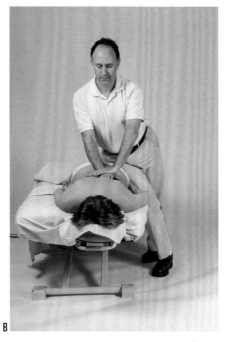 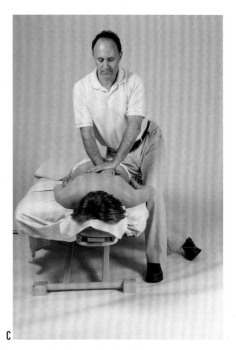

A   B   C

Figure 4-8 Positioning the feet to place the core over the client. **(A)** Begin with both feet parallel to the table. **(B)** By placing the "outer foot" behind the "inner foot," the core naturally positions over the table. **(C)** Alternately, the core can be positioned over the table by placing the "outer foot" in front of the "inner foot" and then adducting the thigh of the inner foot by moving the foot away from the table.

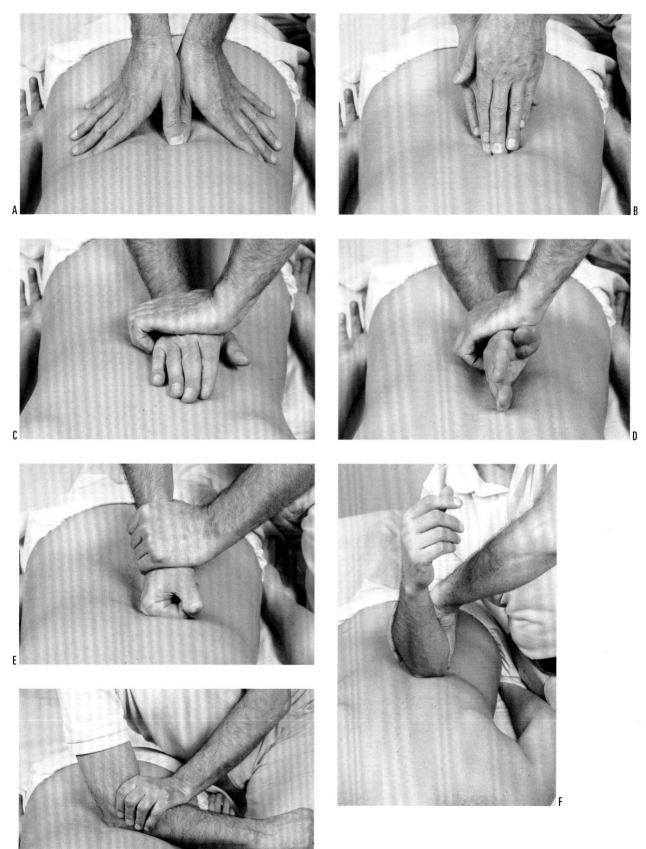

Figure 4-9 Treatment contacts. **(A)** Thumb pad. **(B)** Finger pads. **(C)** Palm. **(D)** "Knife-edge" (ulnar side of hand). **(E)** Fist. **(F)** Elbow. **(G)** Forearm.

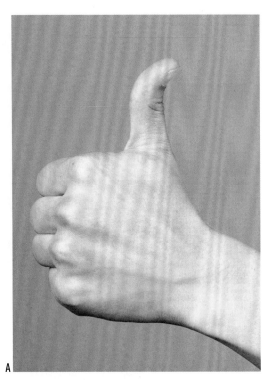
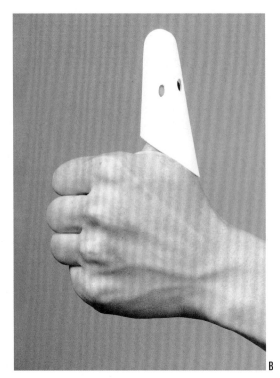

Figure 4-10 Interphalangeal joint of the thumb. **(A)** Hyperextension of the interphalangeal joint of the thumb. **(B)** A brace can be worn to support the thumb's interphalangeal joint. (Reproduced with permission from Muscolino JE. *Advanced Treatment Techniques for the Manual Therapist: Neck.* Baltimore, MD: Lippincott Williams & Wilkins; 2013.)

When thumbs or fingers are used, it is important to contact the client with the pads and not the tips of your thumb or fingers. Applying pressure with the tips of your thumb or fingers will likely feel uncomfortable for the client, especially when you are working deep. To best access the client's tissues with your fingers, you need to change the angulation of the shoulder, elbow, and wrist joints so that the pads naturally meet the client's body. To best access the client's tissues with your thumbs, you slightly extend the thumbs so the pads naturally meet the client's body. However, it is important to not extend the thumb too far or the joints of the thumb will become unstacked and excessive torque will be placed through them. A problem that some therapists have is a hyperextendable interphalangeal joint of the thumb (Fig. 4-10A). If your thumb is mildly hyperextendable, you may be able to do this work with your thumb. There are also supports available that can be worn on the thumb to prevent the interphalangeal joint from collapsing into hyperextension (Fig. 4-10B). But if your thumb is extremely mobile into hyperextension, you may need to employ another contact when doing deep tissue work into the client.

When using the palm as a contact, it is extremely important that the pressure that is exerted into the client is exerted through the base of the palm (heel of the hand), in other words, through the carpal region. If the palm is placed flat on the client and the pressure is exerted through the metacarpals or the fingers, it will usually result in torque being placed into the wrist joint. Figure 4-11 illustrates this concept. In Figure 4-11A, the wrist joint is shown in extension to emphasize that the contact pressure into the client should be at the carpal region. Of course, when actually working on the client, so as not to fatigue the extensors musculature of the forearm, the hand should be relaxed and resting on the client as seen in Figure 4-11B.

Working on the prone client with the palm contact usually requires some bend in the elbow joints so that the wrist joints are not excessively extended. When you lean in with your core to apply pressure into the client, it is extremely important that you stabilize your elbow joint and not allow it to bend any further. The purpose of using your core to lean in is to transfer body weight force through your arm, forearm, and treatment hand contact, and then into the client. If you allow your elbow joint to bend further, even a small amount, you will lose some or all of that core force (Fig. 4-11C, D). This is a common body mechanics error that frustrates many therapists who cannot understand why they are leaning in with their core but the client is still not feeling appreciable pressure.

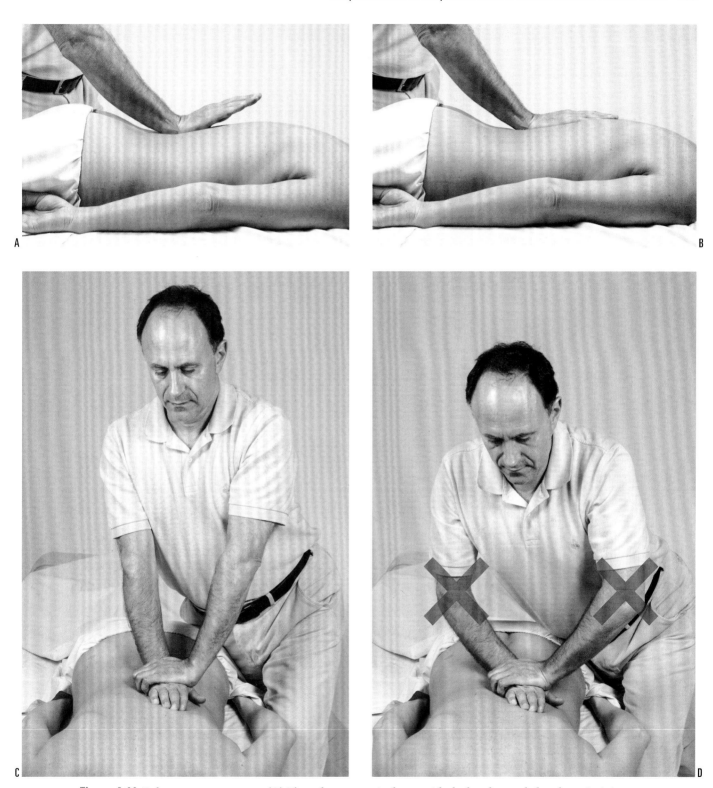

Figure 4-11 Palm treatment contact. **(A)** The palm contact is shown with the hand extended at the wrist joint to illustrate that the pressure should enter the client through the base of the palm. **(B)** When actually working on a client with the palm contact, the hand should be relaxed and resting on the client. **(C, D)** When using core body weight to press into the client with a palm contact, it is important to not let the elbow joints bend further as pressure is applied.

4.3 **THERAPIST TIP**

Transitioning from Palm to Knife-Edge and from Elbow to Forearm

Instead of viewing the palm and knife-edge (ulnar side of hand) as two separate contacts, they can be viewed as the two opposing ends of a continuous spectrum of width, with the palm being the widest and the knife-edge being the narrowest. When working on the client's tissues, if a wide contact is desired, such as when working on the lumbar paraspinal musculature, the palm is best. As you work up the client's back and the paraspinal musculature gradually narrows, it is advantageous to commensurately narrow your contact by gradually supinating the forearm of the contact hand. Supinating the forearm will change the contact surface from being a full flat palm (**Fig. A**) to being the hypothenar eminence of the hand (**Fig. B**); if the fore-

arm is further supinated, the knife-edge contact will be attained (**Fig. C**). Depending on the width of the tissue being worked, the appropriate contact from the full flat palm to the knife-edge can be chosen.

Similarly, the elbow and forearm contacts can be viewed as opposing ends of a continuous spectrum. When more pointed pressure is desired, the olecranon process of the elbow can be used (**Fig. D**). If a slightly wider contact is desired, the elbow joint can be partially extended so that you are contacting the client with the elbow and proximal forearm (**Fig. E**); if you further extend the elbow joint, you will be contacting the client with the full flat forearm, which is the widest contact (**Fig. F**).

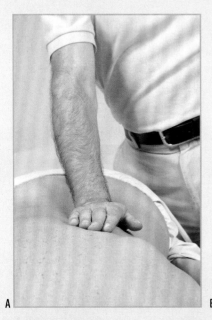

A

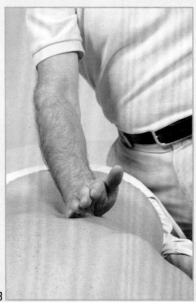

B

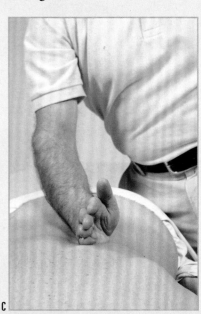

C

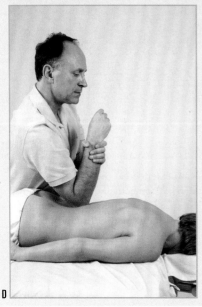

D

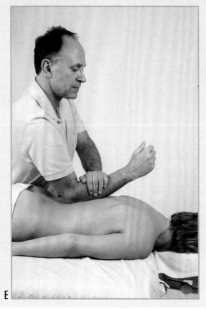

E

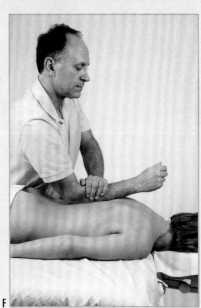

F

Alternating Contacts

Even perfect body mechanics cannot eliminate all physical stress to your body when doing massage. Ideal body mechanics merely minimize the stress. For this reason, when doing massage, it is wise to alternate which contact you use during a session. Given the mass of musculature in the low back and pelvis, it is wise to use larger contacts as much as possible. A good strategy is to begin with smaller contacts such as thumb or finger pads to assess and begin treatment of the lumbar region or pelvis and then switch to a larger contact such as the palm or elbow to deliver deeper pressure.

4.5 Bracing/Supporting Your Treatment Contact

When employing deep pressure, it is extremely important to brace and support the treatment contact that meets the client. This both protects the joints and musculature of the treatment contact as well as allows for the brace hand to contribute to the generation of pressure, thereby increasing the depth of pressure. Bracing the contact means that the two hands must work together instead of each contacting the client separately. Less area of the client's body will be covered this way, but stronger and more efficient pressure will be created at the area that is being worked, which is more important when deep work is needed.

When bracing the contact, the precise location of the brace on the contact is extremely important. The brace should be placed on the contact directly over where the pressure is being exerted into the client. This is where the brace should be to effectively add to the pressure; it is also where the contact will be physically stressed and needs the bracing support to protect it from injury. For example, if a thumb contact is being used, the bracing should be over the distal phalanx of the contact thumb as seen in Figure 4-12A. When the thumb pad presses into the client, the client's body pushes back into the therapist's thumb, tending to hyperextend the thumb at the interphalangeal joint. Placing the brace thumb over the proximal phalanx of the contact thumb or next to the contact thumb as seen in Figures 4-12B and 4-12C will not effectively add to the pressure and will not protect the interphalangeal joint from hyperextension and eventual injury. Although it is common to use the thumb of the other hand as the brace to support the thumb contact, it is not the only body part that can be used as a brace. Any body part that can exert pressure on the distal phalanx of the contact thumb can be used as a brace (see Fig. 4-3). What is important is that the location where pressure is exerted into the client by the contact is braced and supported.

Similar to bracing the thumb pad contact, bracing the finger pads contact should be done over the distal phalanges of the fingers that are contacting the client, usually the index,

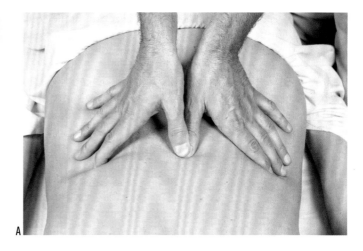

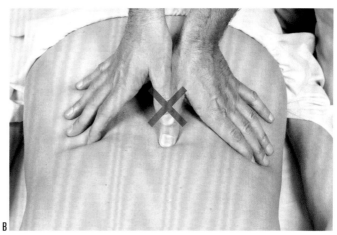

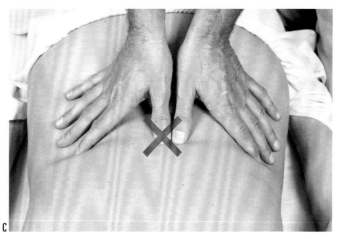

Figure 4-12 Bracing/supporting the thumb pad contact. (**A**) The thumb pad of the other hand braces directly on the distal phalanx of the treatment contact thumb. (**B, C**) Bracing on the proximal phalanx or directly adjacent to the distal phalanx of the treatment contact thumb is not an effective brace.

middle, and ring fingers (see Fig. 4-9B). Finger pads of the other hand work well to brace the finger pads contact.

Proper bracing of the palm contact is extremely important. Because pressure when using the palm contact is exerted through the base of the palm (carpal region), the bracing needs to be placed over the carpal region of the contact hand. Unfortunately, therapists often incorrectly place the brace too far distal on the hand. A common brace for the palm contact is to use the other palm. When using this brace, be sure to place the carpal region of the brace hand directly over the carpal region of the contact hand. In Figure 4-13A, both hands are being held in extension at the wrist joint to clearly illustrate that the pressure from the brace hand is being exerted directly over the carpal contact on the client. Of course, when actually working on a client, it is important to let the hands relax as seen in Figure 4-13B so that the extensor musculature of the forearms is not fatigued.

Another brace for the palm contact that is not used as often but offers a unique advantage over the palm brace is

Figure 4-13 Bracing the palm treatment contact. The palm of the other hand is shown as the brace in **A** and **B**. In **A**, both hands are shown extended at the wrist joint to illustrate that the pressure of the brace should be through the carpal region of the palm contact. When actually working on the client, the hands should be relaxed as seen in **B**. The thumb web of the other hand is shown as the brace in **C** and **D**. In **C**, both hands are shown lifted to illustrate that the pressure of the brace should be through the carpal region of the palm treatment contact. When actually working on the client, the hands should be relaxed as seen in **D**.

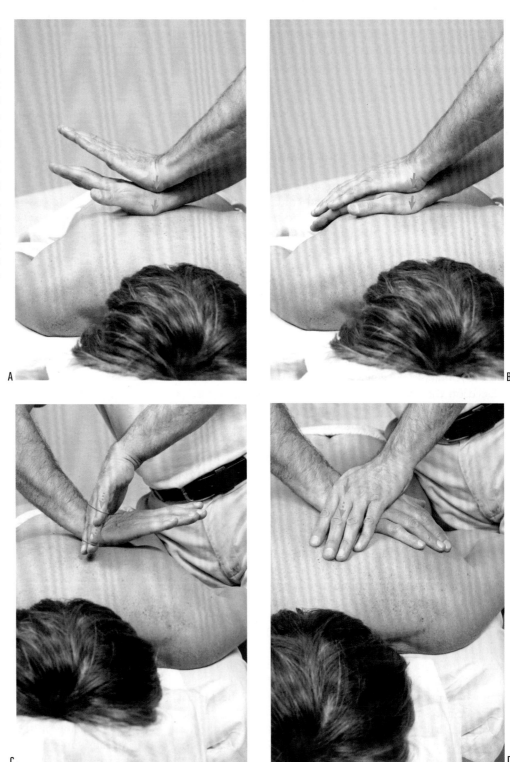

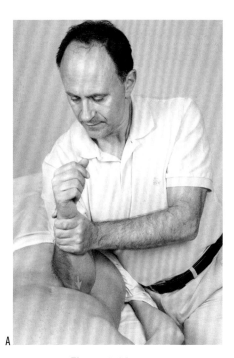 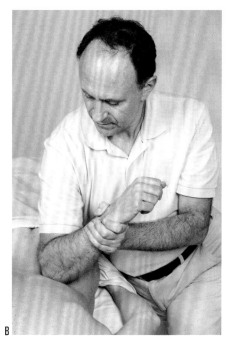 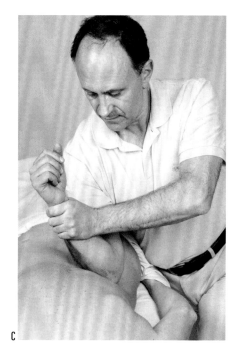

A B C

Figure 4-14 Bracing the elbow contact. Bracing the elbow treatment contact by holding onto the distal forearm allows pivoting of the elbow, which can change the angulation of pressure into the client.

the thumb web. Similar to the illustration of the palm brace, Figure 4-13C illustrates the thumb web brace position with the hands lifted away from the client so that the exact placement and pressure can be easily seen; when working on the client, be sure to let the hands relax as seen in Figure 4-13D. The advantage of the thumb web brace is that it allows for an easy transition when changing from a full flat palm contact to the knife-edge (ulnar side of hand) contact (see Figs. B and C in Therapist Tip 4.3). As the forearm supinates to transition from the full flat palm contact to the knife-edge contact, the thumb web brace can be easily altered to compensate. This allows for the pressure of the brace to always be directly over the contact on the client. The palm brace may work well when the contact palm is flat against the client but is difficult to use when the contact transitions to the hypothenar eminence or the knife-edge.

When using a closed fist to contact the client, the wrist joint can be braced and stabilized with the contact hand (see Fig. 4-9E). Even larger and more powerful than the fist contact are the elbow and forearm contacts. Even though the elbow and forearm contacts are the largest and most efficient for producing deep pressure, use of these contacts can be physically stressful on the shoulder girdle musculature on the contact side because this musculature must function to stabilize the shoulder girdle as pressure is exerted into the client. Bracing that is done by the other side of the body can help to relieve the contact-side shoulder girdle musculature from having to work so hard. Bracing the elbow contact can be done by pressing down on the anterior surface of the elbow joint (see Fig. 4-9F) or by holding onto the distal fore-

arm (Fig. 4-14A). Bracing and pressing down on the anterior elbow region is very effective at adding pressure into the client. Additional pressure can also be exerted when grasping the distal forearm; however, this brace position is especially effective at pivoting the forearm at the elbow joint so that the angulation of pressure into the client can be varied (Fig. 4-14B, C). When working with the forearm contact, bracing is accomplished by holding onto and pressing down onto the forearm (see Fig. 4-9G).

4.6 Stacking the Upper Extremity Joints

Stacked joints are aligned in a straight line; in other words, the joints are extended as in anatomic position. This allows for the force from your core to travel through your upper extremity and into the client with little or no loss of strength. When working on the prone client's low back and pelvis with the thumb or finger pads as the contact, your elbow, wrist, and thumb/finger joints should be stacked (Fig. 4-15A, B). When using the fist, the elbow and wrist joints should be stacked (Fig. 4-15C). The palm contact can be problematic because if the elbow joints are fully stacked/extended, the wrist joints will be extended to nearly 90 degrees (Fig. 4-15D). This can increase torque and perhaps lead to wrist injury. For this reason, it is advisable to slightly bend the elbow joints to protect the wrist joints (Fig. 4-15E). This will require more muscular effort because the triceps brachii musculature will be required to isometrically contract when exerting pressure; but triceps effort is preferable to potential wrist injury.

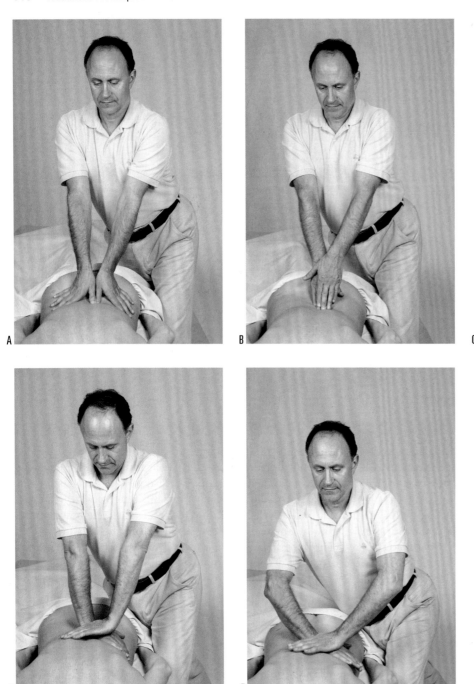

Figure 4-15 Stacking the upper extremity joints when working on the client **(A–C)**. Upper extremity joints stacked with the thumb pad, finger pads, and fist treatment contacts, respectively. **(D)** If the elbow joints are fully extended/stacked when employing the palm contact, the wrist joints may be excessively torqued and injured. **(E)** Partially bending the elbow joints allows the wrist joints to be in a safer posture.

4.7 Aligning Your Core with the Stroke

Now that you have positioned the client on the table, adjusted where and how you are standing, braced your contact, and stacked your joints, it is important to make sure that your core is behind and in line with your stroke. This is accomplished by laterally rotating your arms at the glenohumeral joints so that your elbows are positioned in front of your core (Fig. 4-16A).

Keeping the elbows in is an important aspect of strong and efficient body mechanics that allows you to work from the core. It is not necessary for the elbows to be all the way at the midline of the body, but they should be within the width of your shoulders. If the thumb or finger pads are being used as the contact, then the (upper) arms can be placed against the core/trunk. This will place the elbows just inside (and usually slightly above) your anterior superior iliac spine (ASIS) (Fig. 4-16B).

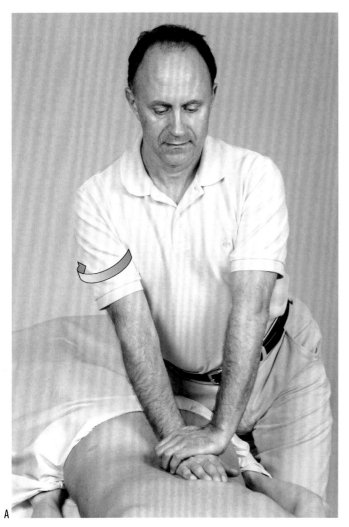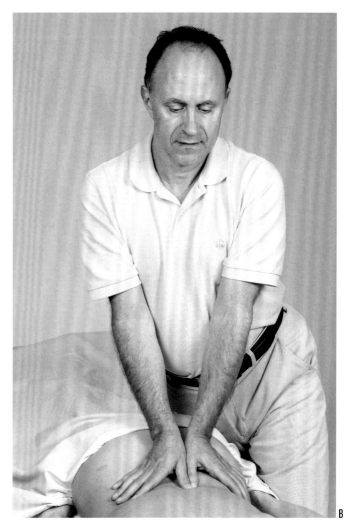

Figure 4-16 Place your upper extremities in front of your core. **(A)** Laterally rotating the arms at the glenohumeral joints helps to keep your elbows in front of your core. **(B)** The (upper) arms can be placed against the core for further support.

As stated, bringing the elbow in and placing the (upper) arm against the core can be extremely efficient for originating power from the core and transferring core strength through the forearm into the client. However, the elbow only needs to be far enough in to be against your core. Do not exaggerate this position and bring the elbow too far in toward the center of your body (see accompanying figure). Doing this would place an outward (valgus) torque force at the medial side of your elbow joint and might result in stress and damage to your flexor musculature common belly/tendon at the medial epicondyle of the humerus, resulting in "golfer's elbow," also known as medial epicondylitis or medial epicondylosis.

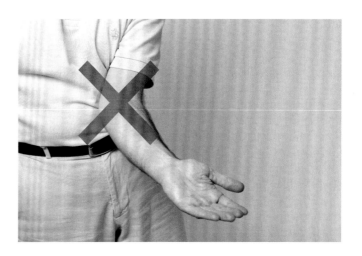

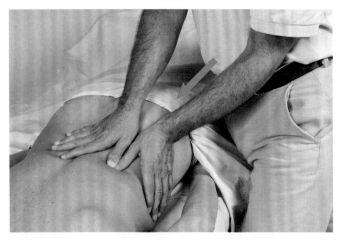

Figure 4-17 Generation of force from the core. Movement of the treatment contact should originate from the core of the therapist's body. The orientation of the core can be visualized by imagining a line that emanates from your belly button.

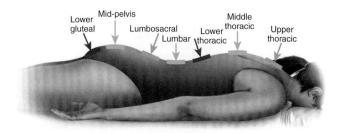

Figure 4-18 Contours of the client's back and pelvis regions. The contours of the posterior surface of the client's body, and perpendicular lines to these contours illustrating ideal lines of force, have been drawn.

When performing the stroke, make sure that whatever motion you create with your core is transferred directly into your upper extremity. In this manner, your core and upper extremity should be one fixed unit so that for each millimeter your core moves, your upper extremity moves the exact same amount, and your hand presses into the client. To make sure that your core is in line with the stroke, you can visually draw a line in the direction that your belly button points and compare it with the line of your stroke, which travels through your forearm (Fig. 4-17). With your core in line with the stroke, it is possible to generate the force of the stroke by using your body weight and larger muscles of the core instead of the smaller muscles of the thumb, hand, forearm, or even shoulder.

4.8 Applying Pressure Perpendicularly

Maximal pressure is achieved if the angle of your force into the client is perpendicular to the contour of the region being worked. To apply this concept of working perpendicularly, the client's back and pelvis can be divided into separate regions based on the curve of the region and therefore where the contour of each region is oriented. Because these regions are all on the posterior side of the body, they are all oriented posteriorly. Therefore, it is important to place as much of your core (posteriorly) above the client as possible so that you are working vertically down (from posterior to anterior) into the client. However, it is important to also determine whether the contour of the region you are working is oriented purely posteriorly, posteriorly and superiorly, or posteriorly and inferiorly. The orientation for each of these regions has been shown in Figure 4-18. In each case, the contour has been outlined, and an arrow that is perpendicular to that contour has also been drawn in. These arrows represent the perpendicular application of force you need to work the client most efficiently.

The upper thoracic and lumbosacral regions are oriented posteriorly and superiorly; therefore, working these regions perpendicularly is best accomplished not only by placing your core above (posterior to) the client but also standing slightly superior to the region (Figs. 4-19A, E). The thoracolumbar and lower gluteal regions are oriented posteriorly and inferiorly; therefore, working these regions perpendicularly is best accomplished by placing your core above (posterior to) the client and standing slightly inferior to the region (Figs. 4-19C, G). The midthoracic, midlumbar, and midgluteal regions are oriented purely posteriorly; therefore, working these regions perpendicularly is best accomplished by standing directly above the region to be worked (Figs. 4-19B, D, F).

If the client is prone and you are working more laterally on the body, then the contour of the region being worked is oriented more laterally. This means that the contour of the region being worked is oriented more vertically, so you need to approach the region with your force oriented more horizontally.

4.9 Dropping Down with Your Core

As stated earlier, force can be generated in two ways: by taking advantage of body weight via the force of gravity or by using muscle contraction. Because gravity is free and takes no effort, it should always be utilized as much as possible. Gravity only goes down, so to take advantage of it, you need to position your body above the client. You can then use your body weight by dropping down into the client. To position your body above the client, the table needs to be very low. The lower the table, the more of your body that you can position above the client, and therefore the more body weight you can use. With your core positioned above the client and in line with your stroke, you can generate deep pressure by dropping down into the client. This is accomplished by dorsiflexing the ankle joints and flexing the knee and hip joints (Fig. 4-20).

4.10 Using Larger Muscles

Dropping down and leaning into the posterior surface of the client with your core primarily involves using your body weight. However, it is often necessary to also contract

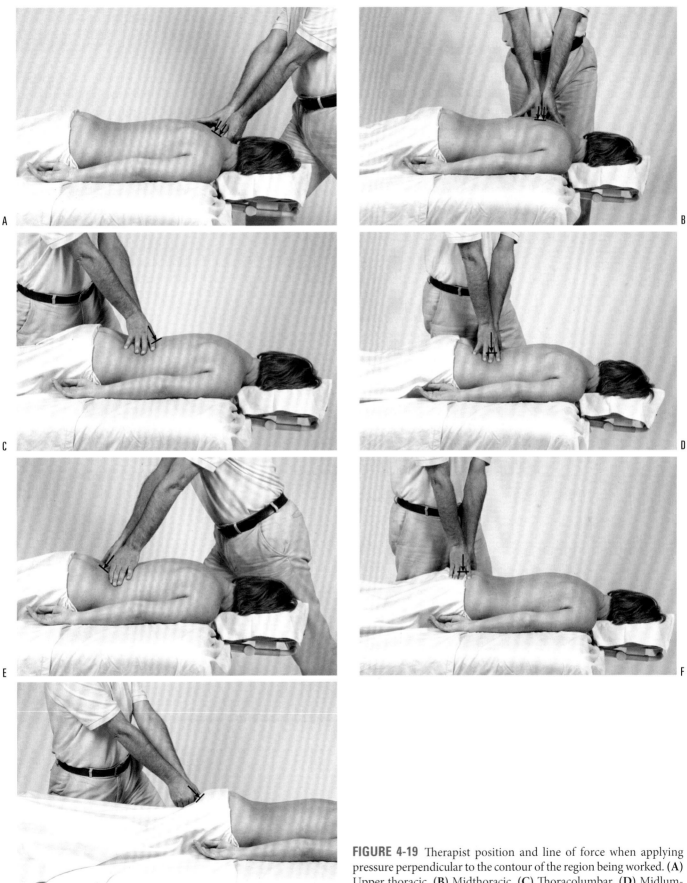

FIGURE 4-19 Therapist position and line of force when applying pressure perpendicular to the contour of the region being worked. (**A**) Upper thoracic. (**B**) Midthoracic. (**C**) Thoracolumbar. (**D**) Midlumbar. (**E**) Lumbosacral. (**F**) Midgluteal. (**G**) Lower gluteal.

The Posture of the Back

When standing and working over the client, there are three possible postures of the back: **stooped back**, **inclined back**, and **vertical back**. A stooped posture (**Fig. A**) is the worst of the three postures because it places the spine in an unstable open-packed position and the back is imbalanced anteriorly, requiring posterior extensor musculature to have to isometrically contract to keep the therapist from falling anteriorly. The inclined posture (**Fig. B**) is better than the stooped posture because the spine is extended and in a more stable closed-packed position; however, the back is still imbalanced anteriorly, requiring isometric contraction of the extensor musculature. The best posture of the back is the vertical posture (**Fig. C**). The spine is extended and in a stable closed-packed position, and it is balanced over the trunk, minimizing the need for spinal extensor musculature to contract. Whenever possible, the therapist should strive to maintain a vertical back posture.

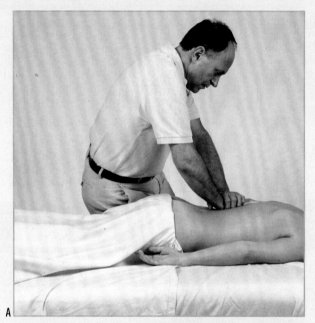

A

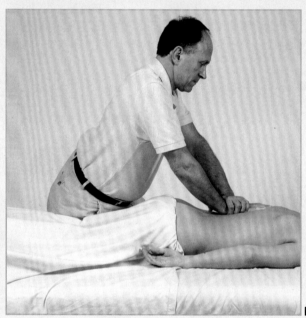

B

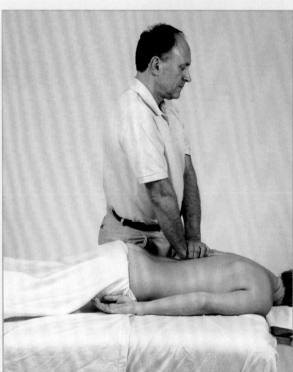

C

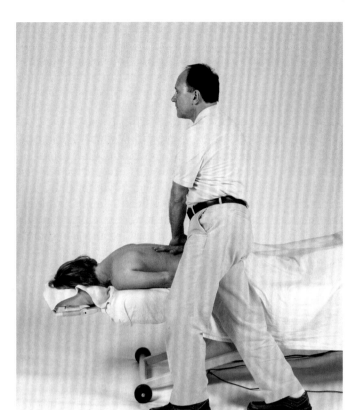
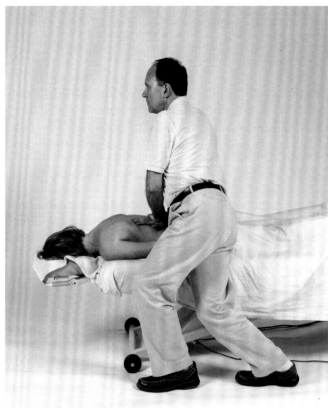

A   B

Figure 4-20 Dropping down into the client with body weight. Core body weight is transferred into the client by dorsiflexing the ankle joints and flexing the knee and hip joints. **(A)** Starting position. **(B)** End position.

| 4.6 | **THERAPIST TIP** |

Using Body Weight

An excellent demonstration of the force that can be generated by using body weight is to lean down onto a bathroom weight scale that is placed on a table that is positioned as various heights. Do not try to exert any force with muscle contraction; simply relax and lean into the scale with your body weight and notice the force that you generate at each height (see accompanying figures). In **Figure A**, the top of the table is at the height of the therapist's knee; in **Figure B**, it is at the height of the therapist's midthigh. The lower the table is positioned, the greater is your force, with no muscular effort.

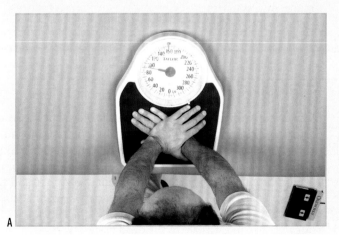
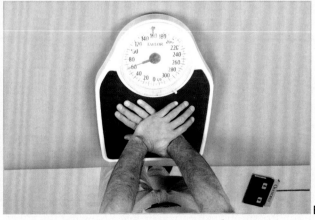

A   B

Letting the Shoulder Girdles Rise

When the table height is too high, it is common for the therapist to have to contract musculature to elevate the shoulder girdles when working on the client. This is considered to be poor posture because it stresses the body by requiring scapular elevation musculature such as the upper trapezius and levator scapulae to overwork by isometrically contracting. For this reason, a general rule of body mechanics is that the shoulder girdles should be relaxed and down. However, there are times when it is fine to have the shoulder girdles elevated. If you are working with deep pressure down into the client with the table adequately low, as you press into the client, the client's body presses back up into your contacts, causing your shoulder girdles to passively rise. In these cases, it is less effortful/stressful for your body to simply let the shoulder girdles rise than to isometrically contract scapular depression musculature to hold them down. The essence of good posture is minimizing stress to the tissues. Having the shoulder girdles relaxed and up is less stressful than contracting to hold them down.

muscles to add to the pressure generated from body weight. When choosing which muscles to contract and use, less effort is expended if you work with the larger, stronger proximal muscles instead of the smaller distal ones. In ascending order of size and strength, the muscles of the upper extremity and axial body that can be used are the muscles of the thumb/fingers, wrist joint, elbow and radioulnar joints, glenohumeral joint, shoulder girdle, and finally the muscles of the core, which comprise the trunk and pelvis. Choosing the larger proximal muscles of your core will decrease fatigue and the possibility of injury.

4.11 Pushing Off with the Lower Extremity

If the surface contour of the client that you are working is oriented somewhat laterally (e.g., the quadratus lumborum or lateral paraspinal musculature), then you need to approach the client more horizontally. A horizontal line of force does not allow for the use of body weight, so muscle contraction is necessary. Less effort is exerted for the same pressure if larger muscles are used. When working somewhat horizontally, it is wise to take advantage of the large musculature of the lower extremity. To do this, the feet should be in a sagittal plane stance, with the rear foot oriented somewhat parallel with the front foot. This allows for the best use of large musculature oriented in the sagittal plane. (If the rear foot is turned outward, as therapists often do, the sagittal plane musculature will not be in line with the stroke, and power will be lost.) Now use the lower

extremity in back to push off the floor and into the client. Many therapists are excellent at using the plantarflexor muscles of the ankle joint but neglect to take advantage of the large musculature of the knee and hip joints. To use these massive muscles, it is important to first assume a somewhat crouched position by flexing the knee and hip joints. Then when you push off into the client by plantarflexing the ankle joint, you simultaneously extend the knee joint with the quadriceps femoris musculature and extend the hip joint with gluteal musculature and hamstrings. To make sure that you do not rise up as you push off, it is necessary to simultaneously dorsiflex the ankle joint and flex the knee and hip joints of the lower extremity that is in front. This allows you to push off forward and also slightly downward into the client (Fig. 4-21).

Pushing a Box

A common error in body mechanics when pushing off with the lower extremity in back is for the therapist to rise up as he pushes off. This is counterproductive to generating pressure into the client because rising upward would move the core of your body away from the client. Your client is in front of you and usually a bit lower. Therefore, it is important to learn to push off with the lower extremity in back and push forward and somewhat downward.

To help get the hang of this motion, it can be useful to picture yourself pushing a large box that is on the floor. When you prepare to push the box, you intuitively crouch down and dorsiflex the ankle joint and flex the knee and hip joints of the lower extremity in back. Then as you push the box, you naturally plantarflex the ankle joint and extend the knee and hip joints in back as you dorsiflex the ankle joint and flex the knee and hip joints in front. As you push the box forward, you would not rise upward. Rather, you would keep the pelvis more level. Practice this when standing; once it feels natural, try to reproduce this motion when working on a client. If any alteration is made, actually drop your pelvis as you push forward so that you push forward and downward into the client.

4.12 Engaging the Tissues

Deep tissue work requires that you engage the client's tissues. This means that you press in until you feel resistance to your pressure. Once resistance is felt, further pressure then needs to be applied for therapeutic deep tissue work to be done. It is important to stay within your client's tolerance and to increase your pressure slowly. For deep tissue work to be successful, however, it is necessary to apply sufficient force for your pressure to translate to the deep tissue layers.

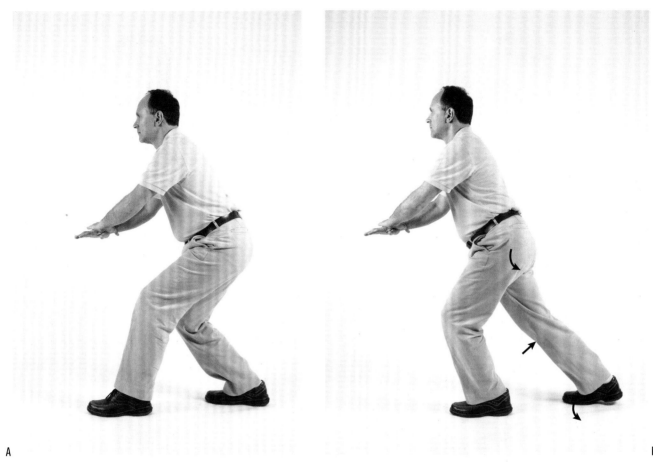

A

B

Figure 4-21 Generating pressure into the client by pushing off with the lower extremity in back. **(A)** Starting position. **(B)** Pushing off involves plantarflexing the ankle joint, extending the knee joint, and extending the hip joint.

Depth of Work

The depth of deep tissue work should always be within the client's range of tolerance. It is never beneficial to force deep pressure on a client or to work beyond the client's tolerance. If this is done, the client may tighten the musculature that you are working on either in response to the pain or in anticipation of pain. Given that one of the principle purposes of massage is to reduce muscle tone, the purpose of the deep pressure is defeated the moment the client tightens up the target muscles being worked on. Further, deep pressure should never be performed in a sudden or abrupt manner. Rather, the client should always be warmed up first with lighter and then moderate depth massage before introducing deep pressure. Even then, it is important to apply deep pressure by slowly and smoothly sinking into the client's musculature. When the client is properly prepared and the deep work is performed appropriately, clients are often comfortable with very strong pressure.

4.13 Focusing the Client's Breathing

It can often be helpful to have the client focus on his or her breathing as the work is done. Ask the client to take in a full breath; as the client relaxes and exhales, slowly begin to sink into the client's tissues. If very deep work is needed, this procedure may be repeated two or three times before the full depth of the pressure is reached.

4.14 Transitioning from Sustained Compression to Short Deep Stroking Massage

All of the guidelines presented thus far are meant to perfect your body mechanics when applying sustained compression into any one spot on the client. This in no way is meant to advocate sustained compression as the treatment technique of choice. It is simply easier to learn how to optimize your body mechanics by focusing on one area of the client at a time. To transition from sustained pressure in one static location to **deep stroking massage**, in which your pressure is moved from one point to another, and maintain proper body mechanics while doing this, it is necessary to glide your treatment contact from the initial point of contact to the adjacent

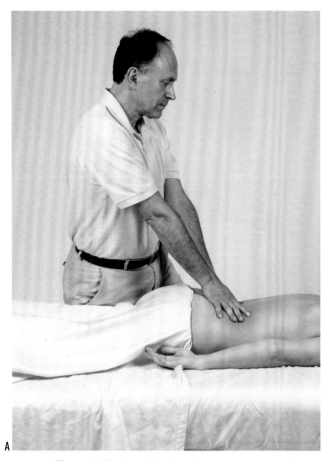
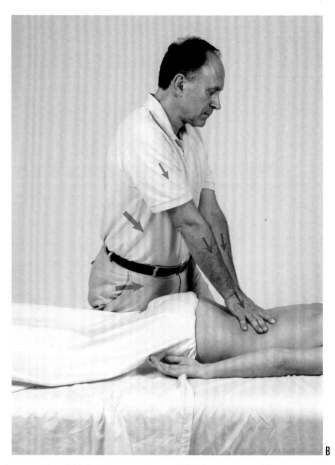

Figure 4-22 Transitioning from static compression to a short stroke. (**A**) Starting position. (**B**) Movement of the stroke should originate from the core.

region. This motion should not come from moving your contact (e.g., your thumb or fingers) but must originate from your core or lower extremities. With stacked joints, this core motion will translate into motion of your treatment contact along the client (Fig. 4-22A, B). However, it is important to keep these strokes short because the farther you reach from your initial point of contact, the more difficult it is to maintain proper body mechanics. Short, deep strokes between 1 and 6 inches in length allow you to preserve optimal body mechanics.

4.1 PRACTICAL APPLICATION

Treating Myofascial Trigger Points

A **trigger point (TrP)** is a small focal area of tenderness that can refer pain or other symptoms to a distant site. When a TrP occurs in muscular tissue, it involves a small area of contraction that is tender and can refer; this is called a **myofascial TrP**, or, in lay terms, a *muscle knot*. Bodywork treatment for TrPs has classically been done with techniques known as **ischemic compression** and **sustained compression**. In ischemic and sustained compression, pressure is applied directly to the TrP and is held for a sustained period of time, usually 10 seconds or more (generally, greater pressure is applied with ischemic compression than sustained compression). However, in recent years, many authorities on TrPs (including Simons and Travell in *Myofascial Pain and Dysfunction: The Trigger Point Manual*, 2nd ed. *Vol 1: Upper Half of Body* [Lippincott Williams & Wilkins, 1999]

and Davies in *The Trigger Point Therapy Workbook: Your Self-treatment Guide for Pain Relief* [New Harbinger Publications, 2004]) have advocated deep stroking massage instead of sustained pressure techniques. Not only is deep stroking usually more comfortable for the client and easier on your thumbs, it seems to do a better job of increasing local arterial circulation, which is needed to truly heal a TrP. Strokes need to be only approximately an inch or two in length and are usually repeated 30 to 60 times in 1 minute. Pressure should be deep, but because the pressure is not constantly held on the TrP, it is usually better tolerated by the client. If you have not yet tried deep stroking massage for the treatment of TrPs, give this approach a try and see how your results compare with those of sustained compression techniques.

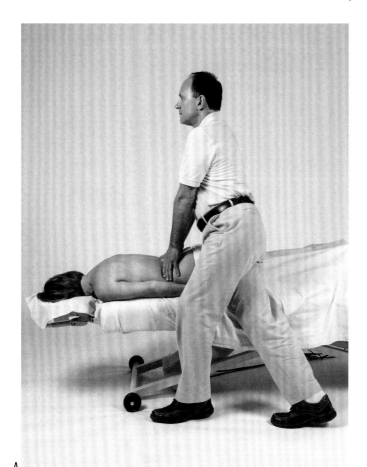
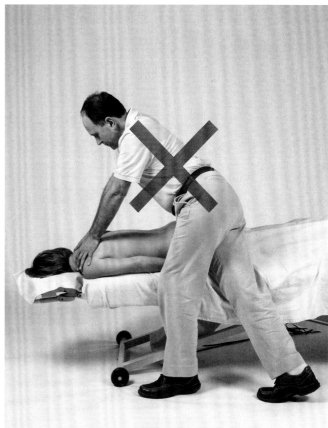

A   B

Figure 4-23 Body mechanics for a long stroke. **(A)** Ideal body mechanics at the beginning of a long stroke. **(B)** If the feet remain planted in the same position as a long stroke is performed, body mechanics will suffer by the end of the stroke.

4.15 Transitioning to Long, Deep Strokes

Good body mechanics are performed by positioning your body as close to the region being worked as possible. This allows you to place your core over the area where pressure is being applied so that body weight can be used (Fig. 4-23A). However, if ideal body positioning and mechanics are used to contact the client at one point on her body and then you remain with your feet planted in the same spot as a long stroke is performed, it is inevitable that your body mechanics will suffer by the end of the stroke. Your trunk will no longer be vertical and positioned over the client's body, you will not have the ability to efficiently generate strength, and you will be in an imbalanced position that requires isometric contraction by back musculature to keep you from falling (Fig. 4-23B). For these reasons, whenever you want to perform a long, deep stroke up the client's back, it is necessary to move your feet as the stroke is performed.

Illustrating this on the client's left side, you begin the stroke with a sagittal stance and your weight balanced over the right (rear) foot (Fig. 4-24A). As you gradually move up the client's back with the stroke, you gradually transfer your weight onto your left (front) foot (Fig. 4-24B). You now reposition your

right foot to be next to the left foot and then shift your weight onto the right foot (Fig. 4-24C). You can now reposition your left foot to be farther in front (Fig. 4-24D). As you continue to gradually move up the client's back with the stroke, you repeat this process, again gradually shifting your weight from the right (rear) foot onto the left (front) foot. If you perform a very long stroke from the client's lumbosacral spine to the top of the thoracic spine, this protocol will usually need to be done approximately two to three times. This protocol allows your core to always be over the region being worked so that you can always take advantage of body weight.

When you reach the top of the client's trunk, if you want to complete the stroke without an interruption in the application of deep pressure, you need to make sure that your core is superior to the client's trunk (just lateral to the face cradle) and you drop/lean backward with your body weight against the top of the client's back/shoulder (see Fig. 4-24D). Whereas for the entire length of the stroke, you were leaning your core body weight forward and down onto the front foot, at the end, you need to lean your core body weight backward and down onto the rear foot. This allows for the stroke to be completed without having to reorient your body 180 degrees around to face the foot end of the table to press onto the top

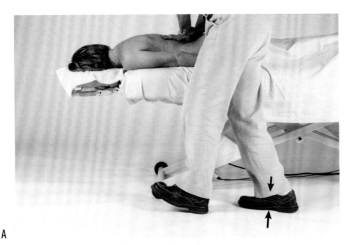

A

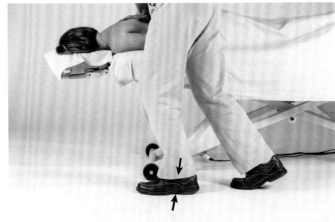

B

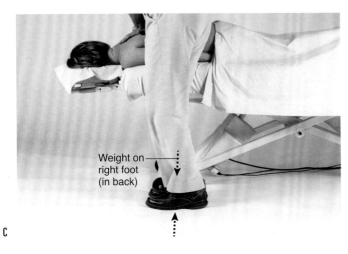

Weight on right foot (in back)

C

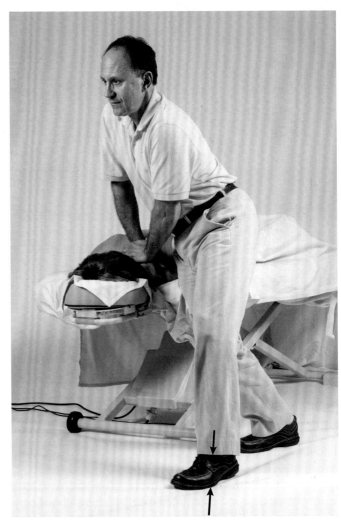

D

Figure 4-24 Ideal body mechanics during a long stroke involve moving the feet and shifting the balance of the body's weight as the stroke is performed. **(A)** At beginning of stroke, the therapist's body weight is balanced over the right (rear) foot. **(B)** Weight is shifted to the left (front) foot. **(C)** Right foot is repositioned to be next to the left foot, and body weight is shifted to the right foot. **(D)** Left foot is repositioned to be farther in front, and body weight is shifted onto the left foot.

of the client's back/shoulder. The more you practice gracefully transferring your body weight from foot to foot as you move your feet up the table, the smoother you can perform one long, deep stroke up the client's back.

4.16 Posture of the Neck and Head

The neck and head do not contribute to the generation of pressure, so their posture should be whatever is most comfortable and least stressful. A common postural pattern that is stressful for the body is to flex the head and upper neck forward to watch the stroke that is being performed (Fig. 4-25A). This should be avoided as much as possible. It is rarely necessary to watch your strokes. And this posture places your head in an imbalanced posture over thin air in front of your trunk, requiring posterior cervical extensor musculature to isometrically contract to hold this posture and prevent your head from falling into flexion until the chin hits the chest. The healthiest posture for the head and neck is to have the head balanced over the vertical trunk so that neck musculature does not have to contract to hold the head in position (Fig. 4-25B).

However, whenever the trunk is not vertical, for example, if it is inclined forward because you are reaching forward to perform a longer stroke, then this posture is not possible. In these cases, it is likely better to relax the head and neck and let the head rest in flexion with the chin at or near the chest (Fig. 4-25C). This affords the opportunity to close the eyes and visualize the structures that are being worked beneath the skin. *Note*: The only disadvantage to letting the head and neck drop into flexion is if this posture is habitually assumed, the fascial tissues of the posterior neck will gradually lengthen, resulting in less passive tension force to hold up the head and neck. In the long run, this could require greater work on the part of the extensor musculature of the neck.

4.10   THERAPIST TIP

Choosing the Right Lubricant

When strokes are performed, to glide along the client's skin without abrading it, a lubricant is needed. Choosing the right lubricant is very important, especially for deep tissue massage. A lubricant allows the therapist to **slide/glide** along the client's skin. However, a lubricant must also provide some **drag** or friction that helps you press down into the client's tissues. Otherwise, the skin will be too slippery, causing you to slide along the surface of the skin without being able to generate pressure into the client's tissues. Each lubricant has a balance of slide and drag. For deep tissue work, it is important to choose a lubricant that offers more drag than slide. Generally, water-based lotions are better than oils for deep tissue work.

The amount of lubricant used is also very important. Too much lubricant increases the slide along the skin, making it difficult to generate pressure down into the tissues. Many therapists have difficulty generating deep pressure not because of a lack of strength but rather because they use too much lubricant. As a general rule, the least amount of lubricant needed to not abrade the client's skin is the amount that should be used.

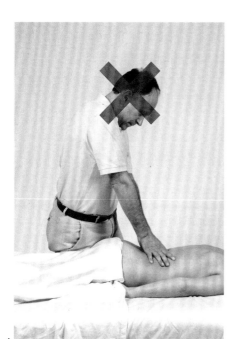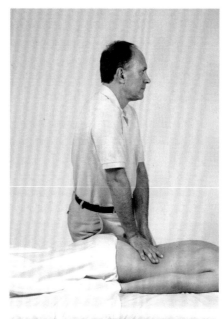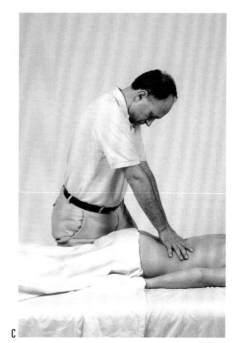

A   B   C

Figure 4-25 Posture of the head and neck. (**A**) Flexing the head and neck to watch the stroke imbalances the head anteriorly, requiring isometric contraction of the posterior cervical extensor musculature. (**B**) Balanced posture of the head over the vertical trunk. (**C**) Relaxing the head and neck into flexion when working with the trunk inclined.

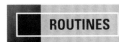
ROUTINES

DEEP TISSUE WORK ROUTINES

There is more than one way to approach working the low back and pelvis. You may choose to do spot work based on your client's needs, or you may choose to perform deep work to the entire region as part of your massage that covers more of the client's body. In either case, you must make sure to always segue into deep tissue work by first working lightly to moderately to prepare the client for the deeper pressure. When performing deep work, remember always to sink slowly into the client's musculature.

The five routines that follow demonstrate body mechanics for deep tissue work to the low back and posterior pelvis (gluteal region). There is no rule as to where to begin when working these regions. The order of the five routines presented here begins at the lumbosacral and lumbar regions, continues up into the thoracic region, and then concludes with the gluteal region.

The order of these routines is an excellent approach, but if you like, you can alter the order of the routines. Also, if desired, once the five routines have been done, a few longer strokes can be done to connect the gluteal, lumbar, and thoracic regions (see "15. Transitioning to Long, Deep Strokes"). The five routines show work to the left side of the low back and pelvis. The right side can be worked in the identical manner by standing on the other side of the table and reversing the roles of your hands.

| 4.11 | **THERAPIST TIP** |

Client Communication

The best measure of the appropriateness of the depth of your pressure should always be the response of the client's tissues to the pressure that you are employing. You should be able to feel this with the finger pads or other treatment contact. In this regard, massage is a two-way street: You are not only exerting pressure into the client, you are also constantly monitoring the response of your client to the pressure. It is also extremely valuable to verbally check in with your client about the depth of the pressure when doing the massage. Even if you feel confident about the depth of pressure given the response from the client's tissues, it is important to communicate directly with the client in a way that shows that you are aware of his or her desires and needs. This can help the client feel at ease and relax, which is especially important when doing deeper work. When asking the client about the pressure, you should not simply ask, "How is the pressure?" This question places your client in the position of having to criticize your massage, which many clients may not feel comfortable doing. As a result, the response is often "Fine," whether it is or not. A better way to phrase the question is, "Would you like more pressure or less pressure?" Now you are specifically inviting the client to ask for a change in what you are doing, and the client has to go out of the way to say that it is fine as is. This phrasing is more likely to elicit an honest and accurate response and to create a massage that the client enjoys and from which the client benefits.

BODY MECHANICS FOR DEEP TISSUE WORK ROUTINES

The following body mechanics for deep tissue work routines are presented in this chapter:

- Routine 4-1—medial low back—paraspinal musculature
- Routine 4-2—lateral low back—quadratus lumborum
- Routine 4-3—middle and upper back—paraspinal musculature

- Routine 4-4—posterior pelvis—gluteal region
- Routine 4-5—lateral pelvis—abductor musculature

Note: For each of the five routines, a specific treatment contact and bracing position has been shown. Other options are possible (see Figs. 4-9 and 4-12 through 4-14).

ROUTINE 4-1: MEDIAL LOW BACK—PARASPINAL MUSCULATURE

Starting Position:

- Have the client prone, if possible, positioned to the left side of the table. Place a bolster under the client's ankles.
- You are standing at the left side of the table, close to the client and adjacent to the client's pelvis (Fig. 4-26A).

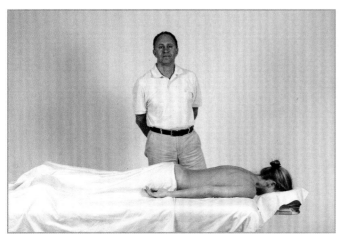

Figure 4-26A

Step 1: Place Contact on the Client's Musculature:

- Your right palm is the treatment contact, and it is placed on the left side of the client's low back, over the dorsal surface of the sacrum.
- Make sure that your forearm is oriented as close as possible perpendicular to the contour of the client's body where you have made contact. Because of the contour of the sacrum at this level, the forearm of the brace/support left hand is actually better aligned to press perpendicularly into the client here (Fig. 4-26B).
- Also, be sure that your core is aligned with your stroke; your belly button should be pointed in line with (or extremely close to and parallel with) the line of your forearm.
- *Note*: Other contacts besides the palm are possible (see Fig. 4-9).

Step 2: Brace/Support the Contact:

- The thumb web of your left hand is the brace that supports palm contact of the right hand (see Fig. 4-26B).
- Your elbows are in front of your body so that you can use your core body weight behind your contact when pressing into the client.
- *Note*: The palm of the left hand can be used as a brace instead of the thumb web (see Fig. 4-13).

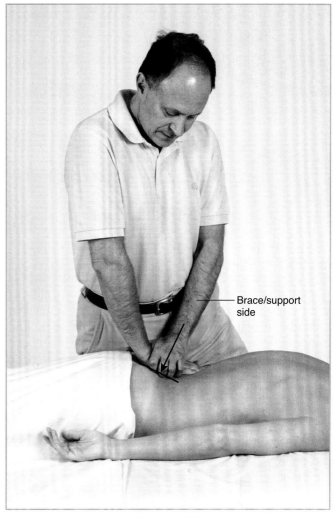

Brace/support side

Figure 4-26B

Step 3: Apply Pressure:

- Slowly press with your palm into the client's musculature over the dorsum of the sacrum, directly lateral to the midline, by shifting your body weight from your right (rear) foot to your left (front) foot.
- This pressure is supplemented by pressure from your left brace hand.
- It is important to slowly sink into the client's tissues and to apply the pressure as close as possible perpendicular to the contour of the client's body that you are working.
- Continue shifting your weight forward, translating this motion into a deep stroke along the client's lumbar paraspinal musculature, close to the spinous processes, from inferior to superior, for a length of approximately 1 to 6 inches (Fig. 4-27A).
- The movement for the stroke should originate from your lower extremities and core.

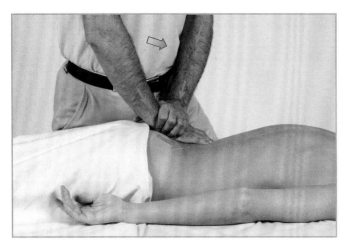

Figure 4-27A

Further Repetitions:

- Repeat this stroke in the same location another two to three times.
- Now move slightly superiorly to the midlumbar to upper lumbar region and perform approximately three to four deep strokes in a similar manner here (Fig. 4-27B).

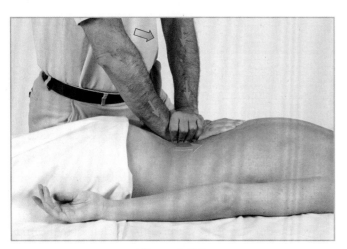

Figure 4-27B

- Repeat further sets of three to four strokes, slightly more laterally on the paraspinal musculature, both in the lumbosacral region and then again in the midlumbar to upper lumbar region (Fig. 4-27C), until the lateral border of the paraspinal musculature has been reached.
- Beginning back at the dorsum of the sacrum again, repeat this entire protocol, this time increasing the depth of pressure.

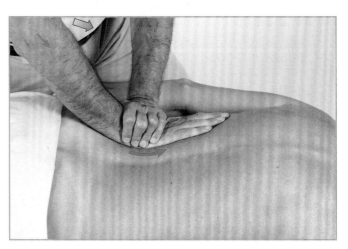

Figure 4-27C

4.2   PRACTICAL APPLICATION

Icing to Increase Depth of Pressure

You never want deep tissue work to be painful and cause the client to tighten in response. However, there are times when the client's musculature is very tender, not allowing you to work sufficiently deep to affect the desired change and improvement. In these cases, it can be helpful to ice an area to numb it so that you can work deeper than you otherwise would have been able to, without causing pain to the client. Sometimes, it also can be beneficial to ice after deep tissue work to decrease the likelihood of post-treatment pain and/or swelling. (*Note:* For more on ice application, see Chapter 11, available online at thePoint. lww.com.)

ROUTINE 4-2: LATERAL LOW BACK—QUADRATUS LUMBORUM

Starting Position:
- Have the client prone, if possible, positioned to the left side of the table. Place a bolster under the client's ankles.
- You are standing at the left side of the table, close to the client and adjacent to the client's lumbar spine, facing across the client (Fig. 4-28A).

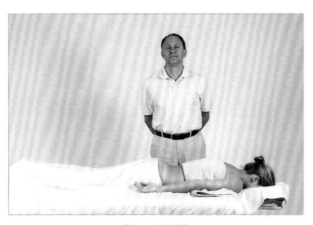

Figure 4-28A

Step 1: Place Contact on the Client's Musculature:
- Your left thumb pad is the treatment contact, and it is placed on the left side of the client's low back over the quadratus lumborum, immediately lateral to the lateral border of the paraspinal (erector spinae) musculature.
- *Note*: To find the lateral border of the erector spinae, ask the client to extend the trunk and look and feel for the contour and borders of the erector spinae to become prominent (Fig. 4-28B).
- Make sure that your forearm and thumb are oriented perpendicularly to the contour of the client's body where you have made contact (Fig. 4-28C).
- Also, be sure that your core is aligned with your stroke; your belly button should be pointed in line with (or extremely close to and parallel with) the line of your forearm.

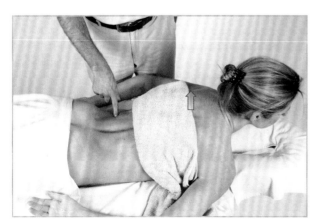

Figure 4-28B

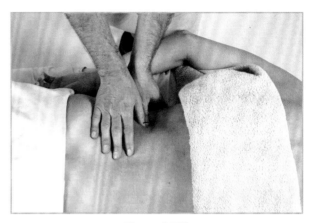

Figure 4-28C

Step 2: Brace/Support the Contact:
- Your right thumb is the brace that supports the thumb pad contact of the left hand (see Fig. 4-28C).
- Your elbows are in front of your body so that you can use your core body weight behind your contact when pressing into the client.

Step 3: Apply Pressure:
- Slowly press into the client's quadratus lumborum (lateral and deep to the erector spinae) with your thumb pad by shifting your body weight from your right (rear) foot to your left (front) foot.
- This pressure is supplemented by pressure from your right brace hand.
- It is important to slowly sink into the client's tissues.
- Press in a medial direction to access the transverse process attachment fibers (Fig. 4-29). Press medial and superior for the 12th rib fibers; press medial and inferior for the iliac crest fibers.
- The movement for the stroke should originate from your lower extremities and core.

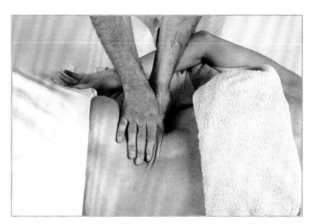

Figure 4-29

4.3   **PRACTICAL APPLICATION**

Working the Quadratus Lumborum Side-Lying

Because of the location of the quadratus lumborum deep to the erector spinae, pressure into this muscle must be directed from lateral to medial. For this reason, side-lying is an excellent position to access this muscle; it also allows for body weight to be used. The client should be as close to the side of the table, positioned either side-lying or side-lying and slightly rotated away from you (toward a prone position), with a small roll between the knees. Place your treatment contact immediately lateral to the erector spinae. Now slowly sink into the quadratus lumborum (see accompanying figure).

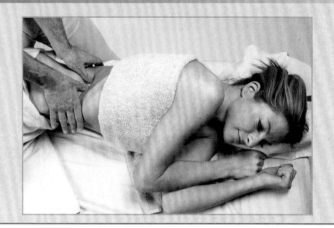

4.4   **PRACTICAL APPLICATION**

Perform Deep Tissue Work on Stretch

Most of the treatment routines in this chapter demonstrate deep tissue work to the back, with the client's spine in a neutral position with respect to flexion or lateral flexion. However, it can also be valuable to work the musculature while on stretch. The advantage to working a muscle on stretch is that it intensifies work into the more superficial musculature. The advantage to working a muscle that is shortened is that it slackens the more superficial musculature, allowing greater access to deeper musculature.

The accompanying figures demonstrate working the lumbar musculature on stretch. In **Figure A**, the prone client's low back is flexed by placing a bolster under the anterior abdominal wall. In **Figure B**, the side-lying client's low back is laterally flexed by placing a bolster under the lateral abdominal wall. In **Figure C**, the side-lying client's low back is laterally flexed by dropping the lower extremity off the side of the table.

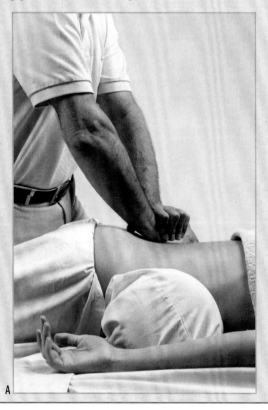

A

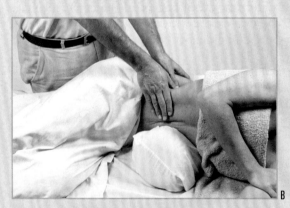

B

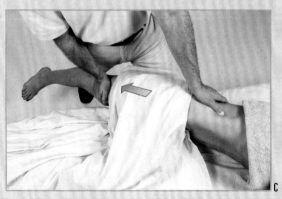

C

ROUTINE 4-3: MIDDLE AND UPPER BACK—PARASPINAL MUSCULATURE

Starting Position:

- Have the client prone, if possible, positioned to the left side of the table. Place a bolster under the client's ankles.
- You are standing at the left side of the table, close to the client and adjacent to the client's lumbar spine (Fig. 4-30).

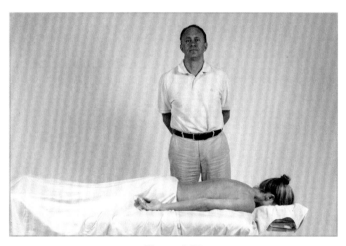

Figure 4-30

Step 1: Place Contact on the Client's Musculature:

- Your right thumb pad is the treatment contact, and it is placed on the left side of the client's lower thoracic spine on the paraspinal musculature.
- Make sure that your forearm and thumb are oriented perpendicularly to the contour of the client's body where you have made contact (Fig. 4-31A).
- Also, be sure that your core is aligned with your stroke; your belly button should be pointed in line with (or extremely close to and parallel with) the line of your forearm.
- *Note*: Other contacts besides the thumb pad are possible (see Fig. 4-9).

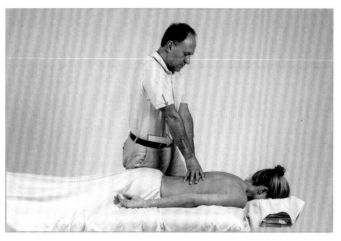

Figure 4-31A

Step 2: Brace/Support the Contact:

- The thumb pad of your left hand is the brace that supports the thumb pad contact of the right hand.
- Your elbows are in front of your body so that you can use your core body weight behind your contact when pressing into the client.
- *Note*: The palm of the left hand can be used as a brace instead of the thumb pad (see Fig. 4-12).

Step 3: Apply Pressure:

- Slowly press with your thumb pad into the client's musculature, directly lateral to the spinous processes, by shifting your body weight from your right (rear) foot to your left (front) foot.
- This pressure is supplemented by pressure from your left brace hand.
- It is important to slowly sink into the client's tissues and to apply the pressure as close as possible perpendicular to the contour of the client's body that you are working.
- Continue shifting your weight forward, translating this motion into a deep stroke along the client's thoracic paraspinal musculature, close to the spinous processes, from inferior to superior, for a length of approximately 1 to 6 inches (see Fig. 4-31A).
- The movement for the stroke should originate from your lower extremities and core.

Further Repetitions:

- Repeat this stroke in the same location another two to three times.
- Now move slightly superiorly to the upper thoracic region and perform approximately three to four deep strokes in a similar manner here (Fig. 4-31B).
- Repeat further sets of three to four strokes, slightly more laterally on the paraspinal musculature, both in the lower thoracic region and then again in the upper thoracic region (Fig. 4-31C), until the medial border of the scapula has been reached.
- Beginning back at the lower thoracic region again, repeat this entire protocol, this time increasing the depth of pressure.

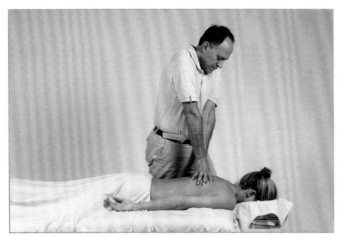

Figure 4-31B

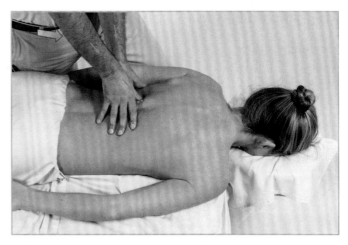

Figure 4-31C

4.5 | **PRACTICAL APPLICATION**

Use the Corner of the Table

When working the thoracic spine, it can be advantageous to work from superior to inferior (instead of inferior to superior) because the therapist can position himself closer to the client's trunk by standing at the head end of the table.

As previously stated, when working from the head of the table, it is unwise to stand above the face cradle because this distances the therapist from the client, making it more difficult to employ efficient body mechanics (see Fig. 4-6D). It is better to choose which side you want to work and then straddle the corner on that side at the head end of the table. This allows you to stand much closer to the client, facilitating positioning the core over the client for more efficient use of body weight.

ROUTINE 4-4: POSTERIOR PELVIS—GLUTEAL REGION

Starting Position:
- Have the client prone, if possible, positioned to the left side of the table. Place a bolster under the client's ankles.
- You are standing at the left side of the table, close to the client and adjacent to the client's pelvis (Fig. 4-32A).

Step 1: Place Contact on the Client's Musculature:
- Your right elbow is the treatment contact, and it is placed on the left side of the client's posterior pelvis over the gluteus maximus, immediately lateral to the apex of the sacrum.
- Make sure that your arm is oriented as close as possible to perpendicular to the contour of the client's body where you have made contact (Fig. 4-32B).
- Make sure that your core body weight is directly above the client.
- *Note*: Other contacts besides the elbow are possible (see Fig. 4-9).

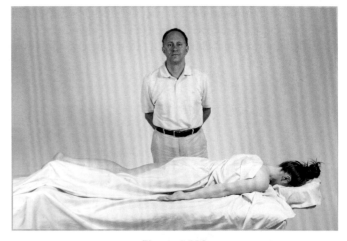

Figure 4-32A

- Continue dropping your weight down, translating this motion into a deep stroke into the gluteal and deep lateral rotator musculature adjacent to the client's sacrum; at the posterior superior iliac spine (PSIS), curve the stroke to then follow along the crest of the ilium (Fig. 4-33A).
- The movement for the stroke should originate from your core.

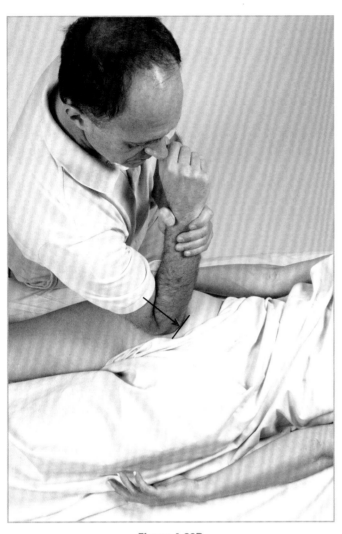

Figure 4-32B

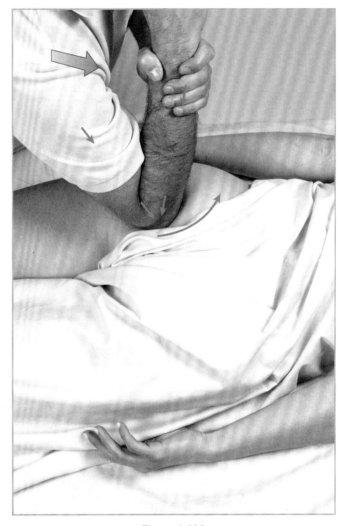

Figure 4-33A

Step 2: Brace/Support the Contact:
- Use your left hand to brace the right upper extremity by grasping the distal forearm (see Fig. 4-32B).
- Your elbows are in front of your body so that you can use your core body weight behind your contact when pressing into the client.
- *Note*: The elbow can also be braced by placing the left hand over the anterior elbow region (see Fig. 4-9F).

Step 3: Apply Pressure:
- Slowly press with your elbow into the client's gluteal and deep lateral rotator musculature, directly lateral to the sacrum, by dropping down with your body weight into the client.
- This pressure is supplemented by pressure from your left brace hand.
- It is important to slowly sink into the client's tissues and to apply the pressure as close as possible perpendicular to the contour of the client's body that you are working.

Further Repetitions:
- Repeat this stroke in the same location another two to three times.
- Repeat another set of three to four strokes, beginning slightly farther lateral from the apex of the sacrum and tracing a path that is parallel with the first stroke (Fig. 4-33B).
- Continue performing sets of parallel strokes, each set successively farther from the sacrum and iliac crest, until the entire buttock has been treated and the greater trochanter

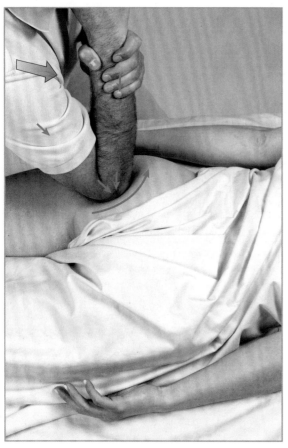

Figure 4-33B

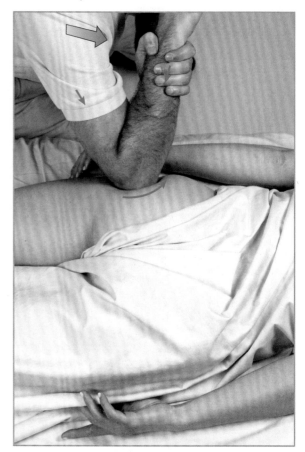

Figure 4-33C

has been reached. The last stroke should begin between the ischial tuberosity and the greater trochanter and should work into the musculature and attachments on the greater trochanter (Fig. 4-33C).

■ Beginning back just lateral to the sacrum again, repeat this entire protocol, this time increasing the depth of pressure.

When applying deep pressure to the gluteal region, be aware that the sciatic nerve exits from the internal pelvis into the buttock close to the sacrum, usually just inferior to the piriformis. It then runs inferiorly/distally between the ischial tuberosity and the greater trochanter.

4.6   PRACTICAL APPLICATION

Pin and Stretch the Piriformis

Pin and stretch is an excellent technique to both increase pressure on the target muscle and to focus the stretch to a particular aspect of the target muscle. It is particularly effective for treating the piriformis. Place an elbow on the gluteal musculature over the piriformis as the pin, and stretch the piriformis by medially rotating the thigh at the hip joint (see accompanying figure). This technique might be contraindicated if the client has an unhealthy knee joint. Using the leg as a lever to move the hip joint places a torque into the knee.

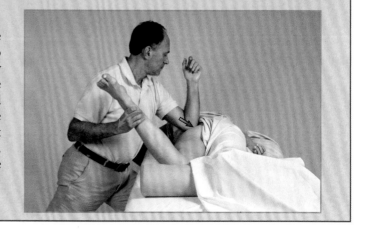

ROUTINE 4-5: LATERAL PELVIS—ABDUCTOR MUSCULATURE

Starting Position:
- Have the client side-lying facing away from you, as close to the side of the table as possible, with a roll placed between the knees.
- You are standing at the side of the table, close to the client and adjacent to the client's pelvis (Fig. 4-34A).

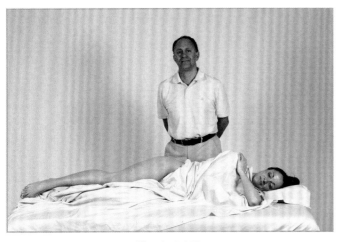

Figure 4-34A

Step 1: Place Contact on the Client's Musculature:
- Your right forearm is the treatment contact, and it is placed on the lateral side of the client's right gluteus medius, immediately distal/inferior to the center of the iliac crest.
- Make sure that your arm is oriented perpendicularly to the contour of the client's body where you have made contact (Fig. 4-34B).
- Make sure that your core body weight is directly above the client.
- *Note*: Other contacts besides the forearm are possible (see Fig. 4-9).

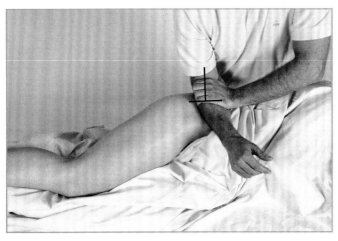

Figure 4-34B

Step 2: Brace/Support the Contact:
- Use your left hand to brace the right upper extremity by grasping the proximal right forearm (see Fig. 4-34B).
- Your elbows are in front of your body so that you can use your core body weight behind your contact when pressing into the client.

Step 3: Apply Pressure:
- Slowly press with your forearm into the client's musculature, just distal/inferior to the iliac crest, by dropping down with your core body weight.
- This pressure is supplemented by pressure from your left brace hand.
- It is important to slowly sink into the client's tissues and to apply the pressure as close as possible perpendicular to the contour of the client's body that you are working.
- Shift your weight from your left (rear) foot onto your right (front) foot, translating this motion into a deep stroke along the client's abductor musculature between the iliac crest and the greater trochanter of the femur, from proximal to distal (superior to inferior), for a length of approximately 1 to 6 inches (Fig. 4-35A).
- The movement for the stroke should originate from your lower extremities and core.

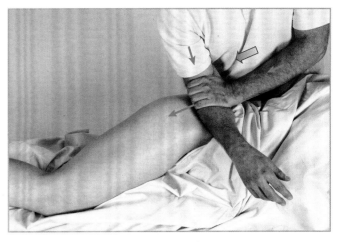

Figure 4-35A

Further Repetitions:
- Repeat this stroke in the same location another two to three times.
- Now move to the anterolateral pelvis and perform approximately three to four deep strokes in a similar manner here (Fig. 4-35B).
- Now move to the posterolateral pelvis and perform approximately three to four deep strokes in a similar manner here (Fig. 4-35C).
- Beginning back at the middle of the lateral pelvis just distal/inferior to the iliac crest again, repeat this entire protocol, this time increasing the depth of pressure.

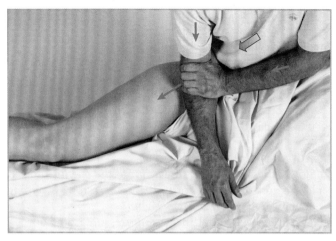

Figure 4-35B

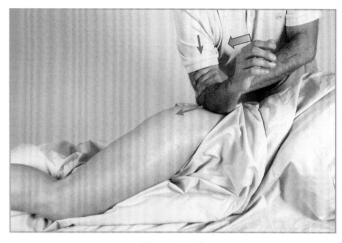

Figure 4-35C

4.7 PRACTICAL APPLICATION

The Iliotibial Band

When working the abductor musculature of the lateral pelvis with the client side-lying, it is an excellent opportunity to continue working distally onto the iliotibial band in the lateral thigh (**Fig. A**). Given the fascial continuity of these regions (the iliotibial band can be looked at as the distal tendinous attachments of the tensor fasciae latae and the gluteus maximus), it is wise to work these regions together. If desired, these regions can also be worked on stretch with the client's thigh adducted off the side of the table (**Fig. B**).

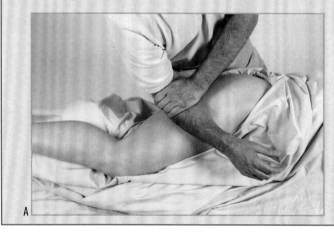

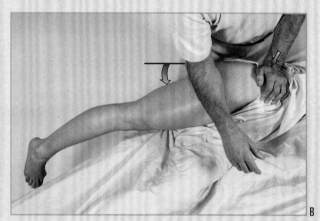

CHAPTER SUMMARY

This chapter has presented the body mechanics for performing deep tissue work into the musculature of the client's low back and pelvis with the least effort possible. When deep work is indicated, proper body mechanics not only facilitate effective work for the client but also accomplish it with less physical stress on the therapist's body. Working deep is a matter of positioning the core of the body in line with the force of the stroke. With the treatment contact braced, the elbow positioned in front of the body, and the upper extremity joints stacked, dropping down with core body weight and/or pushing off with the lower extremities translates pressure through the contact and into the client. In effect, the therapist can work smart instead of working hard.

CASE STUDY

DAN

■ **History and Physical Assessment**

A new client, Dan Canaan, age 53 years, comes to your office complaining of right buttock pain, with occasional tingling into his right thigh. He tells you that he has had nearly constant dull pain in his right buttock for a number of weeks, with no improvement. The thigh tingling is sporadic, occurring approximately once or twice a day, also with no signs of improvement.

You perform a thorough client history. During the history, Dan reports that the pain began shortly after a swing dance competition in which he forcefully threw his right leg out during a dance sequence. At the end of the motion, he felt an immediate twinge of pain in the right buttock. He reports that his discomfort is centered in the middle and lower buttock on the right side. When the tingling occurs, it is located in the posterior thigh, traveling as far as the midthigh (halfway down toward the knee). Dan describes the pain as a fairly constant 3 on a scale of 0 to 10. He cannot discern any postures or motions that aggravate the problem; it is a constant low-grade discomfort/pain. He does not notice any limitation of motion of his low back or lower extremity.

Dan has a history of a lumbar disc problem with left lower extremity referral of pain due to a herniated disc at the L4-L5 level diagnosed on magnetic resonance imaging (MRI) examination approximately 5 years before. After the lumbar disc diagnosis, Dan began a program of Pilates to strengthen his core and has not had a reoccurrence of that problem since. He is an office manager and works at a computer for much of the day. He is also an avid golfer and reports no pain or discomfort when golfing.

Dan first went to an orthopedist who performed a short physical examination and diagnosed Dan's problem as an exacerbation of the disc condition and recommended a cortisone shot. Because Dan has heard that cortisone can have unhealthy side effects, he has come to you to see if you can help him first.

Your assessment shows no range of motion restrictions of his low back or of his thighs at the hip joints. Both active and passive straight leg raise tests and slump test are negative, as are Valsalva maneuver and cough test. Nachlas', Yeoman's, and the medley of sacroiliac joint tests are also negative.

Upon palpatory examination, you find mild tightness in his lumbar paraspinal musculature as well as his superomedial gluteus maximus and his upper gluteus medius bilaterally. The piriformis on the right side is moderately tight, with a TrP present near the greater trochanter attachment. However, pressure upon it does not elicit referral of pain beyond the local area. As you palpate more inferiorly, you find a marked TrP in his right quadratus femoris muscle, immediately lateral to the ischial tuberosity. Pressure to this TrP does result in mild tingling into his proximal posterior thigh. Further, Dan reports that the locations of these two TrPs are where he has been experiencing the pain and discomfort. Due to the presence of the tight piriformis and quadratus femoris, you decide to perform a stretch assessment to the deep lateral rotator musculature (i.e., the piriformis and quadratus femoris). This stretch shows a restriction on the right side, with slight tingling into his proximal right thigh.

■ **Think-It-Through Questions:**

1. Should deep tissue massage be included in your treatment plan for Dan? If so, why? If not, why not?
2. If deep tissue massage would be of value, is it safe to use with him? If yes, how do you know?
3. If deep tissue massage is done, which specific muscles or muscle groups should be worked? Why did you choose the ones you did?

Answers to these Think-It-Through Questions and the Treatment Strategy employed for this client are available online at thePoint.lww.com/MuscolinoLowBack

Massaging the Anterior Abdomen and Pelvis

OBJECTIVES

After completing this chapter, the student should be able to:

1. Explain why assessing and massaging the anterior abdomen is important.
2. Describe in steps an overview of the usual protocol for massaging the anterior abdomen.
3. Describe the usual breathing protocol for the client when massaging the abdomen.
4. State the positions in which the client can be placed when working the abdominal wall.
5. Explain why massaging the anterior abdomen must be performed with caution.
6. Describe the specific caution and contraindication sites of the abdomen and proximal thigh.
7. Explain why placing a roll under the client's knees is beneficial when working into the anterior abdominal wall.
8. Explain how the lateral border of the rectus abdominis can be used as a landmark for locating other muscles of the abdomen.
9. Define each key term in this chapter and explain its relationship to abdominal massage.
10. Perform massage to the abdomen for each of the muscles presented in this chapter.

KEY TERMS

abdomen	**appendix**	**pin and stretch**
abdominal aorta	**femoral neurovascular bundle**	**visceral bodywork**

INTRODUCTION

The **abdomen** is the region of the lower trunk that is inferior to the thorax (which contains the thoracic vertebrae and rib cage) and superior to the pelvis. The lumbar spine is located within the abdomen. The abdomen encircles the entire trunk anteriorly, laterally on each side, and posteriorly. What is often referred to as the *abdomen* in lay terms is actually the anterior abdomen. The anterior wall of the abdomen is composed of four muscles on each side: the rectus abdominis (RA), external abdominal oblique, internal abdominal oblique, and the transversus abdominis (TA). Even though the psoas major is accessed through the anterior abdominal

wall, it sits against the spine and next to the quadratus lumborum and is actually a muscle of the posterior abdominal wall. The diaphragm is also accessed through the anterior abdominal wall but is a muscular partition between the thoracic and abdominopelvic cavities.

Massage to the anterior abdomen merits a separate chapter in this book because many massage therapists do not feel comfortable working therapeutically in this region. The musculature of the posterior trunk, primarily composed of the paraspinal musculature, receives most of the attention, whereas working into the anterior abdominal wall is often glossed over at best. Three reasons may explain this. First, the anterior abdominal wall muscles are not thick layers of musculature like the posterior trunk musculature. Second, the muscles of the anterior abdominal wall are less used posturally to support the trunk than are the posterior trunk muscles, and therefore do not become symptomatic as often. Third, the abdomen has a number of sensitive and fragile

---

Note: In the Technique and Self-Care chapters of this book (Chapters 4 to 12), green arrows indicate movement, red arrows indicate stabilization, and black arrows indicate a position that is statically held.

structures that may cause the therapist to fear venturing into this region. When work is done here, it is often incomplete or so light as to not be therapeutic; this is especially true if the therapist is attempting to access the belly of the psoas major.

Although the anterior abdominal wall musculature will rarely necessitate the depth of pressure used when treating the posterior trunk, it is important to apply enough pressure to properly engage the tissues and work therapeutically. If the psoas major abdominal belly is the target muscle being worked, deep pressure is needed because the muscle is located so deep from the anterior perspective.

This tendency to undertreat the abdomen from the anterior perspective is unfortunate because work in this region is often indicated and needed. This is especially true of the psoas major, a muscle that is crucially important to spinal health. Further, the recent emphasis on core stabilization exercise

has increased the incidence of anterior abdominal wall tightness because of the posture in which the trunk is held when doing core strengthening exercises. For this reason, this book dedicates an entire chapter to treatment options for working into the abdomen and pelvis from the anterior perspective.

BOX 5.1

Abdominal Massage Routines

The following abdominal massage routines are presented in this chapter:

- Routine 5-1—RA
- Routine 5-2—anterolateral abdominal wall (abdominal obliques and TA)
- Routine 5-3—psoas major proximal (abdominal) belly
- Routine 5-4—iliacus proximal (pelvic) belly
- Routine 5-5—iliopsoas distal (femoral) belly/tendon
- Routine 5-6—diaphragm

5.1 THERAPIST TIP

Communication with Client

It is important to pay extra attention to communicating with the client when working the anterior abdominal region. On a physical level, it can be very sensitive. On an emotional level, clients often hold a lot of emotional tension in this region, especially the psoas major. The anterior abdominal area may also have special vulnerability for clients who have gastrointestinal problems. For male and female clients, draping the lower abdomen must be done with modesty given the proximity to the genitalia. For female clients, special attention to modesty must be paid when draping so that the upper abdomen can be exposed while also keeping the breasts covered. Before beginning anterior abdominal work, explain what you will be doing and remind the client to let you know if he or she feels uncomfortable and wants you to discontinue the treatment. Then, begin the work slowly and carefully, checking in every few minutes to make sure the client is comfortable.

BOX 5.2

Strengthening the Anterior Abdominal Wall

Strengthening the anterior abdominal wall is extremely important for a number of reasons. The anterior abdominal wall musculature creates a force of posterior tilt of the pelvis, which is important to prevent the tendency toward excessive anterior tilt due to tight low back extensor and hip flexor muscles. A strong anterior abdominal wall is also a part of core stabilization, increasingly understood to be important both to protect the health of the spine and also to increase the strength of the musculature across the hip joint. When exercises are done to strengthen the anterior abdominal wall, there is a tendency for the strengthened muscles to become tighter. For this reason, strengthening exercises should always be accompanied by stretching exercises. It is important to pay special attention to assessing the anterior abdominal wall and psoas major musculature in clients who do core stabilization (e.g., Pilates) work.

OVERVIEW OF TECHNIQUE

Working the anterior abdomen is not difficult if you are comfortable with locating the muscles that you will be working and if you are aware of the precautions that are necessary as a result of the structures located nearby. The best assurance that your work will be safe and effective is for you to become as familiar as possible with the anatomy of the region. Therefore, before treating the anterior abdomen, it is recommended that you review the anatomy of the region, presented in Chapter 1.

As a quick review for the technique descriptions that follow, the muscles of the abdomen and pelvis that can be worked from the anterior perspective can be divided into the following six muscle/muscle group protocols:

1. Anteromedial abdominal wall (RA)
2. Anterolateral abdominal wall (abdominal obliques and TA)
3. Psoas major proximal (abdominal) belly
4. Iliacus proximal (pelvic) belly
5. Iliopsoas distal (femoral) belly/tendon
6. Diaphragm

The three steps involved in each of the routines for abdominal massage in this chapter are (1) starting position,

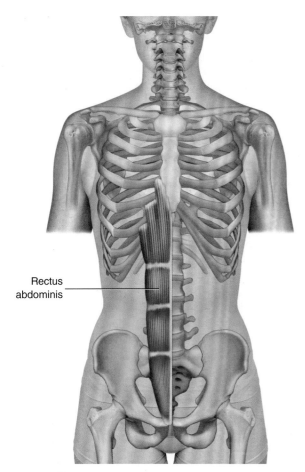

Rectus
abdominis

Figure 5-1 Anterior view of the right RA.

Place a Roll under the Client's Knees

The routines in this chapter demonstrate work into the anterior abdomen with a roll (bolster) under the client's knees. Placing a roll under the knees allows the hip joints to be placed in passive flexion, slackening the hip flexor musculature and allowing the pelvis to relax into posterior tilt. Because the RA and abdominal obliques are posterior tilters of the pelvis, this allows the anterior abdominal wall to relax and slacken, allowing better access into the anterior abdominal wall itself as well as the deeper psoas major, iliacus, and diaphragm. For this reason, whenever working into the anterior abdomen, it is a good idea to place a roll under the client's knees (see accompanying figure). As a rule, the larger the roll, the more the anterior abdominal wall will be slackened and relaxed.

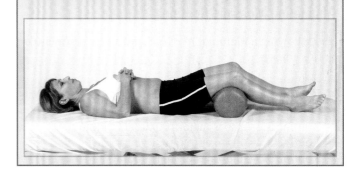

(2) locate target musculature, and (3) perform technique. The following is an overview of anterior abdominal massage presented using the right anteromedial abdominal wall (RA) as the target muscle being worked (Fig. 5-1).

Starting Position:
■ The client is supine with a roll under the knees.
■ You are standing at the right side of the table (Fig. 5-2).

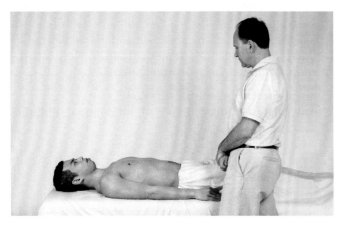

Figure 5-2 Starting position.

Step 1: Locate Target Musculature:
■ To locate the right RA, ask the client to do a small range-of-motion curl-up exercise, being sure to perform this motion entirely from the trunk (not the hip joints), by flexing the spinal column. The RA will contract.
■ If the client is thin and in good shape, the RA will become visible; look for the characteristic boxes of the muscle. If the RA is not visible, feel for its contraction and palpate the muscle from the rib cage to the pubic bone and from the midline of the body to the RA's lateral border (Fig. 5-3).

Step 2: Perform Technique:
■ Now that the right RA has been located, have the client relax and rest on the table.
■ Your right hand is the treatment hand that will work the RA; place your finger pads on the right RA.
■ Your left hand is the brace hand that supports the left hand.
■ Massage the right RA. Depending on the musculature being worked, the type of stroke employed can vary.

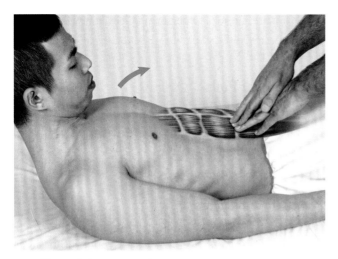

Figure 5-3 Locating the target musculature: the RA.

- An effective method for working the RA is to perform longitudinal strokes from superior to inferior, followed by cross-fiber strokes (Fig. 5-4). When performing cross-fiber strokes, either hand can be used as the treatment/contact hand and the brace hand.

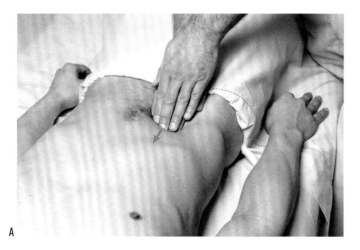

A

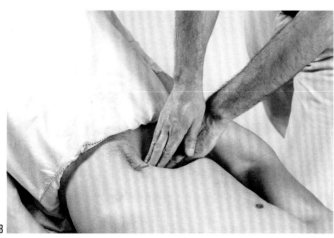

B

Figure 5-4 Performing the technique. **(A)** Longitudinal strokes on the right RA with finger pad contact. **(B)** Cross-fiber strokes across the right RA.

5.2   PRACTICAL APPLICATION

Palpate with the Ulnar Side of the Hand

When palpating toward the pubic bone attachment of the RA, it is important to not overshoot and contact the client's genitalia. Because of this fear, many therapists avoid working the lower portion of the RA. This is unfortunate because it is important to work the entire muscle. An effective method to palpate and safely find the pubic bone attachment of the RA is to use the ulnar side of the hand. Start superiorly on the muscle and gradually make your way inferiorly, pressing with your hand at approximately a 45-degree angle inferiorly and posteriorly (see accompanying figure).

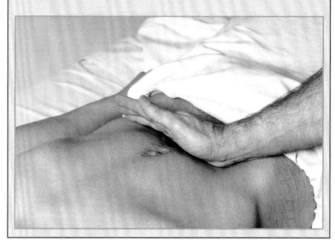

- Work the muscle from the rib cage attachment to the pubic bone attachment.
- *Note*: An open fist contact is also very effective when working the RA (Fig. 5-5).

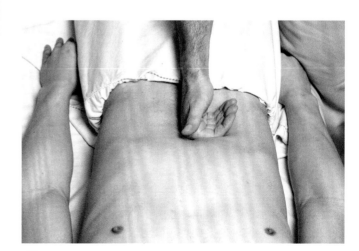

Figure 5-5 An alternate contact to work the RA is the open fist.

PERFORMING THE TECHNIQUE

When working the anterior abdomen, it is important to keep in mind at all times the guidelines that follow. Each point addresses a specific aspect of working this region. Understanding and applying these guidelines will aid in safely and effectively treating the anterior abdomen.

5.1 Lateral Border of Rectus Abdominis as Landmark

It is important that the precise borders of the target muscle being massaged are located. This requires excellent palpatory assessment skills. Although this chapter outlines the specific palpation protocol for each muscle routine, it is worth noting that locating the lateral border of the RA is especially important because it can be used as a landmark for locating and working the muscles of the anterolateral abdominal wall (the external and internal abdominal obliques and TA) and the psoas major muscle (Fig. 5-6).

5.2 Gradually Increase the Pressure

Because the anterior abdominal wall can be very sensitive, it is important to warm up the region before using any appre-

ciable pressure. Be sure to perform at least a few strokes longitudinally as well as cross fiber with gentle pressure before increasing the pressure.

5.3 Use Finger Pads

Finger pads are an excellent treatment contact for the anterior abdomen because they are extremely sensitive. As a rule, the pads of the index, middle, and ring fingers should be used (Fig. 5-7).

5.4 Direction and Number of Strokes

Strokes may be applied longitudinally along the length of the fibers and/or transversely across the direction of the fibers, as there is no one correct or required direction to the strokes used for the muscles of the abdomen. Longitudinal strokes tend to work better when working myofascial trigger points, whereas transverse strokes tend to work better for breaking up fascial adhesions. Mixing the two is recommended. However, it is always best to let the client's needs determine what type of strokes you apply.

The number of strokes applied to the target muscle typically ranges from 3 to 10. As with direction of stroke, it is best to determine the number of strokes based on the client's specific needs.

5.5 Breathing Protocol

There is no single breathing protocol that must be used when working the anterior abdomen. Typically, because the abdomen usually rises when breathing in, it is best to access the region when the client is breathing out and the belly falls. However, because strong exhalation would engage the abdominal wall musculature, it is important to have the client breathe in a quiet and relaxed manner. Because the anterior abdomen is a sensitive region, it can be helpful to

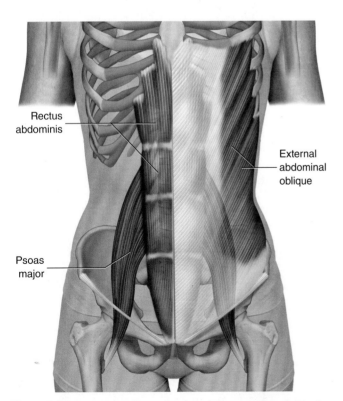

Figure 5-6 The RA muscle as a landmark (anterior view). The lateral border of the RA can be used as a landmark for locating other muscles of the region. The anterolateral abdominal wall muscles (abdominal obliques and TA) are directly lateral to the RA, and accessing the psoas major is best accomplished by sinking into the client's abdomen directly lateral to the lateral border of the RA.

Rectus
abdominis

External
abdominal
oblique

Psoas
major

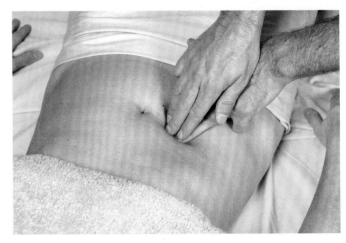

Figure 5-7 Treatment hand contact. Finger pads of the index, middle, and ring fingers provide a sensitive and effective contact for the treatment hand.

have the client focus on the breathing by asking him or her to first inhale, and then exhale as you slowly sink into and work the tissues. This protocol helps the client relax so that he or she allows you to more effectively sink into the musculature of the region. When working the psoas major, because the muscle is so deep, instead of trying to access the muscle on the first exhalation, sink in only part of the way. Now ask the client to take in another breath and sink in farther on the second exhalation. Depending on how relaxed or tight the client is, the psoas major can usually be accessed and worked on the second or third exhalation.

5.6 Proper Draping

Because the musculature of the anterior abdominal wall attaches inferiorly all the way to the pubic bone, proper draping that not only allows full access to the musculature but also preserves the client's modesty is important (Fig. 5-8). A general rule of soft tissue manipulation is that tissue being worked should be visible to the therapist. For the health and safety of the client and therapist, the therapist's hands should not work tissue that is covered and out of sight. Because this requires the draping to be pulled quite low, it is a good idea to first explain to the client what you will be doing and obtain verbal consent before continuing.

Because abdominal wall musculature attaches superiorly all the way onto the rib cage, visual access of abdominal wall

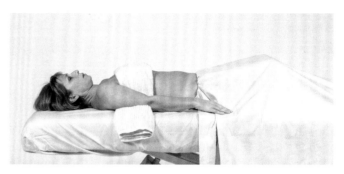

Figure 5-8 Draping for anterior abdominal wall work. It is important to allow full access to musculature being worked while preserving client modesty.

musculature that also preserves client modesty regarding breast tissue must also be considered for the female client. An effective draping method for the breasts is to use a large bath-sized towel that is folded and laid across the client (see Fig. 5-8). Place the towel over the sheet and then carefully remove the sheet from under the towel while making sure that the towel remains securely in place. For extra security, the client can place her arms over the towel at the sides of her body as seen in Figure 5-8. As with draping inferiorly, it is a good idea to explain to the client in advance what you will be doing and first obtain verbal consent.

5.2	THERAPIST TIP

Proper Body Mechanics

The musculature of the anterior abdominal wall rarely requires very deep pressure, so proper body mechanics are not as critically important here as they are elsewhere in the body. However, given the depth of the psoas major, deep pressure is usually required to reach and work effectively this muscle. Regardless of the depth of work, it is optimal to maintain proper body mechanics because they increase the efficiency of your work, decrease the risk of physical stress and injury to your body, and reinforce good habits. Remember to position the core of your body behind and in line with your stroke, checking your alignment by visually drawing a line straight out from your belly button and comparing it with the line of your stroke that travels through your forearm (see accompanying figure). For more detail on using your core and employing proper body mechanics, see Chapter 4.

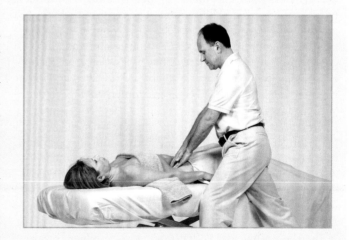

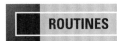

ROUTINES

ABDOMINAL MASSAGE ROUTINES

The routines that follow demonstrate soft tissue massage to the musculature of the abdomen. We begin with the RA; we then use the RA as a landmark to locate and work first the external and internal abdominal obliques and the TA muscle in the anterolateral abdomen. We then demonstrate how to work the proximal (abdominal) belly of the psoas major, the proximal (pelvic) belly of the iliacus, and then the distal common belly/tendon of the iliopsoas in the proximal thigh. The last routine that is demonstrated is working the diaphragm. In each case, massage of the right side is shown. To massage the left-sided musculature, stand to the left side of the table and reverse the treatment and support hands. Individual illustrations and precise attachment and action information for these muscles are given in Chapter 1.

ROUTINE 5-1: RECTUS ABDOMINIS

The RA attaches from the pubic bone inferiorly to the rib cage superiorly. Massage to the right RA was shown in the "Overview of Technique" section at the beginning of this chapter (see Figs. 5-1 through 5-5). For the left RA, work instead from the left side of the table and reverse treatment and support hands.

5.3   **PRACTICAL APPLICATION**

The Effects of Pregnancy on Anterior Abdominal Wall Muscles

As the gravid uterus grows, it moves from a position within the pelvic cavity into the abdominal cavity. At 38 weeks' gestation, the fundus, or the top of the uterus, is inferior to the xiphoid process, inhibiting diaphragm function. To accommodate this growth, the abdominal muscles stretch, often weakening, losing tone, and separating. This separation, called *diastasis recti*, is also encouraged by the release of the hormone relaxin, which softens all the connective tissue in the expectant mother's body to allow for fetal growth and to widen her pelvis for childbirth (**Fig. A**). Since the linea alba is a sheath of connective tissue that separates the right- and left-sided rectus muscles, it also loses its tensile ability and stretches, and trigger points are often created at the attachments of the rectus.

Consequently, this muscular adaptation of pregnancy often leads to lumbar instability, muscle pain and weakness, longer labors, and possibly hernias during postpartum recovery. The loss of abdominal structural integrity also contributes to an exaggerated anterior pelvic tilt, which adds to the lumbar compression and lower back tightness of pregnancy. Massage, although relaxing and soothing, cannot correct the diastasis recti or the structural weakness of the abdominal core. What does help to reduce the size of the diastasis (measured by the number of fingers that fit

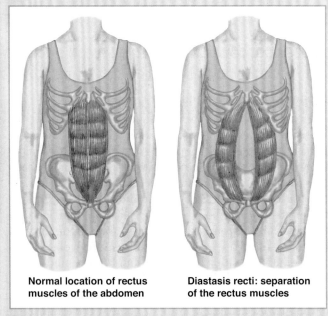

Normal location of rectus muscles of the abdomen

Diastasis recti: separation of the rectus muscles

Figure A   (Reprinted with permission from McKinney ES, James SR, Murray SS, et al. Maternal-Child Nursing. 3rd ed. St. Louis, MO: Mosby; 2009.)

continued

into the space between the sides of the rectus and the depth of the connected tissue) are Tupler Technique exercises that target the deepest abdominal muscle, the TA.

The TA is known as the "girdle" of the body. During pregnancy, a strong TA can support the heavy uterus, minimize the diastasis recti, stabilize the lower spine, reduce back pain, and facilitate labor. Weakness in the TA results in a protruding abdominal wall, a more pronounced separation of the recti, lower back instability and pain, and muscular imbalance. Examining the common attachments of the overlying abdominal muscles (obliques and rectus), it can be seen that contracting the TA pulls the linea alba inward, thereby making the diastasis smaller. Any exercise that puts forward pressure on the weakened connective tissue (i.e., crunches, leg lifts) or that rotates the torso should be avoided until long after the diastasis is healed, if they are done at all.

Manual Therapy Techniques:
The abdominal massage that is provided during pregnancy (after client permission) should be light, slow and rhythmical, clockwise, and an effleurage stroke performed with open hands. Care must be taken to avoid further lateral pulling on the linea alba. In late pregnancy, however, as preparation for birth, techniques that release myofascial restrictions in the abdominal area can be provided. Starting toward the end of the second trimester, myofascial stretching helps maintain pelvic and fascial fluidity and suppleness for the months that follow.

Care must be taken to keep the direction of the stretch horizontal (elongating) but lateral to the uterus—never on it. A pregnant woman's rib cage expands 2 to 3 inches anteriorly and laterally, allowing the baby to grow. However, this expansion can create myofascial restrictions and intercostal tightness. These restrictions can be relieved with gentle finger pad myofascial release and appropriate stretching. This also facilitates diaphragm function and allows the pregnant client to breathe deeper.

Postural shifting in later pregnancy creates hyperextension, causing stretching of most of the muscles in the front of the body, and tightness and compression in muscles of the posterior body. This also includes stretching to the iliopsoas. If the abdominal muscles are weakened, as in pregnancy and diastasis recti, your client may experience lower back instability and pain when walking or lifting her

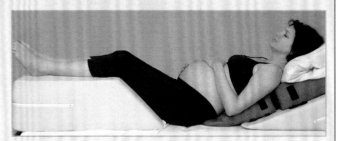

Figure B (Reprinted with permission from Stillerman E. Prenatal Massage: A Textbook of Pregnancy, Labor, and Postpartum Bodywork. St. Louis, MO: Mosby; 2008.)

legs because these motions require contraction of the hip flexors (i.e., iliopsoas).

During pregnancy, psoas balancing can be performed through several noninvasive techniques. For instance, client-initiated posterior pelvic tilts shorten the overstretched iliopsoas. This can also be performed by the massage therapist with the client in a side-lying position: one hand softly covers the client's sacrum, and the other hand cups her anterior superior iliac spine (ASIS). The movement is a gentle stretch with the sacral hand pulling toward the client's feet and the ASIS hand pulling in a posterior direction. Hold the stretch for several seconds and release slowly.

Positional release shortens the iliopsoas: the client is supine with her hip and knee joints bent, she is supported by bolsters or pillows under her lower extremities and trunk so she is not lying flat on her back, and her cervical spine is supported (**Fig. B**). She remains in this position for 15 to 20 minutes.

Rocking in a chair also helps to balance the iliopsoas by affecting proprioception. Another noninvasive technique to balance the iliopsoas comes from Zero Balancing (it is also a part of Native American prenatal care.) Lift the supine client's lower extremity and place the foot on your clavicle. Support her lower extremity under her knee to prevent knee joint hyperextension. Your other hand grabs slightly above her same-side wrist. Following the client's breath, push inward on her foot with your shoulder and pull her upper extremity toward you as she exhales; release on the inhalation. Repeat this for a total of three times before changing sides. This movement, like rocking, affects the proprioceptors and releases the muscle.

Elaine Stillerman, LMT

ROUTINE 5-2: ANTEROLATERAL ABDOMINAL WALL (ABDOMINAL OBLIQUES AND TRANSVERSUS ABDOMINIS)

The three muscles of the anterolateral abdominal wall on each side are the external abdominal oblique, internal abdominal oblique, and the TA. Even though these muscles are thought of as being anterior, as a group, they attach via the thoracolumbar fascia all the way into the transverse processes of the lumbar spine (see Fig. 1-16B). Superiorly, they attach as far as the 5th rib; inferiorly, they attach onto the pubic bone (Fig. 5-9).

Starting Position:
- The client is supine.
- You are standing at the right side of the table, facing diagonally toward the foot end of the table (Fig. 5-10).
- Your right hand is the treatment hand that contacts the client.
- Your left hand is the support hand that braces the contact hand.
- *Note*: The treatment and support hands can be reversed.

Step 1: Locate Target Musculature:
- The anterolateral abdominal muscles are located by using the RA as a landmark.
- Begin by locating the RA as explained in the "Overview of Technique" section (see Figs. 5-1 through 5-5), then find the lateral border of the RA (Fig. 5-11).
- Now drop immediately off the lateral border of the RA (laterally) and you will be on the anterolateral abdominal wall muscles (see Fig. 5-11).

Step 2: Performing the Technique:
- It is important to use the flat surface of the finger pads and not the fingertips, which could be uncomfortable for the client.
- Apply mild to moderate pressure, starting over the lateral rib cage and running inferiorly and medially toward the RA along the length of the fibers of the external abdominal oblique from superolateral to inferomedial (Fig. 5-12A).

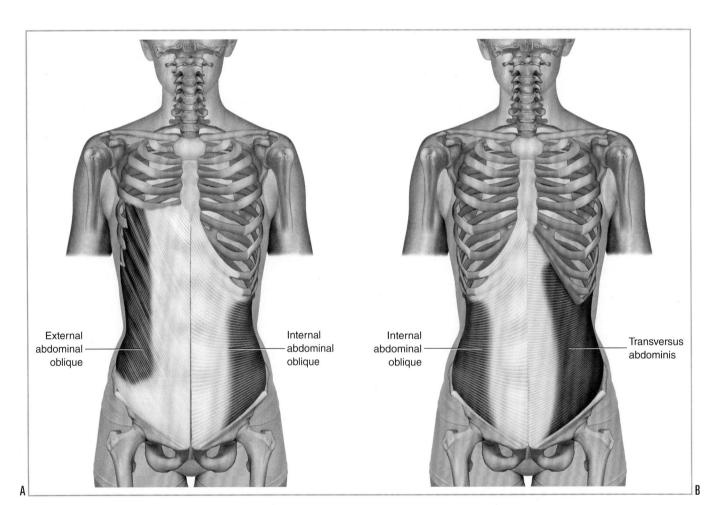

Figure 5-9 Anterior view of the muscles of the anterolateral abdominal wall. **(A)** Superficial view. The external abdominal oblique is shown on the client's right side. The internal abdominal oblique is shown on the client's left side. **(B)** Deeper view. The internal abdominal oblique is shown on the client's right side. The TA is shown on the client's left side.

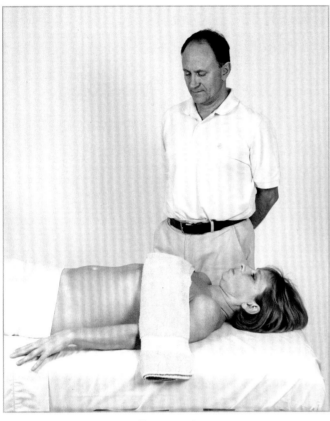

Figure 5-10

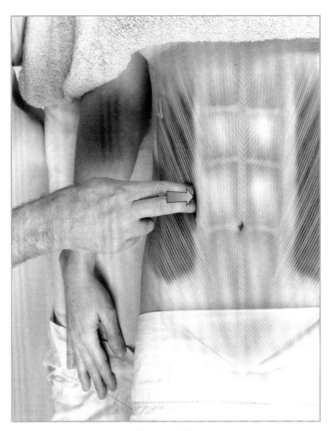

Figure 5-11

Note: Strokes begin over the rib cage wall because the external abdominal oblique attaches as far superiorly as the 5th rib.

■ Repeat this stroke starting slightly more inferiorly each time until the entire width of the anterolateral abdominal wall and lower rib cage has been covered.

■ These strokes work longitudinally along the external abdominal oblique and cross fiber over the internal abdominal oblique (and diagonally across the TA).

■ Now change your orientation to face diagonally toward the head end of the table and work in the opposite direction, from inferolateral to superomedial (Fig. 5-12B).

■ Repeat this stroke until the entire width of the anterolateral abdominal wall and lower rib cage has been covered.

■ These strokes work longitudinally along the internal abdominal oblique and cross fiber over the external abdominal oblique (and diagonally across the TA).

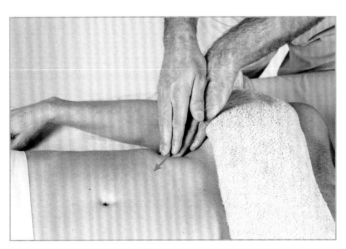

Figure 5-12A

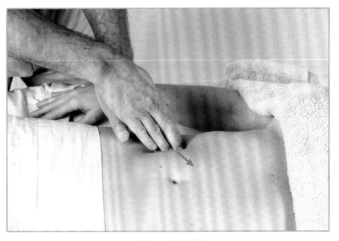

Figure 5-12B

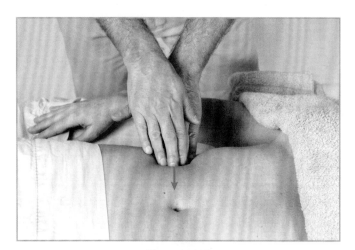

Figure 5-12C

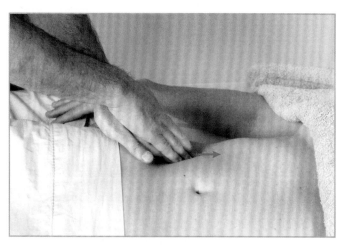

Figure 5-12D

- Now change your orientation to face across the table and work transversely across the anterolateral abdominal wall from lateral to medial (until you reach the lateral border of the RA) (Fig. 5-12C).
- Repeat this stroke until the entire width of the anterolateral abdominal wall has been covered.
- These strokes work longitudinally along the TA (and diagonally across the abdominal obliques).
- Now change your orientation to face toward the head end of the table and work from inferior to superior (until the rib cage is reached) (Fig. 5-12D).

- Repeat this stroke until the entire width of the anterolateral abdominal wall has been covered.
- These strokes work cross fiber over the TA (and diagonally across the abdominal obliques).
- *Note*: It is important to work the entire abdominal wall, including the inguinal ligament at the junction with the thigh. The inguinal ligament is actually a thickening and folding of the fibrous aponeuroses of the abdominal obliques. However, if work is done distal to the inguinal ligament, caution should be used to avoid compressing the femoral artery, vein, and nerve (see Femoral Neurovascular Bundle Precaution on page 154).

5.3 THERAPIST TIP

Digestive Flow

The strokes described in Routine 5-2 for the anterolateral abdominal wall are designed to work longitudinally along and cross fiber across each of the individual muscles of the anterolateral abdominal wall. However, an excellent protocol for the anterior abdominal wall, especially if moderate or deeper pressure is employed, is to work in the physiologic direction of the bowel (colon/large intestine). Bowel flow travels from the lower right abdomen up the right side of the abdomen in the ascending colon, across the upper abdomen in the transverse colon, and then down the left side of the abdomen in the descending colon **(Fig. A)**. Pressure along the bowel and in the direction of the flow may aid in

movement of the bowel contents. This is usually done in three distinct strokes. Begin by working down the descending colon on the client's left side with superior to inferior, vertically oriented strokes. Now work across the transverse colon from right to left. And then finish by working up the ascending colon on the client's right side with inferior to superior, vertically oriented strokes **(Fig. B)**. This order is followed to first clear the descending colon before promoting movement of contents into it from the transverse colon, and the transverse colon is cleared before moving contents into from the ascending colon. In other words, work and clear distally before working proximally.

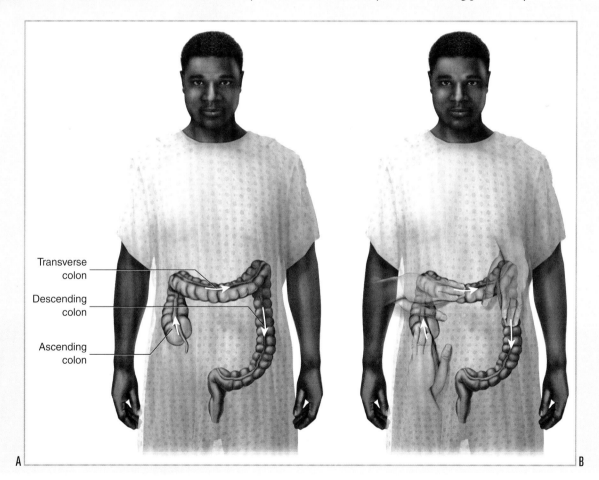

Transverse colon

Descending colon

Ascending colon

A   B

| 5.4 | **PRACTICAL APPLICATION** |

Side-Lying Position

Routine 5-2 describes the abdominal obliques and TA muscles as anterolateral. The term anterolateral is used to emphasize that these muscles are located lateral to the RA, which is located anteromedially. However, this term can be misleading because the obliques and TA are not confined to the anterolateral abdomen; they are also located in the lateral abdominal wall and the posterolateral abdominal wall. Indeed, the internal abdominal oblique and the TA attach all the way posteriorly into the transverse processes of the lumbar spine via their attachment into the thoracolumbar fascia; therefore, their posterior fibers could be considered to be low back musculature (see Figs. 1-26 and 1-27). For this reason, side-lying posture can be an excellent posture to use when working the entirety of these muscles (see accompanying figure).

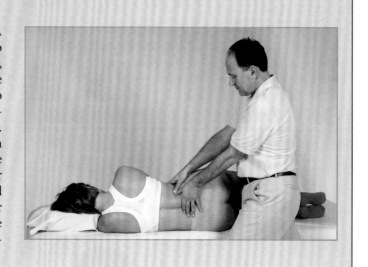

As shown in the figure at right, the **appendix** *is located in the lower abdomen on the right side, approximately halfway between the posterior superior iliac spine (PSIS) and the umbilicus. The appendix is a small extension of the cecum of the large intestine. Exercise caution to avoid working with excessively deep pressure directly on and injuring the appendix.*

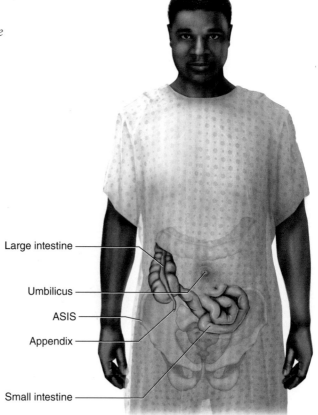

Large intestine

Umbilicus

ASIS

Appendix

Small intestine

ROUTINE 5-3: PSOAS MAJOR PROXIMAL (ABDOMINAL) BELLY

View the video "Psoas Major Abdominal Belly Palpation" online on thePoint.lww.com

The psoas major muscle is rarely assessed or worked. This is unfortunate because this muscle is functionally important as a postural stabilizer of the lumbar spine and often becomes tight due to the principle of adaptive shortening because it is a hip flexor muscle and so much time is spent seated with the hip joints flexed. The psoas major attaches proximally on the anterolateral spine from the levels of T12-L5, and distally onto the lesser trochanter of the femur (Fig. 5-13).

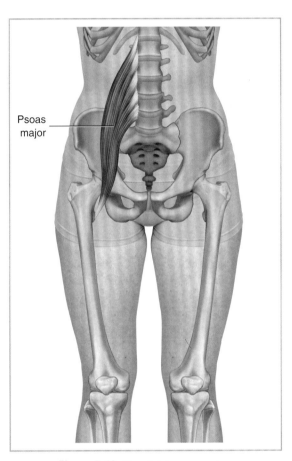

Psoas major

Figure 5-13 The right psoas major.

Starting Position:
- The client is supine with one large roll or a number of smaller rolls under the knees. This relaxes the hip flexor musculature so that the pelvis can drop into posterior tilt, relaxing and slackening the anterior abdominal wall.
- You are standing at the right side of the table (Fig. 5-14).
- The finger pads of your left hand are the treatment contact, and the finger pads of your right hand are the support that braces the left hand treatment contact. *Note*: This could be reversed; the right hand could be the treatment hand and the left hand the support (Fig. 5-15A).

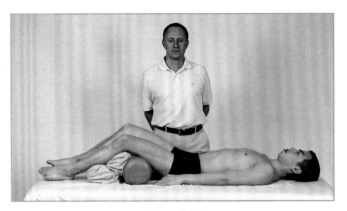

Figure 5-14

| 5.4 | **THERAPIST TIP** |

Placing a Roll under the Bottom Fitted Sheet

A roll is placed under the client's knees to flex the hip joints so the pelvis relaxes into posterior tilt, relaxing and slackening the anterior abdominal wall. If you do not have a large roll or a number of smaller rolls, then you can help the client be relaxed in a position of flexion at the hip joints by placing a roll under the bottom fitted sheet immediately distal to the client's feet. The friction against the table combined with the tension of the fitted sheet are usually sufficient to hold the roll in place, thereby holding the client's feet in position so that the hip joints remain flexed.

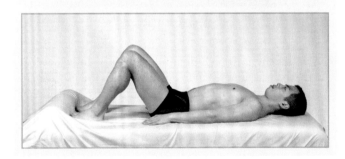

Step 1: Locate Target Musculature:
- Begin by locating the RA as explained in the "Overview of Technique" section (see Figs. 5-1 through 5-5), then find the lateral border of the RA.
- After locating the lateral border of the RA, drop immediately off it (laterally) (see Fig. 5-15A).
- To access and palpate directly on the psoas major, ask the client to take in a breath; as the client gently exhales, slowly sink in toward the spine by pressing into the anterior abdomen in a posterior and slightly medial direction (Fig. 5-15B). Do not try to reach all the way to the psoas major; it is better to take your time to arrive at the muscle.

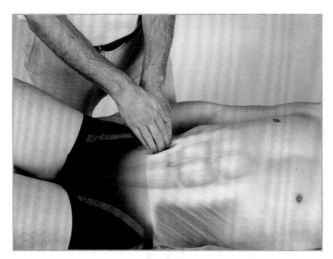

Figure 5-15A

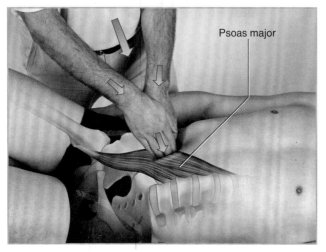

Psoas major

Figure 5-15B

- Ask the client to take in another breath, and as the client exhales again, reach in farther toward the psoas major on the anterolateral bodies and transverse processes of the spine. If necessary, repeat this process a third time to reach in all the way to the muscle. The psoas major can usually be reached on the second or third exhale. Because the psoas major is located deep against the posterior abdominal wall, is rarely worked, and the intestines are located between the therapist's fingers and the psoas major, clients are often sensitive and feel vulnerable here, so pressure should be applied very slowly and gradually.
- Because the psoas major lies directly against the spine, it is usually easy to know when it has been reached because you will feel the firmness of the anterior bodies of the spine deep to them. If you do not feel the firmness of the spine deep to the muscle, you are probably not on the psoas major.
- To confirm that you are on the psoas major, have the client try to gently flex the thigh at the hip joint against the resistance of gravity (Fig. 5-15C). This will cause the psoas major to contract, and you will feel it engage. *Note*: Be sure to ask for only a very small thigh flexion range of

motion; a large range of motion will engage the anterior abdominal wall to stabilize the pelvis from anteriorly tilting. If the anterior abdominal wall engages, it will become difficult to palpate through it to reach the psoas major.

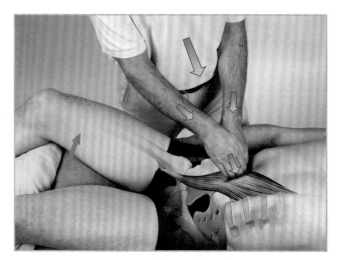

Figure 5-15C

Step 2: Perform the Technique:
- Once you are sure of your placement on the abdominal belly of the psoas major, you can work it by performing short longitudinal strokes running vertically along the musculature with mild to moderate pressure (Fig. 5-16). Strumming transversely across the musculature can also be performed. Circular strokes are also very effective.
- The psoas major attaches along the entire lumbar spine, so once one level has been worked, continue to work the musculature in a similar fashion superiorly as far as possible and then inferiorly as far as possible. As you work inferiorly, keep in mind that the psoas major gradually becomes more superficial, lying closer to the anterior abdominal wall.
- Once the muscle has been worked with mild to moderate pressure, if it is within the client's tolerance, deeper pressure can be used.

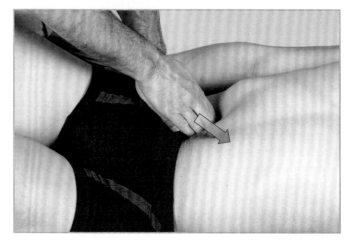

Figure 5-16

*The **abdominal aorta** is located along the midline of the body, over the anterior aspect of the bodies of the lumbar vertebrae, medial to the abdominal belly of the psoas major (see Fig. 1-45A). When sinking into the client's abdomen to assess and treat the psoas major, it is important to aim for the anterolateral aspect of the spine. If the pulse of the aorta is felt, you are too far medial and need to readjust the direction that you are sinking in to be slightly more lateral. Always feel for the pulse of the aorta before exerting deep pressure into the psoas major.*

Because pressure must be exerted through the abdominal contents to reach the psoas major, it is important to make sure that the client will be comfortable. If the client has any type of intestinal condition, has just eaten, or needs to void the bladder, working into the psoas major can be uncomfortable.

5.5 PRACTICAL APPLICATION

Alternate Positions for the Psoas Major

Working the psoas major with the client supine is probably the most common position in which this muscle is worked, perhaps because the client is so often in this position. However, side-lying and seated positions are good alternatives. The advantage of side-lying position is that if the client is overweight and has a large abdomen, it falls away from your palpating fingers, making it easier to access the psoas major. Preferable to pure side-lying position is ¾ side-lying position in which the client is approximately half-way between side-lying and supine. The advantage of this position is that the therapist can better use body weight to drop down into the psoas major (**Fig. A**). When working the psoas major with the client side-lying or ¾ side-lying, it is important to have his hip and knee joints flexed so that the anterior abdominal wall is relaxed and slackened. To confirm that you are on the psoas major, ask the client to perform a small flexion range of motion of the thigh at the hip joint.

Seated position can also be very effective for working the psoas major because it allows the client to slightly flex the trunk to relax and slacken the anterior abdominal wall. Another advantage is that the abdomen also tends to fall out of way in seated position. To confirm that you are on the psoas major, ask the client to perform a very small hip flexion range of motion by lifting the foot slightly off the floor (**Fig. B**). Regardless of the position (supine, side-lying, or seated), be sure to direct your pressure posteriorly and medially toward the anterolateral spine.

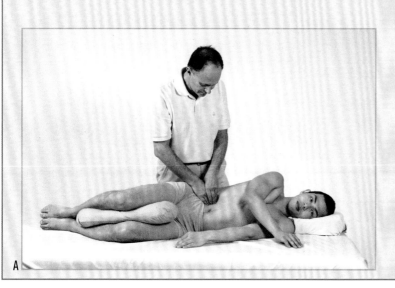
A

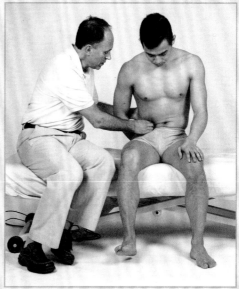
B

| 5.5 | **THERAPIST TIP** |

First Work the Anterior Abdominal Wall

Most clients do not have a tight anterior abdominal wall. However, for the occasional client who does, it is important to first work and loosen the musculature of the anterolateral abdominal wall with moist heat and soft tissue manipulation before attempting to work the psoas major. Otherwise, it will be difficult to penetrate through the abdominal wall to reach the psoas major.

ROUTINE 5-4: ILIACUS PROXIMAL (PELVIC) BELLY

Like the psoas major, the iliacus muscle is also rarely assessed and worked. This is unfortunate because like the psoas major, this muscle often becomes tight due to the principle of adaptive shortening (because it is a hip flexor muscle and so much time is spent seated with the hip joints flexed). The iliacus attaches proximally on the internal (medial) surface of the ilium and distally onto the lesser trochanter of the femur (Fig. 5-17).

Starting Position:

■ The client is supine with one large roll or a number of smaller rolls under the knees. This relaxes the hip flexor musculature so that the pelvis can drop into posterior tilt, relaxing and slackening the anterior abdominal wall.

■ You are standing at the right side of the table (Fig. 5-18).

■ The finger pads of your right hand will be the treatment contact, and the finger pads of your left hand will be the support that braces the right hand treatment contact. *Note*: This could be reversed; the left hand could be the treatment hand and the right hand the support.

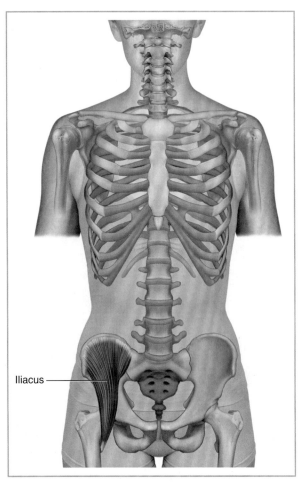

Iliacus

Figure 5-17 The right iliacus.

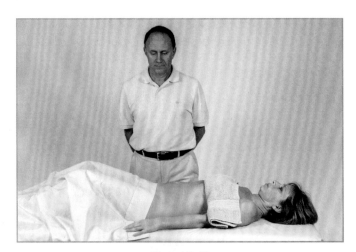

Figure 5-18

Step 1: Locate Target Musculature:

- First, find the ASIS.
- Then drop medial to the ASIS with your finger pads curled around the ilium (Fig. 5-19A).

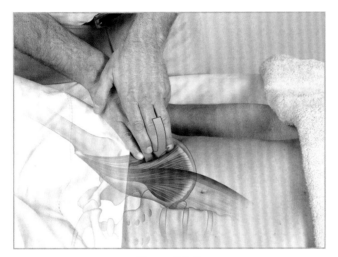

Figure 5-19A

- To access and palpate directly on the iliacus, ask the client to take in a breath; as the client gently exhales, slowly sink in by curling your finger pads toward the internal (medial) surface of the ilium (Fig. 5-19B).

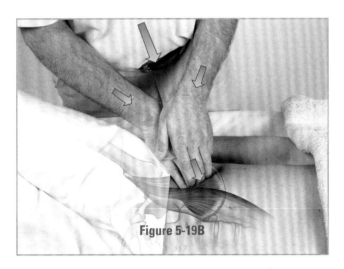

Figure 5-19B

- To confirm that you are on the iliacus, have the client try to gently flex the thigh at the hip joint against the resistance of gravity (Fig. 5-19C). This will cause the iliacus to contract and you will feel it engage. *Note:* Be sure to ask for only a very small thigh flexion range of motion; a large range of motion will engage the anterior abdominal wall to stabilize the pelvis from anteriorly tilting. If the anterior abdominal wall engages, it will become difficult to palpate through it to reach the iliacus.

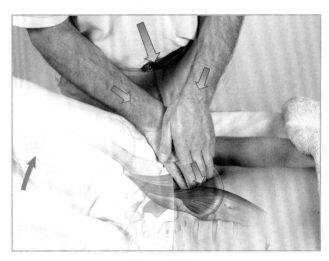

Figure 5-19C

5.6 THERAPIST TIP

Ticklish Clients

Many clients are ticklish when the abdominopelvic and thigh regions are worked. Ticklishness is often a reaction to feeling that personal space is being invaded. It can be helpful to ask the ticklish client to place a hand over your palpating/treatment hand (see figure). This gives the client the sense that he or she is in control of this space and consequently often diminishes sensitivity.

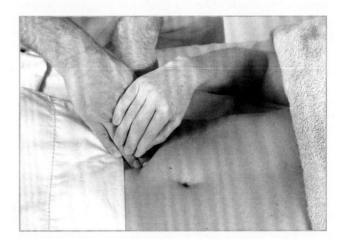

Step 2: Perform the Technique:

■ The iliacus can be worked by performing short longitudinal strokes running vertically along the musculature with moderate to deep pressure (Fig. 5-20A). Strumming transversely across the musculature can also be performed (Fig. 5-20B).

■ The iliacus attaches along the entire internal (medial) surface of the ilium. However, most of it is out of reach and cannot be accessed. Access as much of this muscle as possible by continuing to work the musculature in a similar fashion as far superiorly and inferiorly along the ilium as possible and as far medially as possible.

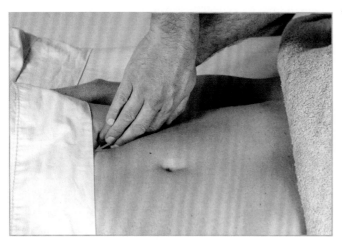

Figure 5-20A

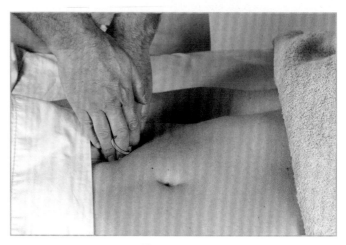

Figure 5-20B

ROUTINE 5-5: ILIOPSOAS DISTAL (FEMORAL) BELLY/TENDON

 View the video "Psoas Major Femoral Belly Palpation" online on thePoint.lww.com

The psoas major and iliacus are separate muscles proximally in the abdominopelvic cavity. However, when they pass deep to the inguinal ligament to enter the thigh, their distal bellies gradually blend into one another, and they attach together and form one common tendon that attaches onto the lesser trochanter of the femur. For this reason, they are often grouped together as one muscle, the iliopsoas (Fig. 5-21).

The iliopsoas is the major flexor of the thigh at the hip joint. Because of the amount of time spent seated with the thighs flexed, the iliopsoas is shortened and often tightens up due to the principle of adaptive shortening. It is generally wise to work a muscle in its entirety from attachment to attachment. Therefore, if the proximal bellies of the iliopsoas (psoas major and iliacus) are worked, the distal belly/tendon in the proximal thigh should also be worked. Routines 5-3 and 5-4 showed protocols for working the proximal bellies of the psoas major and iliacus in the abdominopelvic cavity. This routine shows a protocol for working the distal iliopsoas in the proximal thigh.

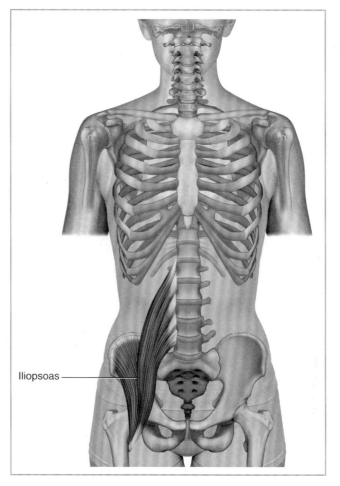

Figure 5-21 The right iliopsoas. The iliopsoas is composed of the psoas major and the iliacus.

Starting Position:

- The client is supine with one large roll or a number of smaller rolls under the knees. This relaxes the hip flexor musculature, allowing better access and deeper work into the iliopsoas.
- You are standing at the right side of the table (Fig. 5-22).
- The finger pads of your left hand will be the treatment contact, and the finger pads of your right hand will be the support that braces the left hand treatment contact. *Note*: This could be reversed; the right hand could be the treatment hand and the left hand the support.

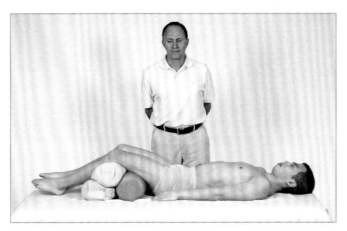

Figure 5-22

Step 1: Locate Target Musculature:

- First, find the ASIS. Then drop off it immediately distal and slightly medially; you should be on the sartorius (Fig. 5-23A).

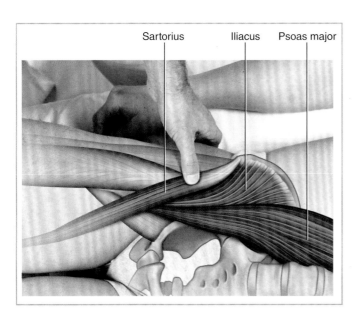

Sartorius   Iliacus   Psoas major

Figure 5-23A

- To confirm that you are on the sartorius, ask the client to laterally rotate the thigh at the hip joint and then flex it. The sartorius will engage, and its contraction can be felt (Fig. 5-23B).

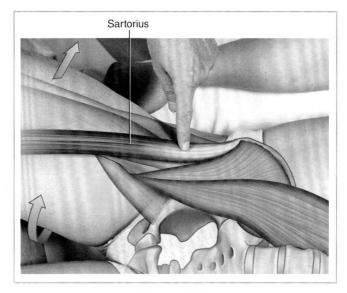

Sartorius

Figure 5-23B

- Once located, drop just off the sartorius medially onto the iliopsoas distal belly/tendon. Strum horizontally across the belly/tendon and feel for its width. The iliacus fibers are more lateral within the common belly/tendon, and the psoas major fibers are more medial (Fig. 5-23C).

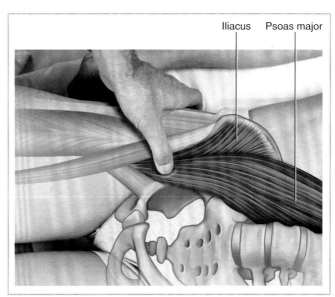

Iliacus   Psoas major

Figure 5-23C

■ You can confirm that you are on the psoas major fibers by asking the client to perform a gentle, small flexion range of motion of the trunk at the spinal joints, in other words, a curl-up. *Note*: This will engage the psoas major fibers but not the iliacus fibers (Fig. 5-23D).

Femoral Neurovascular Bundle
Caution must be exercised when working the distal belly/tendon of the iliopsoas in the proximal thigh because of the presence of the **femoral neurovascular bundle**, *composed of the femoral nerve, artery, and vein in the femoral triangle. These structures usually overlie the iliopsoas and pectineus muscles (see accompanying figure). Before applying any deep pressure in the area, feel for the pulse of the femoral artery. If a pulse is felt, either slightly move your palpating/treatment finger pads or, if possible, try to reach deep to the artery and slightly displace it medially and continue working where you are. Also, be aware that if pressure is placed on the femoral nerve, the client might experience pain, likely a shooting pain, into the anterior thigh. If this occurs, as with the artery, either slightly move your palpating/treatment finger pads or, if possible, slightly displace the nerve and continue working where you are.*

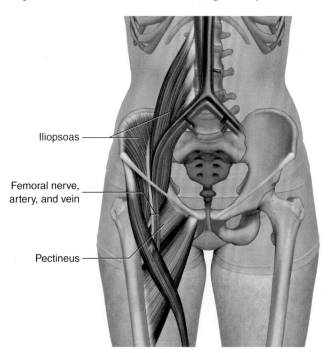

Iliopsoas

Femoral nerve,
artery, and vein

Pectineus

5.7   **THERAPIST TIP**

Fibrous Adhesions in the Inguinal Region

The region of the proximal thigh near the inguinal ligament often accumulates a lot of fibrous adhesions. For this reason, moderate to deep pressure work in this region can be very beneficial to free up and loosen the area.

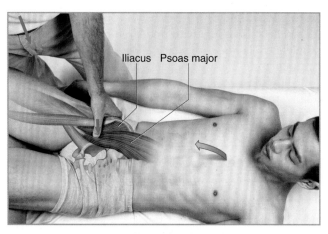

Iliacus   Psoas major

Figure 5-23D

Step 2: Perform the Technique:

■ The distal belly/tendon of the iliopsoas can be worked by performing short longitudinal strokes running vertically from superior to inferior along the musculature with moderate to deep pressure (Fig. 5-24A). Strumming transversely across the musculature can also be performed (Fig. 5-24B).

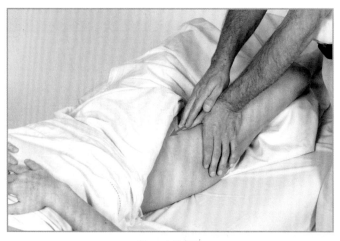

Figure 5-24A

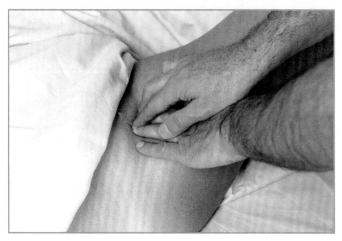

Figure 5-24B

■ When working the iliopsoas in the proximal thigh, it is important to try to access the belly/tendon as far distally toward the lesser trochanter as possible. Depending on the client, this may be very challenging. To facilitate accessing the iliopsoas distally, you can passively support the client's thigh in successively more flexion by grasping under their knee as you reach toward the lesser trochanter attachment (Fig. 5-24C). If it is difficult to support the weight of the client's thigh, then place your right foot on the table and rest their (lower) leg on your thigh.

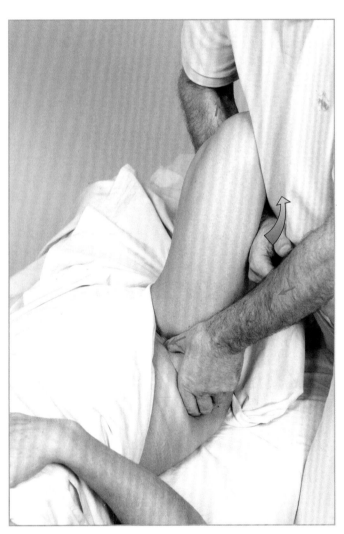

Figure 5-24C

5.6   PRACTICAL APPLICATION

Pin and Stretch the Iliopsoas

Pin and stretch is an extremely effective technique that combines sustained deep pressure with stretching and allows the stretch to be applied to a more specific, focused aspect of the muscle. To perform pin and stretch to the distal belly/tendon of the iliopsoas in the proximal thigh, position the client as close to the side of the table as possible. Support the client's lower extremity up and off the side of the table (**Fig. A**), place your thumb pad treatment contact (finger pads could also be used) onto the iliopsoas with firm pressure to apply the pin, and then lower the client's thigh into extension off the side of the table (**Fig. B**). It is important to maintain the pressure of the thumb pad pin as the stretch is applied. The stretch can be held statically for a short period of time (approximately 1 to 3 seconds) or for longer (5 seconds or more). Now ask the client to remain relaxed and passive as you bring the thigh back up into flexion toward anatomic position. Usually, three to four repetitions are done. This protocol can then be repeated using a different pin location point on the iliopsoas.

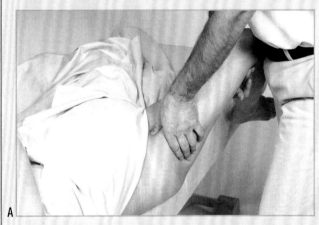

A

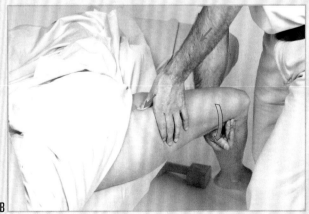

B

ROUTINE 5-6: DIAPHRAGM

Most of the diaphragm cannot be reached for soft tissue work; however, the relatively small part of it that is accessible can sometimes greatly help clients who experience shortness of breath. The diaphragm attaches to the internal surfaces of the sternum and lower six ribs circumferentially around the rib cage as well as to the bodies of L1-L3 (Fig. 5-25).

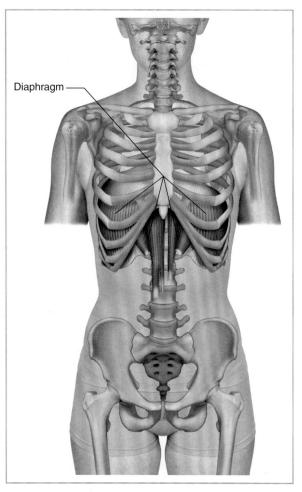

Figure 5-25 The diaphragm.

Starting Position:

- The client is supine with a large roll under the knees. This relaxes the hip flexor musculature so that the pelvis can drop into posterior tilt, relaxing and slackening the anterior abdominal wall.
- You are standing at the right side of the table (Fig. 5-26).
- The finger pads of your right hand will be the treatment contact. If possible, use the finger pads of your left hand as the support that braces the right hand treatment contact.

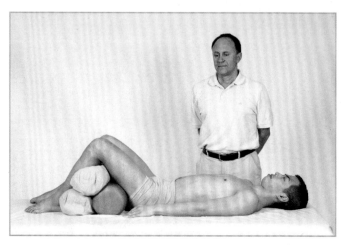

Figure 5-26

Step 1: Locate Target Musculature:

- After finding the inferior border of the rib cage wall, curl your finger pads around the inferior margin of rib cage with the pads of your fingers oriented toward the internal surface of the ribs (Fig. 5-27A).

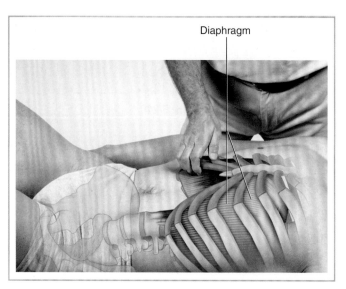

Figure 5-27A

■ Ask the client to take in a breath; as the client gently exhales, slowly sink in by curling your finger pads toward the internal surface of the rib cage (Fig. 5-27B).

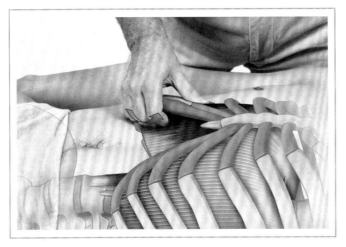

Figure 5-27B

Step 2: Perform the Technique:

■ The diaphragm can be worked by performing short transverse strokes across the musculature with moderate to deep pressure, trapping it against the internal surface of the rib cage.

■ The diaphragm attaches 360 degrees around the entire circumference of the internal surface of the lower rib cage wall (and sternum). Access as much of this muscle as possible by continuing to work the musculature in a similar fashion as far anteriorly toward the midline as possible and then as far posteriorly as possible.

5.8   THERAPIST TIP

Breathing and the Diaphragm

Shortness of breath is usually caused by weakness or deficiency of the heart and vessels of the cardiovascular system, not the pulmonary system (lungs and breathing). However, with age, the pulmonary system can become a limiting factor toward circulating healthy oxygenated blood throughout the body. For this reason, working the diaphragm in elderly clients can often have a beneficial effect on their health. Working the diaphragm is also often beneficial for clients with chronic respiratory conditions (chronic obstructive pulmonary disorders [COPD]) such as emphysema and asthma.

5.7   PRACTICAL APPLICATION

Visceral Massage

Visceral bodywork (visceral massage) refers to working with restrictions in the organs of the thoracic and abdominal cavities. Jean-Pierre Barral, a French osteopath, developed a curriculum called "Visceral Manipulation" that addresses the "mobility" and "motility" of visceral organs and related structures. Mobility refers to the ability of an organ to move relative to the structures around it. Motility refers to the subtle rhythmic motion of an organ that is presumably left over from its movement into position during embryonic development. Work done with mobility is easily felt by the client and can be visibly seen by an observer, whereas motility requires a subtle, almost energetic touch. Both interventions can have a profound impact on the whole system. Barral also works with the cardiovascular structures within and around the visceral organs, as they are structurally and functionally interwoven. Bruno Chikly, also a French osteopath, works with the lymphatics of the viscera. His curriculum is called "Lymph Drainage Therapy."

One of the fundamentals of doing any kind of visceral bodywork is knowing the location of visceral structures. Barral's first admonition to Visceral Manipulation students is, "Know your anatomy." Even though there are as many variations in the *exact* location and shape of specific organs as there are people, a strong understanding of anatomic structure is indispensable. The stomach, for example, probably has the largest amount of variation due to the effects of genetic, congenital, dietary, and age-related influences. It also changes shape and vertical location based simply on how much food is in it. Regardless of these differences, however, it still *feels* like a stomach. It has a stomach's shape, and it has a stomach's texture. It feels texturally very different from a liver or kidney due to the fact that it is hollow while the other two organs are very dense.

It is important to be aware of the way that the "essential" organs are protected by compensations in other body

continued

systems. If one's internal temperature drops, for example, the autonomic nervous system will direct blood flow away from the extremities and toward the internal organs. In other words, the hands and feet will be sacrificed to protect the liver, kidneys, lungs, and so forth. Similarly, there can be fascial strain through a visceral organ due to adhesions or other fascial restrictions within and around the organ. This strain will be compensated for by "folding" the fascial web around the restriction in order to minimize its effect on the organ. Due to the continuity of the fascial web, this means that the whole body's fascial structure will be limited in its expression. These limitations may be as small as a slight reduction in range of motion of a glenohumeral joint or as large as an easily seen and progressively worsening scoliosis. The musculature will likely be involved as the central nervous system inhibits individual muscles in order to limit muscle-induced strain on the organs.

All of these compensations can affect the fascial web because of the restrictions they initiate. Symptoms may appear far away from the original problem, making it difficult to know where or how to start dealing with them. Deducing that a pain in the foot is due to a restriction around the spleen is a Holmesian feat. To deal with this difficulty, Barral uses a technique called "listening" in which the practitioner feels for areas of restriction, that is, where the body folds around a visceral structure. This allows the practitioner to treat visceral causes rather than simply trying to address symptoms. The belief is that only by addressing *core* issues can those that are the result of compensations be truly "cured."

Although some organs or parts of organs are held within fairly strict fascial boundaries, others can slide around within a lubricated cavity. The lungs, for instance, could not function correctly within the pleural cavity if they were adhered to the lining of the ribs, diaphragm, and mediastinum, or if the lobes were adhered to each other. To prevent this, a serous (fluid producing) membrane maintains a steady supply of watery fluid to allow opposing surfaces to glide easily across each other, similar to what happens between two pieces of wet glass. This effect can also be seen inside the pericardium with the heart and in the peritoneal cavity with the stomach, liver, most of the small intestine, and part of the large intestine. If the slippery quality is diminished by disease or surgical adhesions, there can be symptoms such as pain, structural limitation, and organ dysfunction. One of the goals of visceral manipulation is to mobilize the restricted structures so that the normal slippery relationship can be restored.

Some of the organs of the abdomen are outside the peritoneal cavity. This includes the kidneys, spleen, parts of the duodenum and large intestine, and pelvic organs such as the bladder, rectum, uterus, and prostate. Because of their positions behind and below the peritoneum (retroperitoneal), they have no serous covering. They do, however, still need to be able to move within the abdomen the same way that muscles need to be able to change shape within the arms, legs, and so forth. Also, all organs, slippery or not, have ligamentous and fascial relationships to each other, the sternum, the spine, and the diaphragm as well as their respective cavities (pleural, etc.). These connections often require attention the same way that one might address ligamentous restrictions within and around a joint. The lungs, for instance, have suspensory fascia that connects them to the scalenes, cervical spine, and even to the hyoid bone. Due to these fascial relationships, dysfunction in any of the structures of the neck can be directly attributable to pleural restrictions.

Visceral bodywork is necessarily gentle and painless, although it may feel strange and uncomfortable at times. Clients generally are not used to having their internal organs manipulated. It is, however, often profound and long lasting in its effects. That said, it is imperative that a therapist gets appropriate training before performing any visceral bodywork. There are cautions and contraindications to be understood and techniques to be learned in order to fully appreciate the value of this underutilized modality.

Michael Houstle, LMT, Manual Therapist

CHAPTER SUMMARY

Working into the anterior abdominal wall musculature, as well as accessing the psoas major, iliacus, and diaphragm through the anterior abdominal wall, can be very powerful and beneficial to the client. However, it is often skipped during treatment sessions by manual therapists. Although massaging this region requires more caution than massaging the posterior low back, it can be performed safely and effectively if the therapist understands the anatomy of the abdomen and takes the time to practice these techniques. Very deep pressure is rarely appropriate here (except perhaps when working the abdominal belly of the psoas major), but firm, moderate pressure can be carefully and safely applied. For therapists who have not routinely worked the anterior abdomen, the information in this chapter will facilitate including these techniques in their treatment repertoire.

CASE STUDY

VERA

■ History and Physical Assessment

Vera Brasilia, age 48 years, comes to your office complaining of an acute right-sided low back pain. She has been experiencing this pain for 4 days now. She went to her internist who ordered radiographs (x-rays), which were negative for any osseous pathologic condition, and prescribed analgesic prescription medication (pain killers). The medication lessens the severity of the pain but makes it difficult for her to function during the day because it clouds her ability to think, so she is only taking it at night before going to bed. She is concerned because the condition does not seem to be improving.

She states that her pain began after she was moving boxes in the basement; she felt a twinge when bending forward with a box in her hands. She woke up the next morning with moderate pain that increased in intensity as the day went on. She states that the pain is now constant and severe, with sharp twinges whenever she moves. On a scale of 0 to 10, where 0 represents no pain and 10 represents the worst pain that she can imagine, Vera states that her pain ranges from 4 to 9, with the pain at 4 when she is lying down and at 8 to 9 when she first awakens and when she is standing or sitting for longer than 5 to 10 minutes. She describes the pain as feeling very deep, and that her "spine feel very fragile." Further, she is also experiencing pain into her right-sided anterior abdominal wall. She states that she does not have any intestinal conditions. There is no referral of pain into the lower extremity. Hot showers help temporarily to decrease the intensity of the pain.

History reveals that she has experienced low back tightness in the past but has never had overt pain. She has never been involved in an automobile accident and has never had any major physical trauma to her low back. Her job primarily requires seated posture at a desk, with work at a computer. She exercises four to five times per week, doing a combination of cardiovascular exercise, Pilates, and yoga.

Your physical exam reveals a decrease in all six cardinal plane ranges of lumbar spinal motion as well as an increase in pain on these movements. Flexion, extension, and left lateral flexion are most restricted and painful. Bilateral active straight leg raise is positive for local right lumbar pain only. Passive straight leg raise is negative bilaterally. Cough test and Valsalva maneuver are negative (for a review of assessment procedures, see Chapter 3). No orthopedic assessment test creates any lower extremity referral. Nachlas' and Yeoman's tests, as well as the medley of sacroiliac joint tests, are negative for low back pain.

Upon palpation, her erector spinae and quadratus lumborum are moderately tight, but pressure into them does not yield the deep pain that Vera has been experiencing nor does it increase the anterior abdominal wall pain. The musculature of her lower right anterior abdominal wall where she has been experiencing pain, and indeed her entire anterior abdominal wall, is neither tight nor tender to pressure. Her right-sided iliacus is only mildly to moderately tight but also does not reproduce the pain that she has been experiencing. However, deeper palpation of the abdominal belly of the psoas major on the right reveals myofascial trigger points that are extremely painful. Further, Vera states that applying pressure into them increases both the low back and the anterior abdominal wall pain that she has been experiencing.

■ Think-It-Through Questions:

1. Should abdominal massage be included in your treatment plan for Vera? If so, why? If not, why not?
2. If abdominal massage would be of value, is it safe to use with her? If yes, how do you know?
3. If abdominal massage is performed, which specific routines should be done? And why did you choose the ones you did?

Answers to these Think-It-Through Questions and the Treatment Strategy employed for this client are available online at thePoint.lww.com/MuscolinoLowBack

OBJECTIVES

After completing this chapter, the student should be able to:

1. Explain why multiplane stretching is so named.
2. Explain why multiplane stretching is effective.
3. Compare and contrast static and dynamic stretching.
4. Explain how multiplane stretching of a muscle can be reasoned out instead of memorized.
5. Describe how to use your core when stretching the client.
6. Explain the mechanism of multiplane stretching by describing the steps employed in it.
7. Explain why stretching should never be performed too quickly or pushed too far.
8. Describe the roles of the treatment hand and the stabilization hand.
9. Describe the usual breathing protocol for the client during the multiplane stretching technique.
10. Explain how another muscle can be slackened to make the stretch of the target muscle more effective.
11. Define each key term in this chapter and explain its relationship to multiplane stretching.
12. Perform the multiplane stretching technique for each of the muscles and muscle groups presented in this chapter.

KEY TERMS

assisted stretching
classic stretching
creep
dynamic stretching
functional group of muscles
line of tension

multi-cardinal plane stretch
multijoint stretching
multiplane stretching
muscle spindle reflex
presetting the rotation
stabilization hand

static stretching
stretch reflex
stretching
stretching hand
target muscle
target tissue

"the shortest rope"
treatment hand
unassisted stretching

INTRODUCTION

For a joint motion to occur in one direction, soft tissues located on the other side of the joint must lengthen. If any of these soft tissues are tight and resist lengthening, they will restrict proper range of motion of the joint, resulting in loss of joint mobility. These soft tissues may be muscles, ligaments, joint capsules, other fascial planes of tissue, and even skin. Therapeutically, tight soft tissues can be efficiently treated with **stretching**, a treatment modality whose purpose is to lengthen tight/taut tissues.

When stretching of the lumbar spine (LSp) and pelvis is performed, it can be carried out by moving the client's body within one cardinal plane or across multiple cardinal planes (for a review of the planes, see Chapter 1). For example, if the client's trunk is moved forward into flexion, the stretch occurs within one cardinal plane: the sagittal plane. If instead the client's trunk is moved forward into flexion and to the side into either right or left lateral flexion, the stretch occurs within an oblique plane that is across two cardinal planes: sagittal and frontal. Whenever a stretch occurs across two or all three cardinal planes, it is called **multiplane stretching**. The

Note: In the Technique and Self-Care chapters of this book (Chapters 4 to 12), green arrows indicate movement, red arrows indicate stabilization, and black arrows indicate a position that is statically held.

advantage of multiplane stretching is that it allows for more specific and more effective stretching of a target muscle.

Multiplane Stretching Routines

This chapter presents the following multiplane stretch routines:

- Section 1: lumbar spine (LSp) multiplane stretches:
  - Routine 6-1—LSp erector spinae group
  - Routine 6-2—LSp transversospinalis group
  - Routine 6-3—LSp quadratus lumborum
  - Routine 6-4—LSp anterior abdominal wall
- Section 2: hip joint/pelvis multiplane stretches:
  - Routine 6-5—hip abductors
  - Routine 6-6—hip adductors
  - Routine 6-7—hip flexors
  - Routine 6-8—hip extensors: hamstrings
  - Routine 6-9—hip extensors: gluteals
  - Routine 6-10—hip deep lateral rotators

MECHANISM

The essential mechanism of a stretch is simple. When a body part is moved in one direction, it creates a **line of tension** that stretches the muscles (and other soft tissues) located on the other side of the joint. For example, if the trunk is moved anteriorly, the posterior tissues are stretched. Therefore, the direction of motion of a stretch determines which muscles are stretched. Realizing this makes stretching a muscle easy: You simply do the opposite of its action (i.e., you do the antagonistic action to its mover action). For example, if a muscle is a flexor of the trunk, you stretch it by extending the trunk; if it is a right rotator of the trunk, you stretch it by doing left rotation. Stretches of muscles do not need to be memorized. Rather, they can be reasoned out if you know the actions of the muscles that are being stretched.

Stretching Functional Groups

Most therapists stretch their clients' low backs by moving the trunk within a single cardinal plane, such as forward into flexion or backward into extension in the sagittal plane, by flexing laterally to the right or left in the frontal plane or by rotating to the right or left in the transverse plane. As discussed, the target muscles that are stretched are the antagonists of whatever motion you do.

However, moving the client into a cardinal plane motion does not stretch only one specific target muscle; instead, it places a stretching force on an entire functional group of muscles. A **functional group of muscles** comprises muscles that can all perform the same joint motion. For example, if you stretch the client's trunk anteriorly into flexion in the sagittal

Classic Static Stretching Versus Dynamic Stretching

Classic stretching, whether unassisted or assisted, involves movement of a client's body part into a position that elongates the target tissue. Once brought to this position, the client's body part is held statically in that position of stretch for a period of time. The usual recommended period to hold such a stretch ranges from 10 to 30 seconds, although sometimes 2 minutes or more is recommended. Three repetitions are usually done. Because the position of stretch is held statically, this type of stretching is called **static stretching**. The characteristic of soft tissue known as **creep** states that soft tissue will deform based on a sustained force that is placed on it. Therefore, the sustained position of stretch that is held with static stretching efficiently deforms; in other words, stretches/lengthens the target tissue.

Recently, many sources have advocated changing the protocol of stretching from being static in nature to being more dynamic. **Dynamic stretching** is usually performed by the client actively moving the body part to the position of stretch by using the muscles of that body part. Then, instead of statically holding the body part in the position of stretch for a sustained period of time, the client either immediately returns the body part back to the starting position or holds the position of stretch for 1 to 3 seconds at most. By making each stretching repetition only a few seconds long, it is possible for the client to perform more repetitions, usually 8 to 10 or more. The advantages claimed for dynamic stretching are that it not only more effectively stretches the target tissues but that it also warms the tissues, increases blood circulation to the region, lubricates the joints, improves neural control of the motions being performed, and strengthens the muscles being used to bring the body part to the position of stretch. Dynamic stretching is fast becoming the stretching method of choice as recommended by many sources. Because of its other benefits, it is especially recommended as the stretching method that should be done as a warm-up immediately before engaging in any type of strengthening exercise. However, advocates of classic static stretching maintain that to truly change the tension level of a taut soft tissue via the principle of creep, a sustained stretch is necessary.

plane, a stretching force is placed on the entire functional group of trunk extensors. Similarly, stretching the client into right lateral flexion places a stretching force on the entire functional group of left lateral flexors. Although stretching the client in a single cardinal plane might be very effective at stretching an entire functional group of muscles, it is not necessarily effective at isolating the stretch to a specific target muscle within that group. To accomplish this, you need to perform multiplane stretching.

BOX 6.3

Stretching Terms

When a client stretches soft tissues, the stretching may be assisted or unassisted. **Unassisted stretching** is done when the client moves her own tissues into a position of stretch (**Fig. A**). **Assisted stretching** occurs when the therapist helps the client to move the body into the position of stretch (**Fig. B**). The therapist's hand that actually moves the client into the stretch is called the **treatment hand** or **stretching hand**. The other hand is often used to stabilize the rest of the client's body and is called the **stabilization hand**.

The tissue that is to be stretched is termed the **target tissue**. If a muscle is being stretched, it is called the **target muscle**. Although it is important to stretch all taut soft tissues (and all soft tissues are potentially being stretched whenever a stretch is being done), this chapter focuses its consideration and discussion on stretching of muscles.

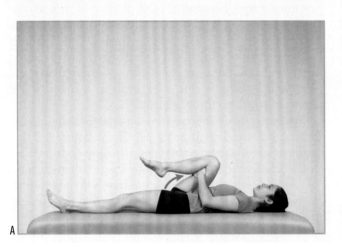

A

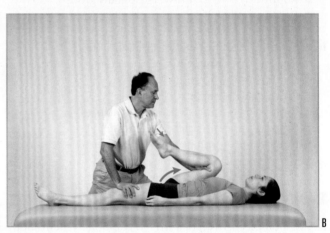

B

6.1   THERAPIST TIP

"The Shortest Rope"

It is important to note that when a stretch is placed on a functional group of muscles, it is extremely unlikely that all the muscles within that group will actually be stretched. A stretching force will be placed on all of them, but they will not all end up being lengthened and pulled taut. In reality, only the shortest (likely the tightest) muscle of the entire group will be lengthened because it will stop the stretching force from increasing to the point where it might cause a stretch of the other muscles. The only way that more than one muscle will end up being stretched when a functional group is stretched is if two or more of the muscles are equally short (tight) and therefore experience the stretch at the same time.

Michael Houstle, a longtime educator in the field of manual therapy describes this phenomenon as **"the shortest rope."** If you are holding the ends of several ropes of differing lengths and you pull simultaneously on all these ropes, will they all be pulled taut? No. Only the shortest rope will actually be stretched. This is analogous to stretching a functional group of muscles. Only the *shortest*, in other words, the *tightest* muscle, will actually be stretched. This is another reason that multiplane stretching is so important. With multiplane stretching, you set up the stretching routine so that your target muscle is the shortest rope.

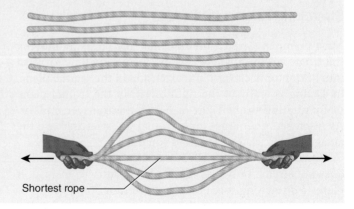

Shortest rope

Multiplane Stretching

Multiplane stretching involves stretching a client's target muscle not in only one cardinal plane but across two or perhaps all three cardinal planes. By involving more than one cardinal plane motion of the target muscle, a more specific and effective stretch can be attained because the target muscle can be lengthened to its maximum extent. For example, if the target muscle is the right erector spinae group, single plane stretching might be accomplished by bringing the client's trunk into flexion in the sagittal plane because the right

---

BOX 6.4

Multi-Cardinal Plane Stretching

It should be noted that stretching the client's low back into two (or all three) cardinal planes is actually motion in a single plane; it is simply motion within a single oblique plane (that has components of multiple cardinal planes). When you say that a stretch is a multiplane stretch, you are really saying that it is a **multi-cardinal plane stretch**. All multiplane stretches presented in this chapter involve motion across multiple cardinal planes, but motion only within one oblique plane. For this reason, multiplane stretching might be better termed multi-cardinal plane stretching.

6.2   THERAPIST TIP

What about the Third Cardinal Plane Action?

Even when a target muscle can be stretched effectively within one plane, if its other plane actions are not at least taken into consideration, the effectiveness of the stretch might be compromised. The right erector spinae group will act as the example again. The right erector spinae group can often be stretched thoroughly by only considering the sagittal and frontal plane components and stretching the client into flexion and left lateral flexion. That being the case, is it truly necessary to add in the transverse plane component to the stretch as well? Perhaps not. However, if you are not at least mindful of the fact that the right erector spinae group has a transverse plane joint action, it might be possible to overlook the rotation of the client's trunk and thereby lose the effectiveness of the stretch. For example, if you let the client right rotate while stretching into flexion and left lateral flexion, the right erector spinae group will be slackened by the right rotation (because it is a right rotator) and the effectiveness of the stretch will be somewhat lost. For this reason, even if you do not intend to stretch the target muscle in all three planes, it is important at least to consider all three cardinal plane components of motion/stretch of the target muscle to make sure that you do not allow it to slacken in one of them.

erector spinae group is an extensor. Or, the client's trunk might be brought into left lateral flexion in the frontal plane because the right erector spinae group is a right lateral flexor. Although either of these single cardinal plane stretches might succeed in stretching the right erector spinae group to some degree, a more effective stretch can be accomplished by moving the client's trunk into a combination of flexion in the sagittal plane and left lateral flexion in the frontal plane because this stretches the right erector spinae group across both planes.

A multiplane stretch of the right erector spinae group that combines the sagittal and frontal plane component actions is more efficient than either the single plane stretch into flexion by itself or left lateral flexion by itself. However, an even more effective stretch would be to consider the transverse plane component action of the right erector spinae group as well. The right erector spinae group, being an ipsilateral rotator, does right rotation of the trunk in the transverse plane. Therefore, to maximize the efficiency of the stretch, the client's trunk should be moved into a combination of flexion, left lateral flexion, and left rotation. Doing the opposite of all three of the right erector spinae group's component cardinal plane actions will achieve the maximum stretch.

OVERVIEW OF TECHNIQUE

The overview of multiplane stretching technique is straightforward. Once you determine what target muscle you want to stretch, simply move the client into the joint actions that are opposite the target muscle's joint actions—in other words, move it into its antagonist actions.

The following is an overview of multiplane stretching using the right erector spinae group as the target muscle being stretched. This overview describes assisted multiplane stretching in which the client is stretched with the assistance of a therapist. However, it is often possible for a client to perform unassisted multiplane stretching without the assistance of a therapist. For more on unassisted multiplane stretching, see Chapter 11 (available online at thePoint.lww.com).

Multiplane Stretching of the Right Erector Spinae Group

Starting Position:
- The client is supine and lying toward the right side of the table. The client flexes both thighs at the hip joints and legs at the knee joints.
- You are standing at the right side of the table.
- Both hands act as treatment hands and are placed on the client's distal posterior thighs.
- No stabilization hand is needed in this protocol. The client's body weight acts to stabilize the upper trunk.
- Keeping your elbows tucked in front of your body enables you to use your core body weight behind your hands when pressing on the client with your treatment hands (Fig. 6-1).

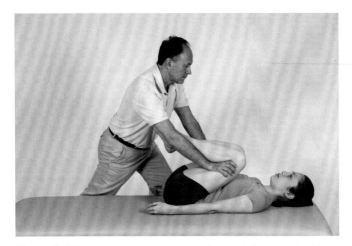

Figure 6-1 Starting position to stretch the right erector spinae group. Note that the therapist's elbows are tucked in to align the core behind the forearms and hands.

■ An alternative starting position is commonly used:
  ▪ Position your body on the table. Hold the client's distal posterior thighs as before but place the client's feet on your right clavicle (Fig. 6-2). The advantage to this position is that it is even easier to use your core body weight, so your shoulder musculature does not have to work as hard.

Stretching the Client:

■ Simultaneously stretch the client's pelvis and lower trunk up into posterior tilt and flexion away from the table and left lateral flexion and a small amount of left rotation toward the opposite side of the body until you meet tissue resistance (Fig. 6-3). (*Note*: These actions were chosen because they are the opposite actions of the mover actions of the right erector spinae group. For more on this, see Box 6.5.)
■ Add a little more pressure to increase the intensity of the stretch.

<table>
<tr><td>**6.3**</td><td>**THERAPIST TIP**</td></tr>
</table>

Body Mechanics and Stretching

Like other manual therapies, stretching is a physical endeavor and can be hard work. In fact, when the client is much larger or much taller than the therapist, stretching can be much more physically taxing than soft tissue manipulation because the client's body parts need to be moved, lifted, and stabilized. For this reason, good body mechanics are essential (see Chapter 4 for the principles of body mechanics).

The first tenet of good body mechanics is to work from the core; this involves keeping the elbows in front of the body. It may seem uncomfortable at first to tuck your elbows in front of your body. However, with a little practice, this position will become comfortable. It is well worth the effort because the advantage of this position is that you can use your core weight and strength to press into and stretch the client and to stabilize the client's trunk and/or pelvis instead of overtaxing the musculature of your glenohumeral joints. For overweight and large-breasted female therapists, if it is difficult to tuck your elbows in front of your body, the closer you can place them to being in front of your core, the better. If you find that it is difficult to get both of your elbows in front, then focus on getting the one in front that requires the most effort. With some clients, this may be the treatment hand; with other clients, it may be the stabilization hand. Consciously laterally rotating your arms at the glenohumeral joints helps you to keep your elbows in. Once you have practiced this position for a little while, it will come naturally.

Skipping using your hands entirely and having the client contact you directly on your trunk (as seen in Fig. 6-2) allows for an even more efficient use of your core because all that you need to do to generate the force of the stretch is to lean in.

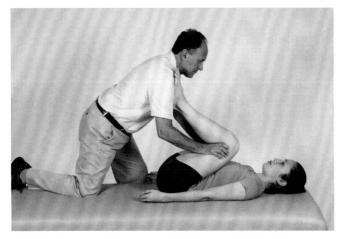

Figure 6-2 Alternate position to stretch the right erector spinae group.

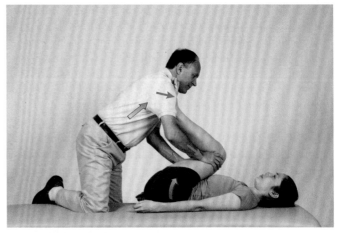

Figure 6-3 The right erector spinae group is stretched into flexion, left lateral flexion, and left rotation.

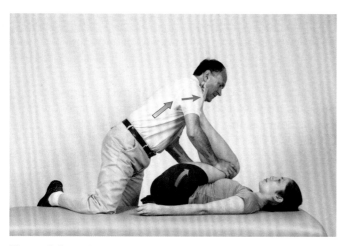

Figure 6-4 With successive repetitions, the right erector spinae musculature can be stretched farther.

■ Hold the position of the stretch anywhere between 3 and 30 seconds.

■ After the repetition is done, return the client to the starting position and have the client relax for a few seconds.

Further Repetitions:

■ The number of repetitions performed is usually determined by how long you hold the stretch for each individual repetition.

■ If you hold each repetition for 10 to 20 seconds or longer, three repetitions typically are done.

■ If you hold each stretch for less time (e.g., 2 to 3 seconds), then it is typical to perform more repetitions, often as many as 10 or more.

■ As with all clinical orthopedic manual therapy, the response of the client's tissues should be the final determinant for exactly how you carry out the stretching protocol.

■ Each successive repetition should increase the degree of stretch of the client's muscles (Fig. 6-4).

■ Repeat for the other side; Figure 6-5 illustrates stretching of the left-sided erector spinae group.

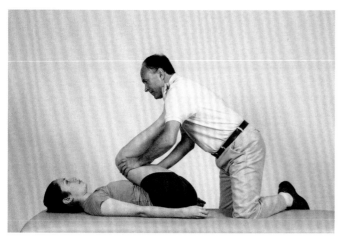

Figure 6-5 The left erector spinae group is stretched.

6.1   PRACTICAL APPLICATION

Alternative Position for Stretching the Low Back

In this section, the erector spinae group was stretched with the client supine and the pelvis and lower trunk moved up toward a stabilized upper trunk. However, the erector spinae and other low back musculature can also be stretched in the opposite direction; that is, moving the (upper) thoracolumbar trunk down toward the (stabilized) pelvis. To stretch the right erector spinae group in this manner, have the client seated at the end of the table (or on a bench or chair) with her feet flat on the floor for stability. Stand behind the client and to her left side. Both hands are used as treatment hands; no stabilization hand is needed because the pelvis is stabilized by body weight and contact with the table as well as the feet being planted on the floor. Your treatment hands can both be placed on the right side of the client's back. Alternately, you can place your right hand on the right side of the client's back while your left hand supports the client's left shoulder/ upper trunk (see accompanying figure). Bring the client down into flexion, to the left into left lateral flexion, and rotated into left rotation. These seated stretches are excellent to recommend to the client for self-care (for more on client self-care, see Chapter 11, available online at thePoint.lww.com). *Note*: This stretch can also be done with the client seated on the floor, but if her hamstrings are tight, it makes it difficult to perform the stretch.

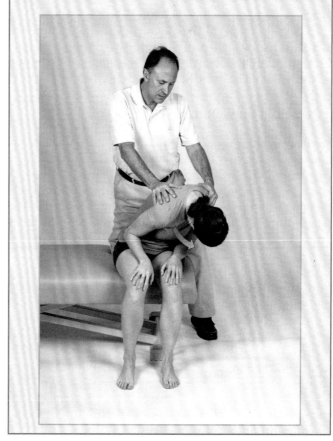

BOX	6.5

Reverse Actions

The low back can be stretched two ways. One way is to stabilize the pelvis and move the upper trunk toward the stabilized pelvis. The second way is to stabilize the upper trunk and move the pelvis and lower trunk toward the stabilized upper trunk. Figuring out what actions to perform to stretch the low back when moving the upper trunk toward the stabilized pelvis is straightforward. For example, to stretch the right erector spinae group, because its actions are extension, right lateral flexion, and right rotation, you stretch it by moving the client's upper trunk into flexion, left lateral flexion, and left rotation. However, it can be a bit challenging to figure out how to stretch the low back when moving the pelvis and lower trunk toward the stabilized upper trunk because you need to create the reverse actions of the actions you did when moving the upper trunk. Reverse actions in the sagittal and frontal planes are the same: namely, flexion and left lateral flexion. However, the transverse plane reverse action is different. Whereas you would have performed left rotation of the upper trunk to stretch the right erector spinae group musculature, you need to perform right rotation of the pelvis and lower trunk. (For more on this, see Table 1-3 in Chapter 1.)

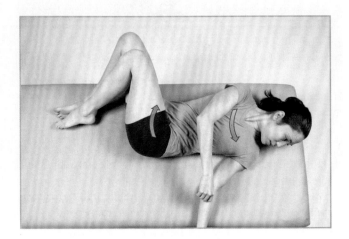

PERFORMING THE TECHNIQUE

When performing multiplane stretching, it is important to keep the following guidelines in mind. Each point addresses a specific aspect of the multiplane stretching technique. Understanding and applying these guidelines will help you perform multiplane stretches more effectively.

6.1 Stretch: Slow and Easy

When stretching the client's target musculature, whether it is the first repetition or the last, it is extremely important that you perform the stretch slowly and never force it. If a target muscle is stretched too fast or too far, the **muscle spindle reflex** (also known as the **stretch reflex**) may be triggered. The muscle spindle reflex is a neurologic reflex whose function is protective. When a muscle is stretched either too fast or too far, the muscle spindle reflex directs that muscle to contract in order to prevent it from possibly being overstretched and torn. This will cause a spasm of the target muscle, defeating the purpose of the stretch. Therefore, stretching should always be performed slowly and within the client's comfort zone. It is important to emphasize that when you begin to feel the client's target tissues offering resistance to your stretch, you should add only a small amount of additional pressure to the stretch. Because you will be performing a number of repetitions, increasing the stretch by a small increment with each repetition will allow for a more effective stretch by the end of the stretching protocol.

6.2 Treatment Hand

As with all stretching techniques, it is important that you place the treatment hand in a comfortable manner for the client. To do this, offer as broad a contact with your hand as possible so that the pressure of your hand against the client is distributed as evenly as possible (Fig. 6-6). Try to avoid pincering in with your fingertips.

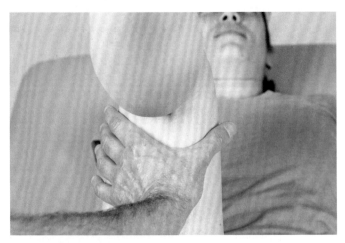

Figure 6-6 Treatment hand. Use a broad contact with your hand for client comfort.

6.3 Stabilization Hand

As a general rule with each stretching routine, both the treatment hand and stabilization hand are needed. However, when stretching the client's LSp by bringing the client's lower body up toward the upper body, the body weight and contact of the client's trunk against the table provide sufficient stabilization of the upper body so no stabilization hand is needed. For this reason, no stabilization hand was shown in the "Overview of Technique" section for the erector spinae group.

However, in Section 2 of the stretching routines, where multiplane stretches of the hip joint are demonstrated, a stabilization hand will usually be needed to hold down the pelvis. In these cases, the position of your stabilization hand is critical. Unless it is properly positioned, the client's pelvis will often move and lift off the table, slackening the target muscle and losing the effectiveness of the stretch across the hip joint, and, in some instances, causing an unhealthy torque (rotary force) to be placed into the LSp. Like the treatment hand, placement of your stabilization hand should also be comfortable for the client and offer as broad a contact as possible.

6.4 Breathing

When performing multiplane stretching, it is customary for the client to inhale before each repetition and then slowly exhale as you move them into the stretch.

6.5 Direction of Stretch

The direction in which a multiplane stretch is carried out is critically important to the technique's effectiveness. Indeed, the entire purpose of a multiplane stretch is to determine the ideal direction in which to move the client so as to achieve the optimal stretch of the target muscle across all three planes. Because a multiplane stretch is performed by doing the opposite (antagonist) actions of the target muscle, being able to reason out and perform multiplane stretching is dependent on a solid knowledge of all of the actions of the target muscle.

6.6 Length of Time and Repetitions

There is controversy regarding how long to hold a stretch. Classic static stretching advocates anywhere from 10 seconds to 2 minutes or more; usually three repetitions

---

6.2   PRACTICAL APPLICATION

Keep the Stretch in the Lumbar Spine

No stabilization hand was needed when stretching the erector spinae with the client supine because the client's upper trunk is stabilized by body weight and contact with the table. However, the exact direction in which you press the client's pelvis and lower trunk can make a big difference to what aspect of the client's spine is stabilized and therefore where the stretch is experienced. If your pressure on the client's thighs is oriented too horizontally (parallel with the table) in the cephalad/cranial direction, the client's entire LSp will lift off the table, and the tension will move into the thoracic spine, resulting in a loss of much of the stretch to the LSp **(Fig. A)**. To prevent this, it is necessary to press the client's thighs more downward into her chest **(Fig. B)**. However, if this is done excessively, the client may experience discomfort or pain in the anterior hip joint region (groin). Optimal is to press as little into the client's chest as possible (i.e., as much horizontally parallel to the table in the cephalad/cranial direction as possible) and still keep part or all of the client's LSp down on the table. The ideal balance between these two directions will vary from client to client.

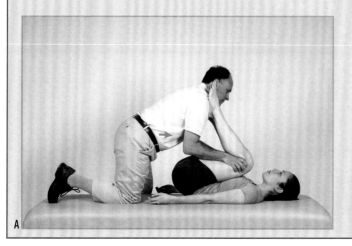

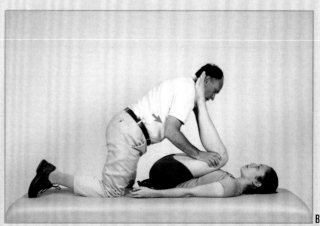

A

B

are done. Recently, advocates of dynamic stretching have recommended shorter times to hold the stretch, between 1 and 3 seconds but a greater number of repetitions (between 8 and 10 or more). What works best for one client will likely not work best for another. Try both methods and see what is most effective for each client. Many therapists like to use a combination of the two methods wherein they perform a number of shorter-held repetitions and then finish with a longer-held repetition.

6.7 Lumbar Spine and Rotation

When performing a multiplane stretch in all three planes of the LSp, keep in mind that there is not very much rotation possible in the LSp. On average, there is only approximately one degree of rotation possible at each lumbar segmental joint level in each direction (see Chapter 1 for ranges of motion). Therefore, the rotation component of a multiplane stretch for the LSp will be the least important aspect of the direction of the stretch.

6.8 Electric Lift Table

When stretching the low back and pelvis/hip joint, the value of an electric lift table cannot be overstated. Stretching can be much more physically demanding than soft tissue manipulation, especially if the differential in size between the therapist and client is large. If the therapist is small and/or short or the client is large and/or tall, stretching can be challenging. For good body mechanics, it is extremely important for the table height to be appropri-

ate. For many of the stretching routines presented in this chapter, such as the stretch of the LSp erector spinae or hip adductor or hamstring groups, the table needs to be low so that the therapist can use his or her core body weight. For other routines, such as the hip flexor or hip abductor groups, the table must be high enough so that the client's stretch is not obstructed by his or her foot hitting the floor. Therefore, to be able to perform multiple stretching routines to the LSp and pelvis/hip joint, the therapist must be able to change the height of the table, and having the client continually get off and back on the table while the height is adjusted manually is not logistically feasible. For these reasons, an electric lift table is essential for clinical orthopedic work.

6.9 Be Creative

There is a science to stretching: Move the client's body part into the joint actions that are the opposite of the joint actions of the target muscle. But there is also an art to stretching. It is important to be creative when stretching the client, altering the direction of the stretching force based on where you feel tension in the client's tissues. Each different line of stretch that you create will optimally stretch different fibers of the muscles and soft tissues that you are treating. As long as you are not forcing the body into positions that are not within the ranges of motion of the joint being stretched and as long as you are mindful of the cautions and contraindications, there is no such thing as a bad stretch. Play with the stretching angles. Feel for the response of the client's tissues. Be therapeutic. Be creative. Have fun.

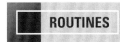

MULTIPLANE STRETCHING ROUTINES

The routines that follow demonstrate multiplane stretching for the major muscles and muscle groups of the LSp and also for the major muscles and muscle groups of the pelvis that cross the hip joint.

SECTION 1: LUMBAR SPINE MULTIPLANE STRETCHES

Stretching the lumbar spine (LSp) can be performed in more than one position. The client can be lying down; in which case, the upper trunk is stabilized while the pelvis and lower trunk are moved to create the stretch. Alternately, the client can be seated; in which case, the pelvis is stabilized while the upper (thoracolumbar) trunk is moved to create the stretch.

As a general rule, stabilization of the part of the body that is not moving is accomplished by the client's body weight and contact with the table. As a result, there is often no need for one of the therapist's hands to be used to stabilize the client.

Lumbar Spine Multiplane Stretches

This section provides four LSp multiplane stretching routines.
- Routine 6-1—LSp erector spinae group
- Routine 6-2—LSp transversospinalis group
- Routine 6-3—LSp quadratus lumborum
- Routine 6-4—LSp anterior abdominal wall

6.4   THERAPIST TIP

Transitioning to the Thoracic Spine

The focus of this book is on the low back, in other words, the LSp and pelvis. However, it can be extremely valuable to stretch the thoracic spine as well. Each of the stretches presented here for the LSp can be transitioned to become an efficient stretch of the thoracic spine if the movement and/or stabilization are changed so that the line of tension of the stretch enters and is focused on the thoracic region.

ROUTINE 6-1: LUMBAR SPINE ERECTOR SPINAE GROUP

Figure 6-7 shows the erector spinae muscle group. The erector spinae group is composed of three subgroups: the iliocostalis, longissimus, and spinalis. Multiplane stretching of the erector spinae group is performed by simultaneously stretching the client's pelvis and lower LSp into posterior tilt and flexion in the sagittal plane (the pelvis into posterior tilt and the LSp into flexion), lateral flexion to the opposite side in the frontal plane, and contralateral rotation in the transverse plane. Therefore, the right erector spinae is stretched with posterior tilt and flexion, left lateral flexion, and left rotation. The left erector spinae is stretched with posterior tilt and flexion, right lateral flexion, and right rotation. Multiplane stretching of the right- and left-sided lumbar erector spinae musculature was demonstrated in the "Overview of Technique" section, Figures 6-1 through 6-5.

As a group, the erector spinae extends, laterally flexes, and ipsilaterally rotates the trunk at the spinal joints. It also anteriorly tilts and contralaterally rotates the pelvis and elevates the same-side pelvis at the lumbosacral joint.

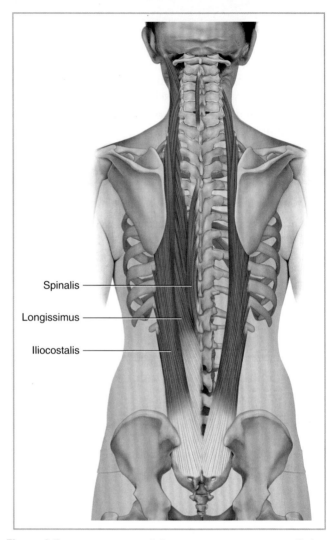

Figure 6-7 Posterior view of the erector spinae group. All three subgroups are shown on the left side; only the iliocostalis is shown on the right side.

ROUTINE 6-2: LUMBAR SPINE TRANSVERSOSPINALIS GROUP

Figure 6-8 shows the transversospinalis group. The transversospinalis group is composed of three subgroups: the semispinalis, multifidus, and rotatores. The semispinalis does not attach into the LSp. Stretching the transversospinalis group is extremely similar to stretching the erector spinae group in that flexion and opposite-side lateral flexion are performed. The difference is that the transversospinalis musculature does contralateral rotation so it is stretched with ipsilateral rotation (whereas the erector spinae does ipsilateral rotation so it is stretched with contralateral rotation). Following are two methods for stretching the transversospinalis group: The first is with the client supine; the second is with the client seated.

As a group, the transversospinalis extends, laterally flexes, and contralaterally rotates the trunk at the spinal joints. It also anteriorly tilts and ipsilaterally rotates the pelvis and elevates the same-side pelvis at the lumbosacral joint.

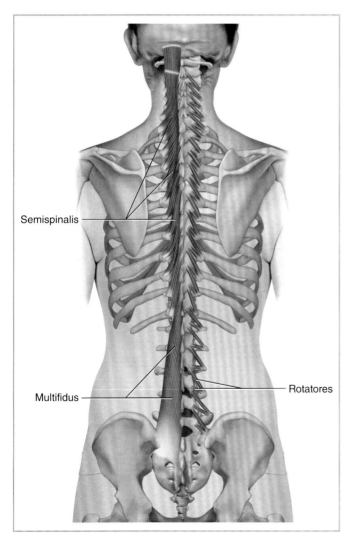

Figure 6-8 Posterior view of the transversospinalis group. The multifidus and semispinalis are shown on the left side, and the rotatores are shown on the right side.

Multiplane Stretching of the Right Transversospinalis Group: Stretch #1

- The client is supine.
- You are standing to the side of the client.
- Stretch the client's pelvis and LSp into posterior tilt and flexion, lateral flexion to the opposite (left) side, and ipsilateral (right) rotation.
- The client's upper trunk is stabilized by body weight and contact with the table.
- Therefore, the right transversospinalis group is stretched with posterior tilt and flexion, left lateral flexion, and right rotation (left rotation of the pelvis and lower LSp, which is equivalent to right rotation of the upper spine) (Fig. 6-9A).

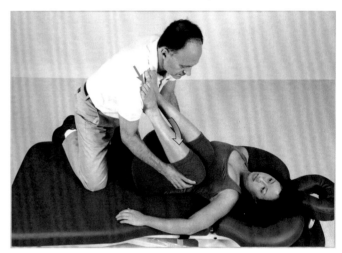

Figure 6-9A

- The left transversospinalis group is stretched with posterior tilt and flexion, right lateral flexion, and left rotation (right rotation of the pelvis and lower LSp, which is equivalent to left rotation of the upper spine) (Fig. 6-9B).

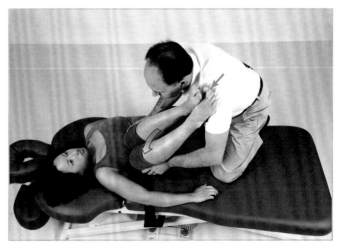

Figure 6-9B

Multiplane Stretching of the Right Transversospinalis Group: Stretch #2

- Have the client seated.
- Stand behind and to the side of the client.
- Bring the client's (upper) thoracolumbar trunk down toward her lower trunk and pelvis.
- The client's upper trunk is stretched into flexion, opposite-side (left) lateral flexion, and ipsilateral (right) rotation.

- Therefore, the right transversospinalis group is stretched with flexion, left lateral flexion, and right rotation (Fig. 6-10A).
- Stretch the left transversospinalis group with flexion, right lateral flexion, and left rotation (Fig. 6-10B).

 Whenever stretching the LSp with the client seated, it is important to have the client's feet flat on the floor not only for stabilization for the stretch but also to prevent the client from possibly falling.

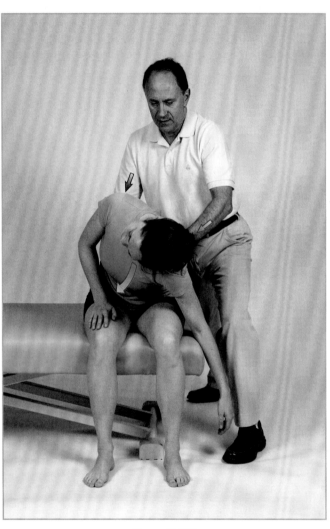

Figure 6-10A

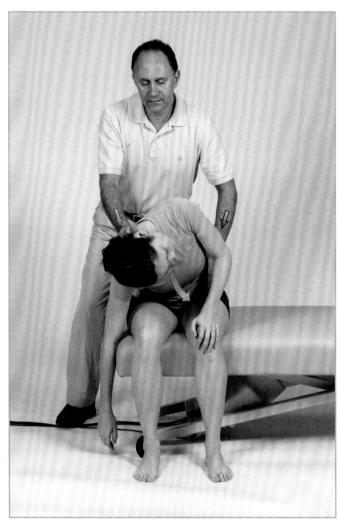

Figure 6-10B

ROUTINE 6-3: LUMBAR SPINE QUADRATUS LUMBORUM

Figure 6-11 shows the quadratus lumborum. Following are two methods for stretching the quadratus lumborum. The first method is performed with the client seated; the second method is performed with the client side-lying.

> *The quadratus lumborum elevates the same-side pelvis and anteriorly tilts the pelvis at the lumbosacral joint and extends and laterally flexes the trunk at the spinal joints. It also depresses the 12th rib at the costovertebral joint.*

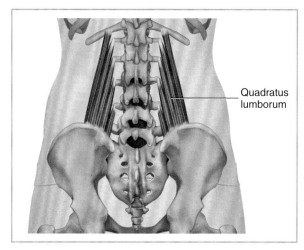

Quadratus lumborum

FIGURE 6-11 Posterior view of the right and left quadratus lumborum muscles.

Multiplane Stretching of the Right Quadratus Lumborum: Stretch #1

- Stretching the quadratus lumborum is similar to stretching the erector spinae and transversospinalis musculature in that flexion and opposite-side lateral flexion are performed. However, for the quadratus lumborum, the lateral flexion frontal plane component is more important than the flexion sagittal plane component, and no transverse plane rotation component needs to be added in.
- Have the client seated at the end of the table with her feet flat on the floor.
- Stand behind and to the left side of the client.
- Stretch the client into left lateral flexion and flexion; the lateral flexion component should be greater than the flexion component.
- Therefore, the right quadratus lumborum is stretched with left lateral flexion and flexion (Fig. 6-12A).
- The left quadratus lumborum is stretched with right lateral flexion and flexion (Fig. 6-12B).

Multiplane Stretching of the Right Quadratus Lumborum: Stretch #2

- An alternate position to stretch the quadratus lumborum is to have the client in side-lying position, oriented diagonally on the table so that her thigh that is away from the table can be dropped off the backside of the table without its path obstructed by the table.
- When the thigh drops into adduction, the pelvis on that side will be pulled into depression, stretching the quadratus lumborum on that side. You can press the thigh further into adduction to increase the stretch.

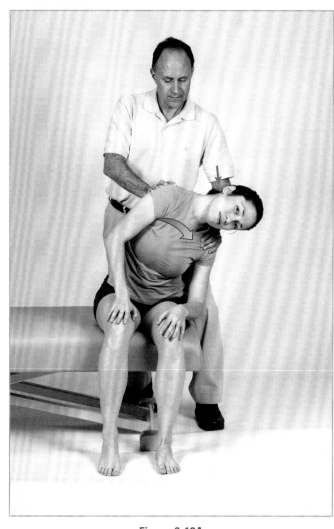

Figure 6-12A

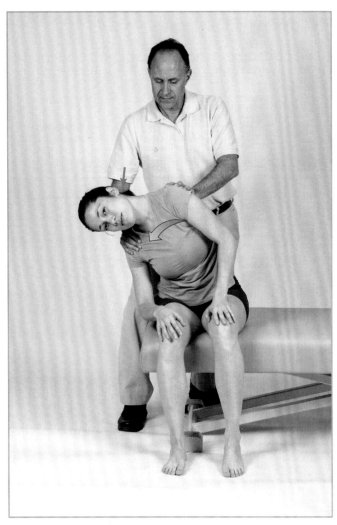

Figure 6-12B

- The client's rib cage is stabilized with your other hand; be careful to spread out the stabilization pressure across the rib cage with a cushion.
- Therefore, to stretch the right quadratus lumborum, have the client side-lying on the left and stretch the client's right thigh into adduction and right-side pelvis into depression (Fig. 6-13A).

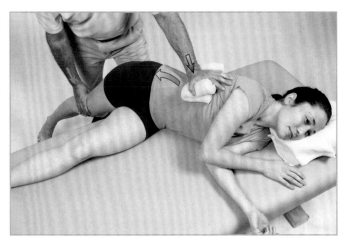

Figure 6-13A

- To stretch the left quadratus lumborum, have the client side-lying on the right and stretch the client's left thigh into adduction and left-side pelvis into depression (Fig. 6-13B).
- *Note:* Technically, this is not a multiplane stretch because the stretch is only in the frontal plane.

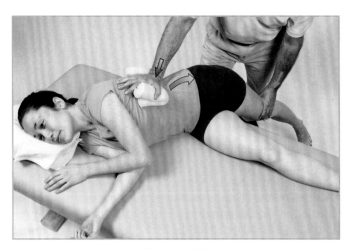

Figure 6-13B

ROUTINE 6-4: LUMBAR SPINE ANTERIOR ABDOMINAL WALL

The anterior abdominal wall is composed of four muscles: the rectus abdominis (RA), external abdominal oblique (EAO), internal abdominal oblique (IAO), and transversus abdominis (TA). The muscles of the anterior abdominal wall are shown in Figure 6-14.

Clients do not often present with an excessively tight anterior abdominal wall. However, when they do, it is important to know how to stretch the region. Stretching the anterior abdominal wall involves having the client prone and moving her into extension. Whenever the client's spine is brought into extension, be sure that this position is comfortable and healthy for the client's spine.

Following are five stretching protocols for the anterior abdominal wall. The first three stretches involve the therapist having to climb up onto the table and either hover over or sit on the client and lift the client's upper body into extension. This brings up a number of issues.

1. Professional modesty. Both you and the client must be comfortable with these boundaries.
2. Therapist agility. You must be agile enough to be able to climb onto the table.
3. Safety. The table must be secure enough to support the combined weight of you and the client.

The fourth stretch avoids the therapist having to climb onto the table; instead, the therapist stands at the head of the table and lifts the client's upper body into extension. The fifth stretch demonstrated has the therapist using the client's thigh to bring the client's lower spine into extension as well as opposite-side lateral flexion and ipsilateral rotation.

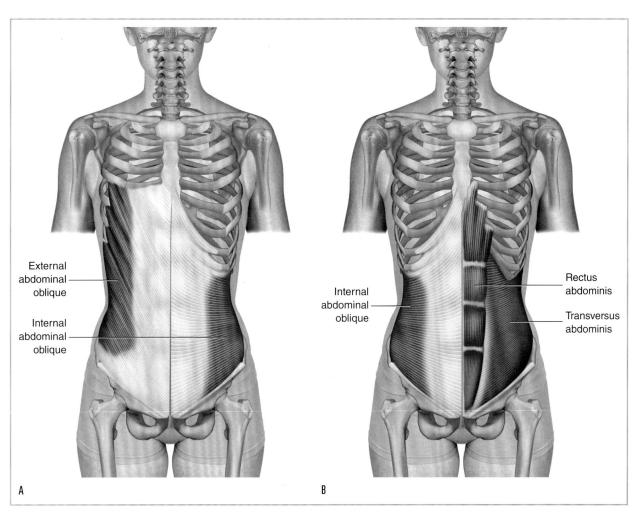

Figure 6-14 The anterior abdominal wall. **(A)** Superficial view. The EAO is shown on the client's right side; the IAO is shown on the client's left side. **(B)** Deeper view. The IAO is shown on the client's right side; the RA and TA are shown on the client's left side.

The RA flexes and laterally flexes the trunk at the spinal joints and posteriorly tilts the pelvis at the lumbosacral joint. It also compresses the abdominal contents.

 The EAO flexes, laterally flexes, and contralaterally rotates the trunk at the spinal joints. It also posteriorly tilts and ipsilaterally rotates the pelvis and elevates the same-side pelvis at the lumbosacral joint. It also compresses the abdominal contents.

The IAO flexes, laterally flexes, and ipsilaterally rotates the trunk at the spinal joints. It also posteriorly tilts and contralaterally rotates the pelvis and elevates the same-side pelvis at the lumbosacral joint. It also compresses the abdominal contents.

The TA compresses the abdominal contents.

Multiplane Stretching of the Anterior Abdominal Wall: Stretch #1

- Have the client prone with her hands clasped together on the back of her head.
- Climb onto the table and position yourself on the client's buttocks (using a cushion between you and the client can increase both comfort and modesty); grasp the client's arms.
- Stretch the client into extension by leaning back with your body weight (Fig. 6-15A). This stretch is a uniplanar stretch in the sagittal plane.

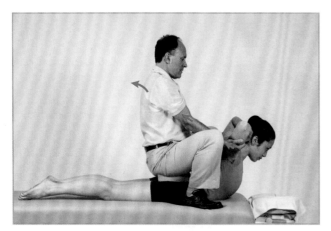

Figure 6-15A

- The client's pelvis is stabilized by your body weight on the buttocks.
- Now add in a frontal plane component by extending and right laterally flexing the client's spine (Fig. 6-15B). This is now a multiplane stretch that preferentially stretches the left side anterior abdominal wall muscles.

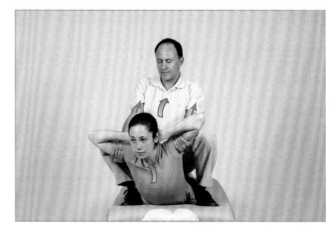

Figure 6-15B

- If right rotation in the transverse plane is added to the extension and right lateral flexion, the stretch becomes focused on the left-sided IAO (Fig. 6-15C).

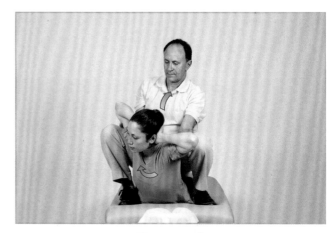

Figure 6-15C

- If left rotation in the transverse plane is added to the extension and right lateral flexion, the stretch becomes focused on the left-sided EAO (Fig. 6-15D).

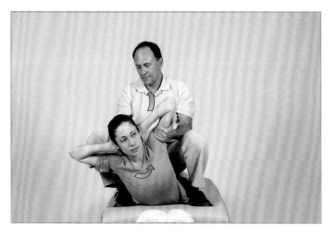

Figure 6-15D

■ Now repeat for the other side combining left lateral flexion with extension. If desired, rotation to the right or to the left can be combined with the left lateral flexion. Figure 6-15E demonstrates extension with left lateral flexion and left rotation.

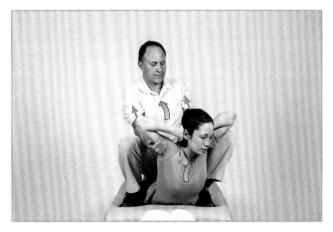

Figure 6-15E

■ Focusing the stretch to the TA is challenging because of the horizontal direction of its fibers. The best position to stretch the TA unilaterally or bilaterally is slight extension with rotation to one side and then the other (Fig. 6-15F,G).

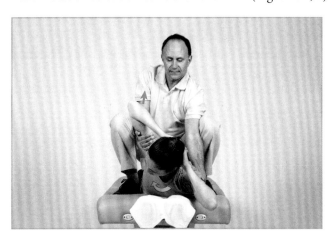

Figure 6-15F

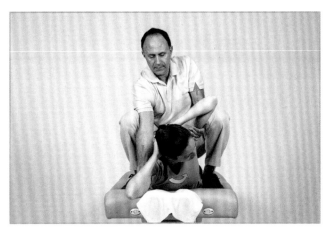

Figure 6-15G

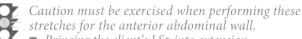

Caution must be exercised when performing these stretches for the anterior abdominal wall.

■ *Bringing the client's LSp into extension approximates the facet joints and narrows the intervertebral foramina and is therefore contraindicated if the client has facet syndrome or a space-occupying lesion, such as pathologic disc or a large bone spur.*

■ *The client's glenohumeral joints must be healthy enough to reach behind him or her and have a stretching force placed through them.*

■ *Positioning your body weight on the client's buttocks is important. If you sit too far superiorly on the pelvis, it can push it excessively into anterior tilt, increasing the client's lumbar lordosis. If you sit too far inferiorly, the pelvis will not be adequately stabilized.*

Multiplane Stretching of the Anterior Abdominal Wall: Stretch #2

■ With the client prone, have the client arms extended behind her. You grasp her arms and she grasps your arms as you lean back with core body weight (Fig. 6-16A).

■ Similar to stretch #1, this stretch can also be transitioned into a multiplane stretch by adding lateral flexion and/or rotation to either side (Fig. 6-16B).

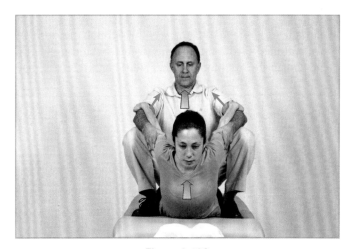

Figure 6-16A

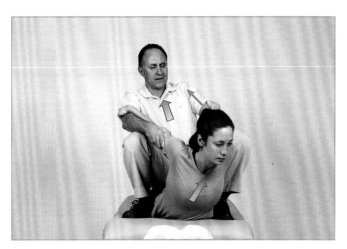

Figure 6-16B

Multiplane Stretching of the Anterior Abdominal Wall: Stretch #3

- The client is prone with her knee joints flexed to 90 degrees, and her arms extended behind her. You sit on her feet and grasp her arms, and she grasps your arms as you lean back with core body weight (Fig. 6-17A).

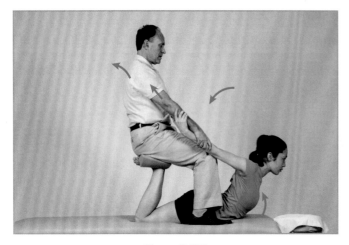

Figure 6-17A

- Similar to stretches #1 and #2, this stretch can also be transitioned into a multiplane stretch by adding lateral flexion and/or rotation to either side (Fig. 6-17B).

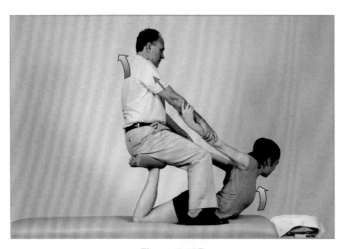

Figure 6-17B

Multiplane Stretching of the Anterior Abdominal Wall: Stretch #4

- Have the client prone with her hands placed on the back of her head.
- You stand at the head of the table; grasping her elbows, lift her upper body into extension.
- No stabilization hand is used. The client's pelvis is stabilized by body weight and contact with the table.
- The client can relax her head and neck into flexion with gravity if desired (Fig. 6-18A). However, if the client lifts her head and neck into extension, the tension force of the stretch into the anterior abdominal wall will be increased (Fig. 6-18B).

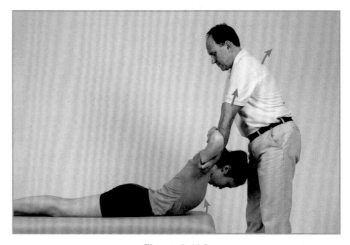

Figure 6-18A

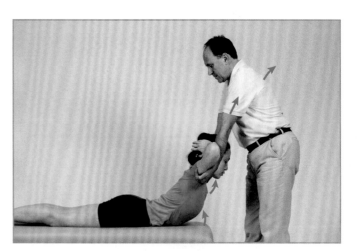

Figure 6-18B

■ This stretch can be transitioned into a multiplane stretch by adding in a component of lateral flexion and/or rotation (Fig. 6-18C).

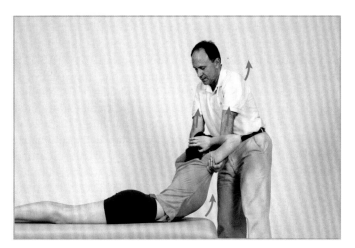

Figure 6-18C

Multiplane Stretching of the Anterior Abdominal Wall: Stretch #5

■ Following is the protocol for stretching the left side anterior abdominal wall.

■ Have the client prone.

■ Standing at the right side of the table, use your left hand to grasp under the client's distal left thigh and pull on the thigh and bring the client's pelvis and lower trunk into anterior tilt and extension, right lateral flexion, and left rotation (Fig. 6-19A).

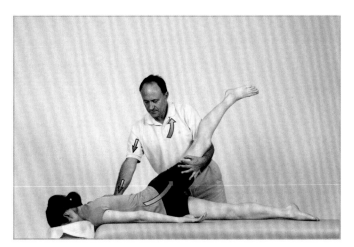

Figure 6-19A

■ Your right hand is the stabilization hand and holds down the client's upper trunk.

■ This protocol stretches the left side anterior abdominal wall, but because of the left rotation of the pelvis and lower LSp, it preferentially stretches the left IAO.

■ Now repeat this stretch for the other side (Fig. 6-19B).

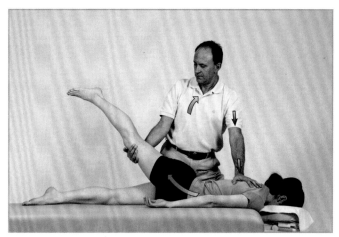

Figure 6-19B

SECTION 2: HIP JOINT/PELVIS MULTIPLANE STRETCHES

Including stretches of the muscles of the hip joint in a book on the low back and pelvis is done for two reasons. First, the bellies of many of the muscles that cross the hip joint are located in the pelvis. Second, all muscles of the hip joint exert their pull on the pelvis as well as the thigh. Therefore, if hip joint musculature becomes tight, it can and usually will affect the posture of the pelvis, which will then affect the posture of the LSp. Therefore, knowing how to stretch the hip joint is essential to the health of the low back.

Therapist-assisted stretching of the hip joint can be performed with the client in many positions. Depending on the musculature being stretched, the client will be prone, supine, or side-lying. As a rule, the client's thigh will be moved relative to the stabilized pelvis. For this to be adequately and safely done, the therapist's stabilization contact must firmly, but comfortably, hold down the pelvis and prevent it from moving. If the pelvis is allowed to move, the line of tension of the stretch will move into the LSp, resulting in a loss of the stretch to the hip joint and perhaps an unhealthy torqueing of the LSp.

Bony landmarks of the pelvic bone are used to stabilize the pelvis. Anteriorly, the anterior superior iliac spine (ASIS) is used; posteriorly, the posterior superior iliac spine (PSIS), or perhaps the ischial tuberosity is used; and laterally, the iliac crest is used. To broaden and make the stabilization hand more comfortable to the client, a cushion should be used.

Each of the routines presented will start with a uniplanar stretch of an entire functional group of musculature. Transitioning this stretch to a multiplane stretch will then be shown, indicating which specific muscles within the functional group are targeted with each additional plane of stretch.

6.3   PRACTICAL APPLICATION

How to Stabilize the Pelvis

Placement of the stabilization hand on the client's pelvis and the proper direction of your stabilization hand's pressure can be reasoned by understanding how the treatment stretch force on her thigh would move the pelvis if it were not stabilized. In whichever direction the pelvis would move, you need to exert stabilization pressure in the opposite direction. In other words, if the pelvis would depress, then your pressure must be toward elevation (**Fig. A**); if it were to rotate to the left, then your pressure must be toward right rotation (**Fig. B**), and so forth. Instead of the hand, there are times when using the forearm to stabilize the client's pelvis is preferred (see Fig. A). The advantages of using the forearm are that it is a larger, more powerful contact and that it broadens out the stabilization pressure on the client. However, be sure that the ridge (medial border) of the ulna is not digging into the client; pronating the forearm exposes the soft anterior surface of the forearm to contact the client.

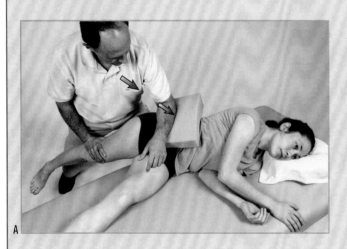

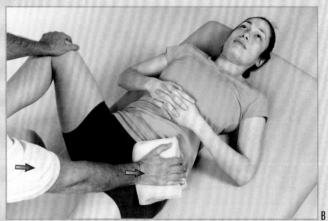

A   B

continued

An alternative to using your hand or forearm to stabilize the client's pelvis is to use a strap or seat belt that wraps around the table and holds down the client's pelvis. Some type of cushioning is needed to spread out the compression stabilization force so that it is comfortable for the client **(Fig. C, D)**. The advantage of this method of stabilization is that it frees your upper extremity/hand. The disadvantage is that it can take a couple of minutes to set up the strap/belt, so unless you will be using it for at least a few stretches, it might not be worth the time.

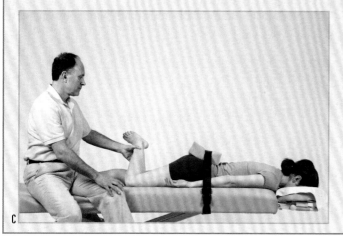

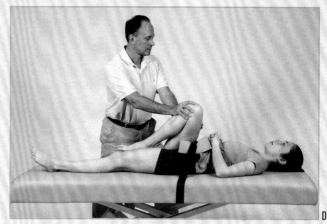

BOX **6.7**

Hip Joint/Pelvis Multiplane Stretches

This section provides six hip joint multiplane stretching routines.

- Routine 6-5—hip abductors
- Routine 6-6—hip adductors
- Routine 6-7—hip flexors
- Routine 6-8—hip extensors: hamstrings
- Routine 6-9—hip extensors: gluteals
- Routine 6-10—hip deep lateral rotators

- *If the client reports any discomfort in the LSp during a stretch of the hip joint, most likely you are not adequately stabilizing his or her pelvis. In that case, go back to the starting position of the stretching protocol and increase your stabilization pressure on the pelvis (making sure it is still comfortable to the client) before rebeginning the stretch.*
- *Caution must also be exercised for clients with pathologic conditions of the hip joint such as degenerative joint disease (also known as osteoarthritis). Exercise special caution with clients who have had hip replacements, especially when stretching the hip joint toward flexion, adduction, and/or medial rotation.*
- *Also, because most of the hip joint stretches require the client to be positioned far to the side of the table, it is important to reassure the client before the stretch begins that he or she will not fall off the table. To be sure that the client cannot fall off the table, have a strong and stable lower body posture with pressure of your lower extremity against the table so that the client would have to fall through you to fall off the table.*
- *Moving the client's thigh relative to the stabilized pelvis can often be accomplished with contact on the client's thigh or leg. Contacting the leg often offers greater leverage for the stretch; however, it also places physical stress through the client's knee joint. If the client has an unhealthy knee joint, avoid contacting the client's leg during the stretching procedures; instead, be sure to place your contact on the client's thigh.*

ROUTINE 6-5: HIP ABDUCTORS

Figure 6-20 shows the abductor musculature of the hip joint. The abductors of the hip joint are the gluteus medius and minimus, upper fibers of the gluteus maximus, tensor fasciae latae (TFL), and sartorius. Abductors of the hip joint cross the hip joint laterally with a vertical direction to their fibers. Following are two methods for stretching the abductor group: The first method is with the client side-lying; the second is with the client supine.

Hip abductors do abduction of the thigh at the hip joint. They also depress the same-side pelvis at the hip joint. These actions occur within the frontal plane. The more anteriorly located hip abductors also flex the thigh and anteriorly tilt the pelvis at the hip joint in the sagittal plane and medially rotate the thigh (and ipsilaterally rotate the pelvis) at the hip joint in the transverse plane. The more posteriorly located hip abductors also extend the thigh and posteriorly tilt the pelvis at the hip joint in the sagittal plane and laterally rotate the thigh (and contralaterally rotate the pelvis) at the hip joint in the transverse plane.

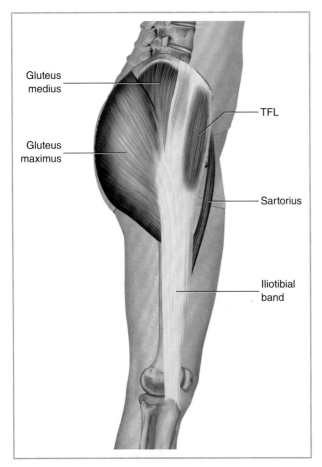

Figure 6-20   Lateral view of the hip joint abductor musculature of the right pelvis and thigh. The gluteus minimus is not seen.

Multiplane Stretching of the Right Hip Joint Abductor Musculature: Stretch #1

■ Have the client side-lying on her left side with her bottom as close to the near (your) side of the table as possible and her left shoulder as far to the opposite side of the table as possible. This positions the client diagonally on the table so that her right thigh can be dropped off the side of the table into adduction without its path being obstructed by the table (Fig. 6-21A).

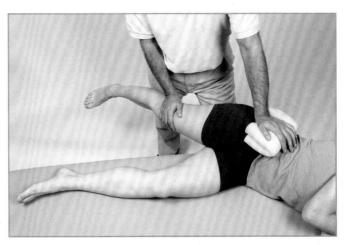

Figure 6-21A

■ Stand behind the client.
■ Your right hand is the treatment hand and is placed on the lateral surface of the client's distal right thigh.
■ Your left hand is the stabilization hand and is placed on the client's iliac crest. It is important to press on the pelvis in a cephalad/cranial direction; that is, pressing toward elevation of pelvis on that side (to prevent it from depressing during the stretch).
■ Stretch the client's right thigh down into adduction off the side of the table by dropping down with your core body weight (Fig. 6-21B).

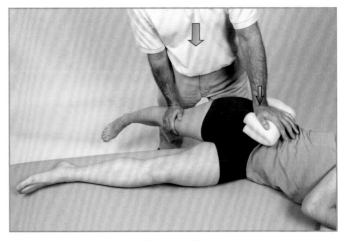

Figure 6-21B

CHAPTER 6

Multiplane Stretching **183**

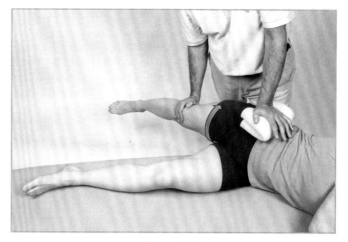

Figure 6-21D

Where to Position Your Core

Having your core body weight behind your line of force is the most efficient way to work and a guideline of good body mechanics. However, when performing most stretching routines, there are two lines of force: the line of force of your treatment hand and the line of force of your stabilization hand. So behind which one do you position your core? The answer is wherever the greater effort is needed. This can vary based on the body part being stretched and from client to client but is often behind the stabilization hand. For most hip joint stretches, more effort is needed to stabilize the client's pelvis than to move the client's thigh into the position of the stretch.

- This stretch is essentially uniplanar in the frontal plane. Because the thigh is dropped off the backside of the table, there is a small sagittal plane component of thigh extension, which would slightly and preferentially stretch the anteriorly located abductor musculature that also does flexion.
- To further transition this stretch to be multiplanar, the following additions can be made to the stretching protocol.
  - If the client's thigh is brought into more extension as it is adducted, the stretch for the anterior abductor musculature will be increased (Fig. 6-21C). These muscles are the TFL, sartorius, and the anterior fibers of the gluteus medius and minimus.

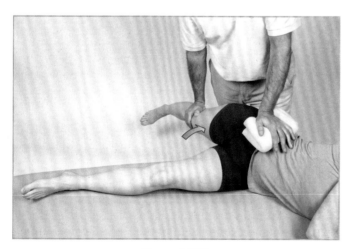

Figure 6-21C

- If the client's thigh is brought into lateral rotation as it is adducted, the stretch will focus more on the abductor musculature that also does medial rotation (Fig. 6-21D). These muscles are the TFL and the anterior fibers of the gluteus medius and minimus.

- Similarly, if the client's thigh is brought into medial rotation as it is adducted, the stretch will focus more on the abductor musculature that also does lateral rotation (Fig. 6-21E). These muscles are the sartorius, gluteus maximus, and the posterior fibers of the gluteus medius and minimus.

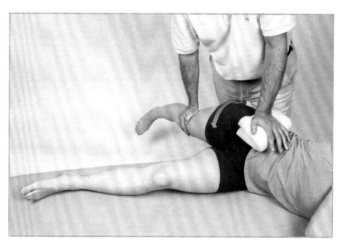

Figure 6-21E

- It is also possible to combine either rotation (lateral or medial) with extension.
- *Note*: When the stretching routine is completed, be sure to ask the client to completely relax the thigh as you passively return it to the table.
- After performing the appropriate stretches as indicated for the right side, switch to the left side of the client's body and perform these stretches there.

Multiplane Stretching of the Right Hip Joint Abductor Musculature: Stretch #2

- Have the client supine. To stretch the right-sided abductors, cross the client's left leg over the right leg.
- Stand to the left side of the client and grasp the distal right leg. Placing a small towel/cushion between the dorsal surface of your hand and their left leg can add to client comfort.
- Stabilize the left side of the client's pelvis and pull the right thigh into adduction (Fig. 6-22A).

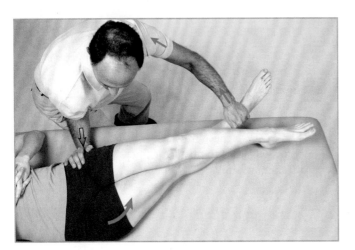

Figure 6-22A

- The more challenging body mechanics aspect of this stretch is usually the stabilization, so be sure that your right elbow is in so that your core is in line with your right hand/forearm.
- A possible alternate stabilization for the pelvis is shown in Figure 6-22B.

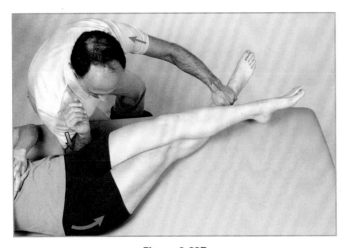

Figure 6-22B

- If the client is tall and you cannot reach her distal leg, a towel can be used to extend your reach (Fig. 6-22C).

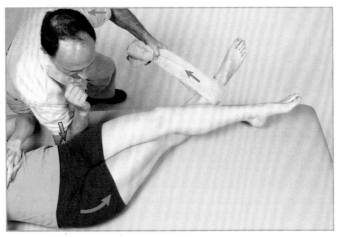

Figure 6-22C

- Repeat for the other side (Fig. 6-22D).

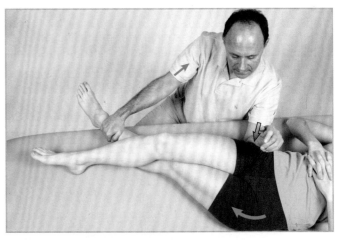

Figure 6-22D

6.5   **THERAPIST TIP**

Presetting the Rotation

When performing multiplane stretching that involves rotation in the transverse plane, it is often easier to incorporate the rotation component of the stretch by presetting it. **Presetting the rotation** means that you place the client's thigh into the rotation position before you perform the stretch. Using stretch #1 of the abductor group as an example, while the client is still in the starting position, before you begin the actual stretch itself, place the client's thigh into medial or lateral rotation, then stretch the client into adduction, being mindful to keep the client's thigh in the position of rotation as much as possible as you perform the stretch.

ROUTINE 6-6: HIP ADDUCTORS

Figure 6-23 shows the adductor musculature of the hip joint. The muscles of the adductor group are the adductors longus, brevis and magnus, and the pectineus and gracilis. The quadratus femoris and the lower fibers of the gluteus maximus also do adduction of the thigh at the hip joint. Adductors of the hip joint cross the hip joint medially, below the center of the joint. The first stretch of this routine does start with a multiplane stretch; the client's thigh is both abducted and laterally rotated, optimally stretching the muscles of the adductor group because they do adduction and medial rotation. The degree of flexion or extension can vary to optimally stretch different aspects of the adductor group. The second stretch of this routine is performed with the thigh abducted and laterally rotated, but the knee joint extended so that the gracilis (which is also a flexor of the knee joint) is preferentially stretched.

As a group, the adductor group muscles adduct, flex, and medially rotate the thigh at the hip joint and anteriorly tilt and ipsilaterally rotate (and elevate the same-side) pelvis at the hip joint. The adductor magnus extends the thigh and posteriorly tilts the pelvis at the hip joint. The gracilis can flex the leg (and/or thigh) at the knee joint.

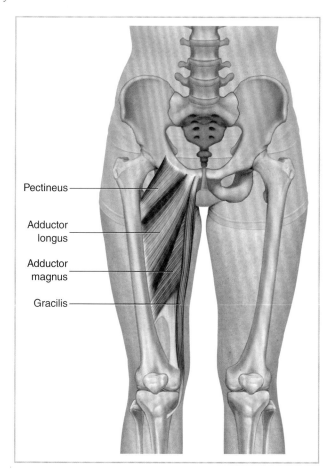

Figure 6-23 Anterior view of the muscles of the adductor group of the right pelvis and thigh. The adductor brevis is not seen.

Multiplane Stretching of the Right Hip Joint Adductor Musculature: Stretch #1

■ Have the client supine toward the right side of the table. His right hip joint is abducted and laterally rotated at the hip joint, his right leg is flexed at the knee joint, and his right foot is placed on your left ASIS (Fig. 6-24A). (*Note:* If the client's adductor musculature is tight, it is likely that he will need to also flex the right thigh at the hip joint to attain this position.)

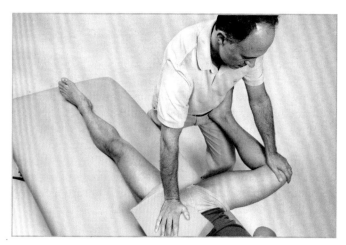

Figure 6-24A

■ Stand to the side of the client. Your left hand is the treatment hand and is placed on the medial side of the client's right knee. Your left side pelvis (ASIS) is also a treatment contact and is placed against the client's right foot.
■ Your right hand is the stabilization hand and is placed on the client's left ASIS. *Note:* A cushion is used to spread out and soften the contact pressure on the client.
■ First, press downward toward the floor on the client's right knee by dropping with your core body weight. This motion is horizontal abduction (also known as horizontal extension) of the thigh at the hip joint and, because of the position of the client's thigh, stretches the more anteriorly placed fibers of the adductor group. During this stretch, the pelvis will tend to rotate to the right, so your stabilization pressure must be oriented toward left rotation (Fig. 6-24B).

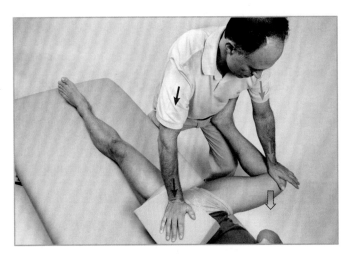

Figure 6-24B

■ Now lean in with your pelvis against the client's foot, further stretching the client's thigh into abduction. Because of the position of the client's thigh, this focuses the stretch to the more posteriorly oriented fibers of the adductor group. During this stretch, the pelvis will tend to depress on the left side (and elevate on the right side), so your stabilization pressure must be oriented toward elevation of the left side of the pelvis (Fig. 6-24C).

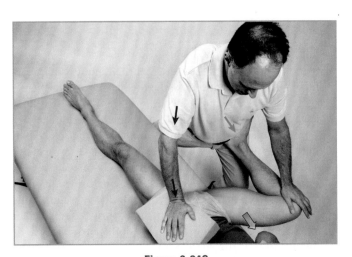

Figure 6-24C

■ Now combine these two stretching motions by dropping down on the medial knee and also leaning in and pressing against the client's foot. Be sure to stabilize the client's left-side pelvis toward both left rotation and elevation simultaneously (Fig. 6-24D).

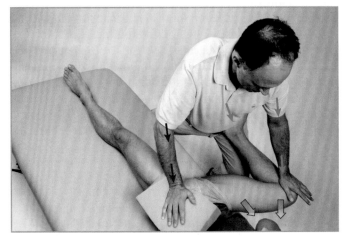

Figure 6-24D

■ To focus the stretch on the gracilis, you have to also consider the knee joint because the gracilis crosses this joint, too. The gracilis is a flexor of the knee joint, so to stretch the gracilis, the client's knee joint must be extended as you abduct and laterally rotate the thigh at the hip joint (Fig. 6-24E).

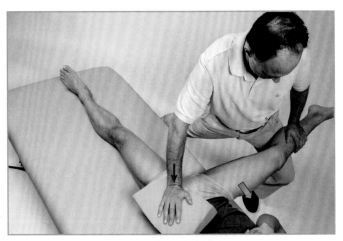

Figure 6-24E

■ After performing the appropriate stretches as indicated for the right side, switch to the left side of the client's body and perform these stretches there (Fig. 6-24F).

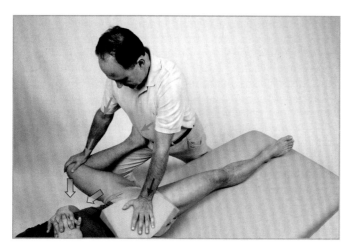

Figure 6-24F

Multiplane Stretching of the Right Hip Joint Adductor Musculature: Stretch #2

■ Have the client supine toward the right side of the table. His right thigh is abducted and laterally rotated at the hip joint, and his right leg is extended at the knee joint.
■ Stand to the side of the client, facing the head end of the table. Your left hand is the treatment hand and grasps his right leg, pulling his thigh into abduction.

■ Your pelvis is the stabilization contact and is placed against the side of the client's pelvis. Your right hand assists in stabilization by contacting the client's opposite (left) side upper trunk/shoulder girdle. *Note*: A cushion can be used to spread out and soften the contact pressure of your hand's contact on the client.
■ Now lean forward with your body weight, bringing the client's right thigh farther into abduction as you continue to stabilize his pelvis and trunk (Fig. 6-25).
■ *Note*: Because the knee joint is extended, this adductor stretch primarily focuses on the gracilis.

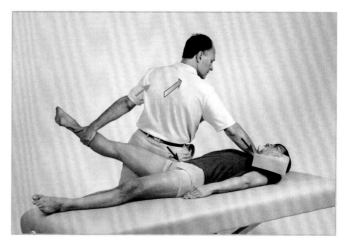

Figure 6-25

ROUTINE 6-7: HIP FLEXORS

Figure 6-26 shows the flexor musculature of the hip joint. Flexors of the hip all cross the hip joint anteriorly with a vertical direction to their fibers. The flexors of the hip joint are (from lateral to medial) the anterior fibers of the gluteus medius and minimus, TFL, rectus femoris, sartorius, iliacus, psoas major, pectineus, adductor longus and brevis, and gracilis. Following are six methods for stretching the hip flexor group. The first two methods are performed with the client supine. The next three methods have the client side-lying, and the last method has the client prone. Each position and method of stretch has unique advantages and disadvantages.

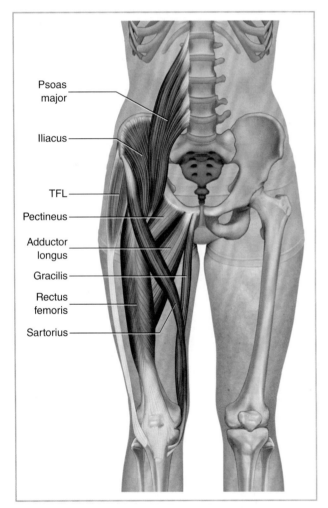

Figure 6-26 Anterior view of the hip joint flexor musculature of the right pelvis and thigh. *Note*: Not all muscles are seen.

 As a functional group, the flexors all flex the thigh at the hip joint and anteriorly tilt the pelvis at the hip joint. The more laterally located hip flexors (gluteus medius and minimus, TFL, and sartorius) also abduct the thigh or depress the same-side pelvis at the hip joint. The more medially located hip flexors (adductor group muscles) also adduct the thigh and elevate the same-side pelvis at the hip joint. The sartorius, psoas major, and iliacus can also laterally rotate the thigh (and contralaterally rotate the pelvis) at the hip joint. The anterior fibers of gluteus medius and minimus, TFL, and adductor group can also medially rotate the thigh (and ipsilaterally rotate the pelvis) at the hip joint.

Multiplane Stretching of the Right Hip Joint Flexor Musculature: Stretch #1

- Have the client supine as far to the right side of the table as possible.
- Stand to the right side of the client. Your right hand is the treatment hand and is initially placed on the posterior surface of the client's distal right thigh.
- Your left hand is the stabilization hand and is placed on the client's left ASIS. *Note*: A cushion is used to spread out and soften the contact pressure on the client (Fig. 6-27A).

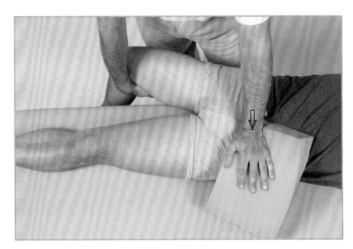

Figure 6-27A

- *Note*: The client needs to be positioned far enough to the right side so that his right thigh can be slightly abducted off the table and then dropped down into extension without the table obstructing its path. The table must also be set high enough so that the excursion of the client's thigh is not blocked by his foot hitting the floor.
- Switch the placement of your right hand to be on the anterior surface of the client's distal right thigh and gently press the client's right thigh farther downward into extension (toward the floor) by dropping with your core body weight. During this stretch, the pelvis will tend to anteriorly tilt and rotate to the right, so your stabilization pressure must be oriented toward posterior tilt and left rotation (Fig. 6-27B).

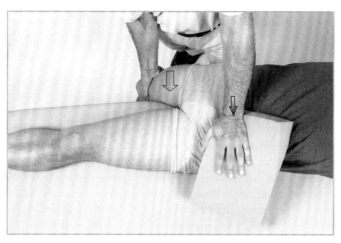

Figure 6-27B

- This stretch can be transitioned to be multiplanar by adding in abduction or adduction in the frontal plane or medial rotation or lateral rotation in the transverse plane.
- Abduction increases the stretch to the more medially located flexors (Fig. 6-27C). Adduction increases the stretch to the more laterally located flexors.

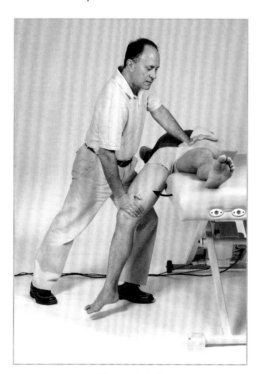

Figure 6-27C

- Lateral rotation increases the stretch to the flexors that do medial rotation (Fig. 6-27D).
- Medial rotation increases the stretch to the flexors that do lateral rotation.
- These frontal and transverse plane components can be combined to focus the stretch more specifically.
- *Note*: When the stretching routine is completed, be sure to ask the client to completely relax the thigh as you passively return it to the table.

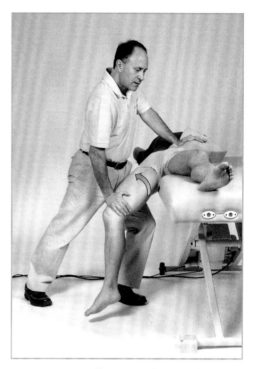

Figure 6-27D

- After performing the appropriate stretches as indicated for the right side, switch to the left side of the client's body and perform these stretches there (Fig. 6-27E).
- The advantage to this stretch is that the client is often in a supine position, so setting up this stretch is easy to do. The disadvantage is that it places a torque into the sacroiliac joints, so it may be contraindicated for clients with an unhealthy sacroiliac joint.

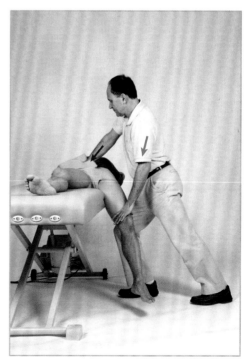

Figure 6-27E

Multijoint Stretching

This chapter discusses the idea that a target muscle can be optimally stretched if you consider all of the planes of its actions to figure out the most effective stretch. Considering all the planes of a target muscle is called *multiplane stretching*. However, this concept can be expanded. When a muscle crosses more than one joint, if you want to optimally stretch it, you need to consider its actions across all the joints that it crosses; this might be called **multijoint stretching**. An excellent example is the rectus femoris of the quadriceps femoris group. It crosses and flexes the hip joint and also crosses and extends the knee joint. Therefore, to optimally stretch it, you need to consider both joints,

extending the thigh at the hip joint and flexing the leg at the knee joint, to lengthen the muscle across both joints **(Fig. A)**. You can also use this information and reasoning to figure out how to eliminate a muscle from a stretching routine so that other muscles in the functional group are more efficiently stretched. Use the rectus femoris again as your example. It is often one of the tighter hip flexors and therefore commonly limits the extension stretch of the hip joint, preventing other hip flexors from being adequately stretched. To slacken and stop the rectus femoris from limiting the stretch, make sure that the client's knee joint is extended **(Fig. B)**.

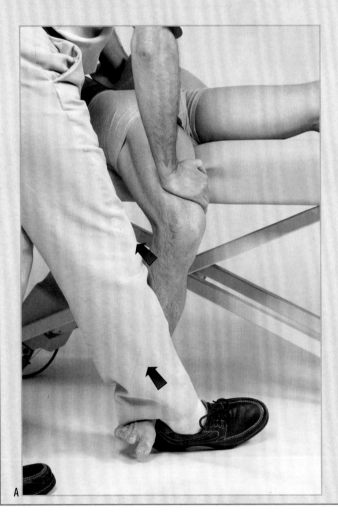

A

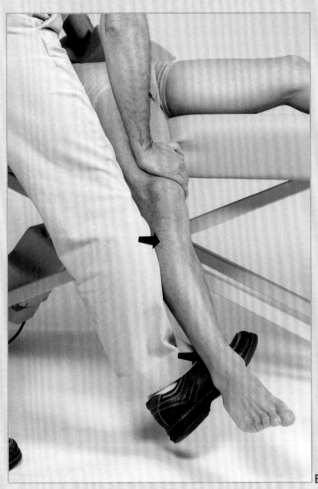

B

Multiplane Stretching of the Right Hip Joint Flexor Musculature: Stretch #2

Following are the directions for stretching the right-sided hip flexor group at the end of the table:

- Ask the client to stand facing away from the end of the table, place his tailbone (coccyx) at the top of the table, and lean back onto the table to lie supine hugging his left thigh into his chest.
- You stand facing the client at the end of the table, placing your right hand on his distal posterior left thigh to assist in stabilizing his pelvis and your left hand on his anterior right thigh.
- To perform the stretch, gently drop down with body weight, pushing his right thigh into extension (Fig. 6-28A).

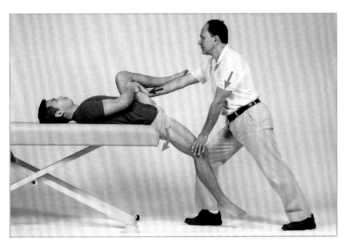

Figure 6-28A

- An alternative stabilization position is to place his left foot on your clavicle (Fig. 6-28B).

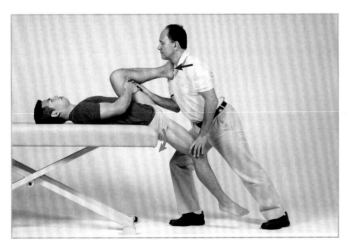

Figure 6-28B

- The stretch can be focused toward specific muscles in the hip flexor group by adding in adduction or abduction and/or medial or lateral rotation to the extension (abduction and lateral rotation are shown in Fig. 6-28C).

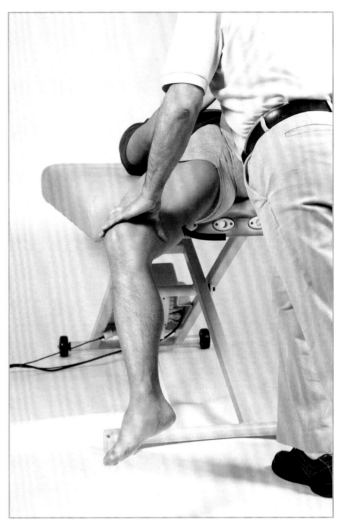

Figure 6-28C

- Now perform this stretch for the client's left side.
- This is a powerful stretch for the hip flexor region. Its disadvantage is that draping is challenging, so it might be best to perform this stretch at the end of the session after the client has dressed.

 It is healthier for the client's knee joint if the knee is hugged into the chest with pressure against the posterior distal thigh (see Fig. 6-28A) instead of the proximal anterior leg as is often done.

Multiplane Stretching of the Right Hip Joint Flexor Musculature: Stretch #3

- To stretch the client side-lying, have the client side-lying as close to the side of the table as possible, facing away from you.
- Use your right hand to bring the client's right thigh back into extension as your left hand stabilizes his pelvis (Fig. 6-29A).

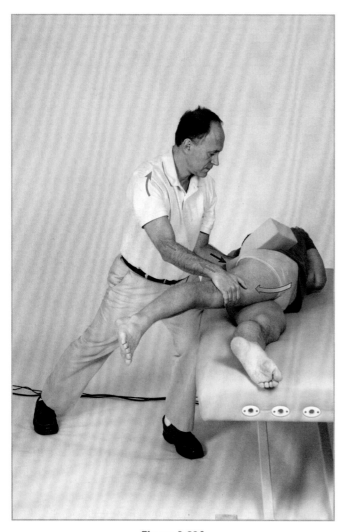

Figure 6-29A

- Now perform this stretch method for the client's left side.
- The disadvantage to this method is that if the client is heavy, it can be difficult to lift and support his thigh. Also, stabilization of his pelvis can be challenging; an alternative stabilization is shown in Figure 6-29B. The advantage to this side-lying method is that it can be done with the table low, whereas the supine methods required the table to be higher.

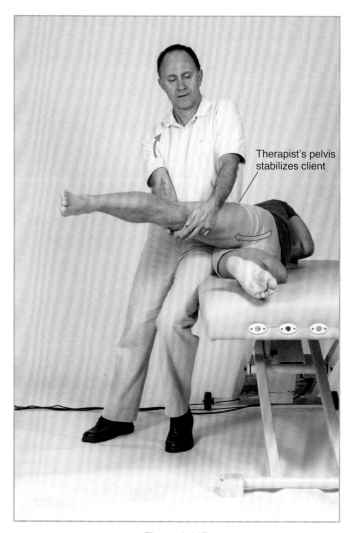

Therapist's pelvis stabilizes client

Figure 6-29B

Multiplane Stretching of the Right Hip Joint Flexor Musculature: Stretch #4

- An alternative position for the therapist with the client side-lying method is to position yourself between the client's distal thighs, facing toward their head.
- You then use your left thigh and pelvis to push the client's right thigh into extension as you stabilize his pelvis by contacting his right PSIS with both hands, pulling anteriorly on it as you lean back with body weight (Fig. 6-30).
- After performing for one side, repeat for the other side.
- The advantage of this side-lying method compared to the first is that it saves you from having to lift the weight of his thigh. But stabilizing the pelvis can be challenging, and the positioning of you and the client can be an issue regarding modesty.

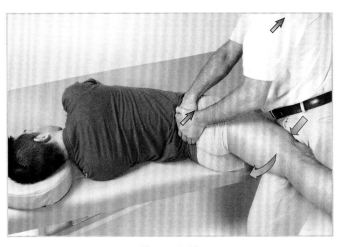

Figure 6-30

Multiplane Stretching of the Right Hip Joint Flexor Musculature: Stretch #5

▧ Yet another alternative position for the therapist with the client side-lying method is to stand facing away from the client's lower extremities. Use your left hand to stretch the client's thigh into extension; your pelvis/trunk stabilizes the client's pelvis, and your right hand stabilizes the client's upper body (Fig. 6-31A).

▧ If you grasp the client's leg to move his thigh into extension, his knee joint will be flexed and his rectus femoris will be preferentially stretched (Fig. 6-31B). If you can reach to grasp his thigh instead, then the knee joint can be held in extension as the stretch is done so that other flexors of the hip joint will be preferentially stretched (see Fig. 6-31A).

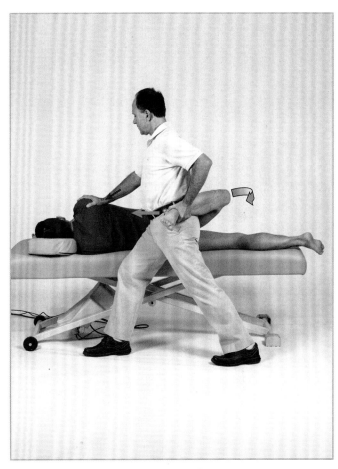

Figure 6-31B

▧ The actual stretch is accomplished by leaning forward with body weight to pull the client's thigh into extension as you continue to lean against and stabilize his pelvis (see Fig. 6-31B).

▧ After performing for one side, repeat for the other side.

▧ The advantage of this side-lying method compared is that stabilizing the pelvis is easier. You also do not have to support the weight of the lower extremity. The disadvantage is that it is more challenging to keep the knee joint in extension.

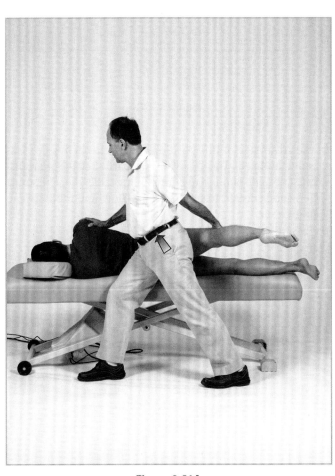

Figure 6-31A

Multiplane Stretching of the Right Hip Joint Flexor Musculature: Stretch #6

- Probably the most powerful method to stretch the client's hip flexor group is to have the client prone, with you sitting on his buttocks (a cushion can be placed between you and the client both for comfort and modesty).
- Interlace your fingers and lift his thigh up into extension by using body weight to lean back (Fig. 6-32A).

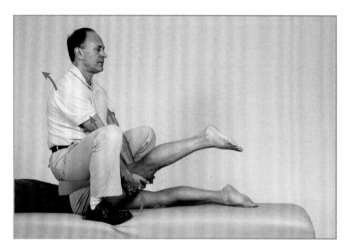

Figure 6-32A

- This stretch can be easily transitioned into a multiplane stretch by adding in a component of abduction/adduction and/or rotation (Fig. 6-32B).

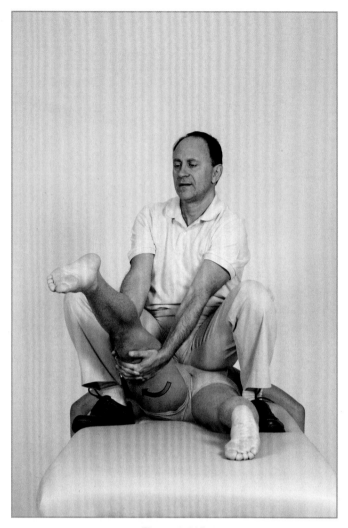

Figure 6-32B

- The advantage of this position is that the client's pelvis is well stabilized. The disadvantages are that the therapist must be agile enough to climb on the table, the table must be strong enough to support the weight, and modesty can be an issue.

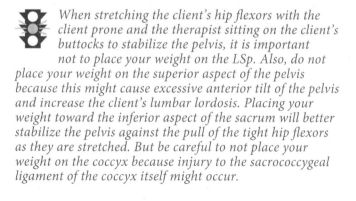
When stretching the client's hip flexors with the client prone and the therapist sitting on the client's buttocks to stabilize the pelvis, it is important not to place your weight on the LSp. Also, do not place your weight on the superior aspect of the pelvis because this might cause excessive anterior tilt of the pelvis and increase the client's lumbar lordosis. Placing your weight toward the inferior aspect of the sacrum will better stabilize the pelvis against the pull of the tight hip flexors as they are stretched. But be careful to not place your weight on the coccyx because injury to the sacrococcygeal ligament of the coccyx itself might occur.

ROUTINE 6-8: HIP EXTENSORS: HAMSTRINGS

 View the video "Multiplane Stretching of the Hamstring Group" online on thePoint.lww.com

Figure 6-33 shows the muscles of the hamstring group. The hamstring group is composed of the semitendinosus and semimembranosus medially and the long and short heads of the biceps femoris laterally. The hamstrings cross the hip and knee joints posteriorly with a vertical direction to their fibers. Because the hamstrings cross the hip joint posteriorly, they do hip extension. Therefore, the hip joint must be flexed for them to be stretched. Because the hamstrings cross the knee joint posteriorly, they also do knee flexion so the knee joint must be extended for them to be stretched.

*As a group, the hamstrings extend the thigh and posteriorly tilt the pelvis at the hip joint. They also flex the leg (and/or thigh) at the knee joint. (**Note**: The short head of the biceps femoris does not cross the hip joint and therefore has no action at that joint.)*

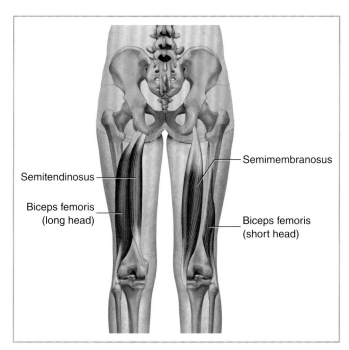

Figure 6-33 Posterior view of the hamstring group. The semitendinosus and long head of biceps femoris are shown in the superficial view on the left; the semimembranosus and short head of biceps femoris are shown in the deep view on the right.

Multiplane Stretching of the Right Hamstring Group

■ Have the client supine toward the right side of the table.

■ Position yourself at the right side of the table. Place the client's right leg on your right shoulder. Position your hands on the client's distal anterior right thigh to help keep the knee joint extended.

■ Your right leg is the stabilization contact and is placed on the client's left anterior thigh (Fig. 6-34A). *Note*: Stretching the client's right hamstrings into extension will cause a posterior tilt tension force on the client's pelvis, pulling the pelvis into posterior tilt, which will cause the left thigh to lift from the table. Your right leg holds down the client's left thigh, preventing this from occurring.

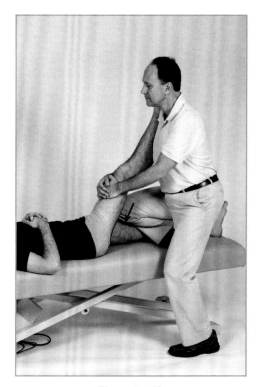

Figure 6-34A

- Using core body weight, gently lean into the client, pressing his right thigh farther into flexion (Fig. 6-34B). Make sure that his right knee joint remains fully extended (without being hyperextended).

- This stretch can be transitioned to be multiplanar by adding in abduction or adduction of the thigh in the frontal plane or medial rotation or lateral rotation in the transverse plane.

- Abduction increases the stretch to the more medially located hamstrings (Fig. 6-34C).

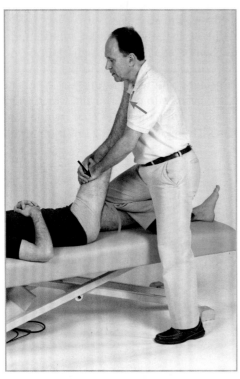

Figure 6-34B

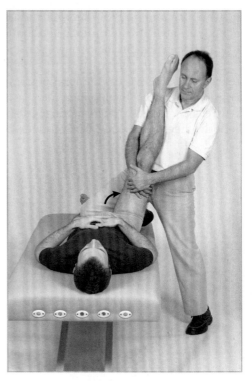

Figure 6-34C

- Adduction increases the stretch to the more laterally located hamstrings (Fig. 6-34D).

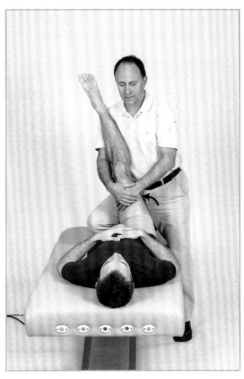

Figure 6-34D

- Medial rotation increases the stretch to the hamstrings that do lateral rotation.
- Lateral rotation increases the stretch to the hamstrings that do medial rotation.
- Frontal and transverse plane components can be combined to focus the stretch more specifically toward certain fibers.
- After performing the appropriate stretches as indicated for the right side, switch to the left side of the client's body and perform these stretches there (Fig. 6-34E).

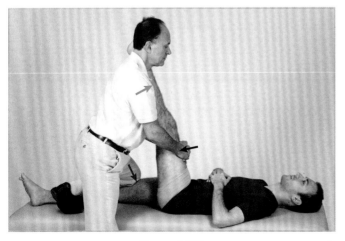

Figure 6-34E

| 6.6 | **THERAPIST TIP** |

Align the Core

Best practice body mechanics is to have the core in line with the force being generated. To facilitate this, the therapist can position himself on the table instead of standing at the side of the table. Be sure that the table can support the weight of you and the client.

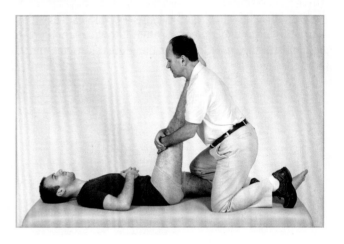

When stretching the client's hamstrings, it is important that the knee joint is not allowed to flex or the stretch will be lost. However, be sure not to push on the client's leg so forcefully that you cause the knee joint to hyperextend.

ROUTINE 6-9: HIP EXTENSORS: GLUTEALS

Extensors of the hip joint comprise the hamstrings, gluteal muscles (gluteus maximus and posterior fibers of the gluteus medius and minimus), and the adductor magnus. Stretching the hamstrings was shown in Routine 6-8. The gluteals and adductor magnus are being given a separate routine because they do not cross the knee joint, whereas the hamstrings do. Focusing the stretch on the gluteal and adductor magnus muscles is accomplished by slackening the hamstrings; this is accomplished by flexing the client's knee joint. The stretch routine used for the gluteals is often known as the *knee-to-chest stretch*. Figure 6-35 shows the gluteal muscles and the adductor magnus.

 The gluteus maximus extends, laterally rotates, abducts (upper fibers), and adducts (lower fibers) the thigh at the hip joint. It also posteriorly tilts and contralaterally rotates the pelvis at the hip joint.

The entire gluteus medius and minimus abduct the thigh at the hip joint and depress the same-side pelvis at the hip joint. The anterior fibers also flex and medially rotate the thigh and anteriorly tilt and ipsilaterally rotate the pelvis at the hip joint; the posterior fibers also extend and laterally rotate the thigh and posteriorly tilt and contralaterally rotate the pelvis at the hip joint.

The adductor magnus extends the thigh and posteriorly tilts the pelvis at the hip joint.

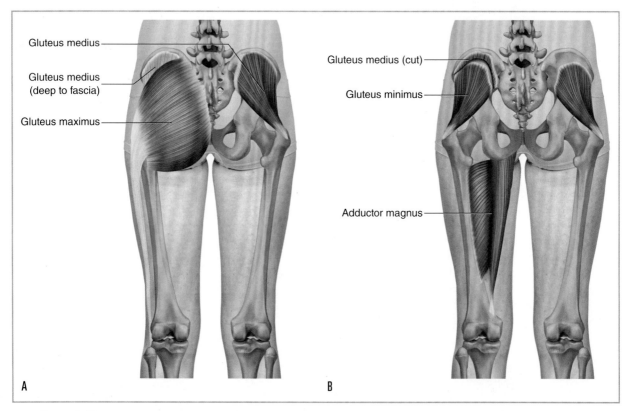

Figure 6-35 Posterior view of the gluteal muscles and the adductor magnus. **(A)** Gluteus maximus and gluteus medius. **(B)** Gluteus minimus and adductor magnus.

Multiplane Stretching of the Right Gluteal Group

- Have the client supine toward the right side of the table.
- Position yourself at the right side of the table.
- Bring the client's right hip and knee joints into flexion and grasp the client's distal posterior right thigh with both hands. *Note:* As with similar positioned stretches, an alternate position is to place the client's right foot on your clavicle.
- Your right leg or right hand is the stabilization contact and is placed on the client's left anterior thigh to stabilize her pelvis (Fig. 6-36A).

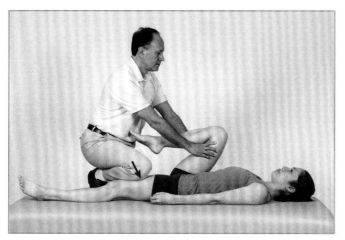

Figure 6-36A

- Using core body weight, gently lean into the client, bringing her knee to her chest by pressing her right thigh farther into flexion (Fig. 6-36B).

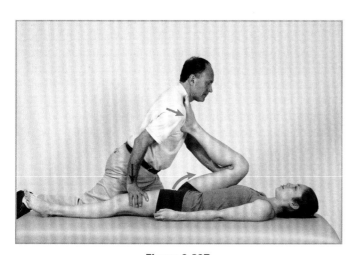

Figure 6-36B

- This stretch can be transitioned to be multiplanar by adding in abduction or adduction in the frontal plane or medial rotation or lateral rotation in the transverse plane.
- Abduction increases the stretch to the more medially located fibers (Fig. 6-36C).

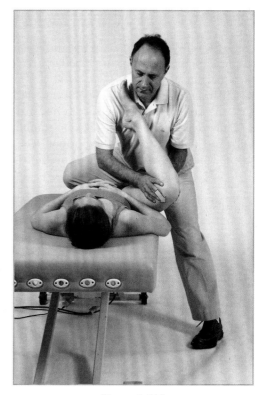

Figure 6-36C

- Adduction increases the stretch to the more laterally located fibers (Fig. 6-36D).

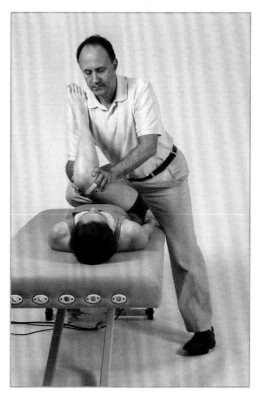

Figure 6-36D

- If medial rotation is added, it increases the stretch to the gluteal muscles.
- If lateral rotation is added, it decreases the stretch to the gluteal muscles, thereby allowing a better stretch of the adductor magnus.
- Frontal and transverse plane components can be combined to focus the stretch more specifically toward certain fibers. Figure 6-36E demonstrates flexion combined with adduction and medial rotation. This position preferentially stretches the upper fibers of the gluteus maximus.

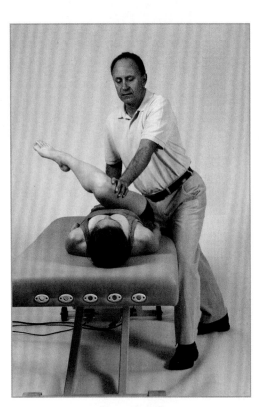

Figure 6-36E

- *Note*: If knee-to-chest stretch is performed and transitioned into a multiplanar stretch by adding in adduction, lateral rotation, or both, it begins to target the deep lateral rotator group of the hip joint (see Routine 6-10).
- After performing the appropriate stretches as indicated for the right side, switch to the left side of the client's body and perform these stretches there. Figure 6-36F demonstrates the initial stretch to the gluteal group performed on the client's left side.

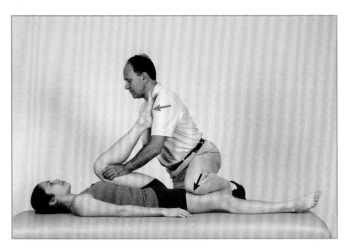

Figure 6-36F

6.7	THERAPIST TIP

Stretching the Hip Joint Ligaments

This chapter concerns itself primarily with stretching musculature. But, as stated previously, stretches create a line of tension that lengthens all soft tissues. As a whole, the ligament complex of the hip joint is pulled taut with extension as well as medial rotation and abduction. Therefore, if you do a multiplane stretch of the hip joint into these motions, you will be placing a stretch into the ligament complex. If the hip joints' ability to move into these ranges of motion is limited because the ligaments of the joint are taut, this stretch could be a very beneficial toward restoring healthy range of motion.

ROUTINE 6-10: HIP DEEP LATERAL ROTATORS

The deep lateral rotator group of the hip joint is composed of the piriformis, superior and inferior gemelli, obturator internus and externus, and the quadratus femoris (Fig. 6-37). This group is located on the posterior side of the pelvis, crossing the hip joint with a horizontal direction to their fibers to attach to the femur.

You can generalize and say that the gluteal musculature runs primarily vertically, and for that reason, it is oriented differently from the fiber direction of the deep lateral rotators; therefore, a separate stretching routine is presented here. However, they really are not that different; rather, there is a gradual transition in fiber direction from the gluteals to the deep lateral rotators (see the relationship of the posterior fibers of the gluteus medius and the piriformis; Fig. 1-16). This is evidenced by the fact that, as mentioned previously, the knee-to-chest stretch for the gluteals easily transitions into a stretch for the deep lateral rotators (see Fig. 6-36).

Following are two routines for stretching the right-sided deep lateral rotator group using horizontal adduction of the thigh and the Figure 4 stretch.

*As a group, the deep lateral rotators laterally rotate the thigh at the hip joint and contralaterally rotate the pelvis at the hip joint. If the thigh is first flexed to 90 degrees, the deep lateral rotators can horizontally abduct (horizontally extend) the thigh at the hip joint. **Note:** If the thigh is first flexed (approximately 60 degrees of more), the piriformis changes to become a medial rotator of the thigh at the hip joint instead of a lateral rotator.*

Stretch #1: Horizontal Adduction

- Have the client supine toward the left side of the table.
- Position yourself at the left side of the table.
- Bring the client's right hip and knee joints into flexion and then horizontally adduct the right thigh at the hip joint and trap the client's right knee between your trunk and right arm, in other words, under your right axillary region.
- No stabilization hand is necessary; the client's body weight and contact with the table stabilizes his pelvis.
- Using core body weight, gently lean into the client, bringing his thigh down and across his chest, farther into horizontal adduction (Fig. 6-38A). Be sure that the client's pelvis remains stabilized down onto the table.
- It is beneficial to purposely vary the exact degree of flexion versus horizontal adduction of the client's thigh to catch as many angles as possible between a pure flexion knee-to-chest stretch and a pure horizontal adduction stretch across the client's body (Fig. 6-38B, C). Each different angle will preferentially stretch different directions of fibers of the deep lateral rotator group and musculature of the posterior buttock in general.
- After performing the appropriate stretches as indicated for the right side, switch to the left side of the client's body and perform these stretches there (Fig. 6-38D).

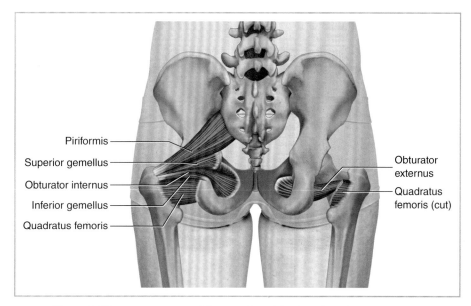

Figure 6-37 Posterior view of the muscles of the deep lateral rotator group.

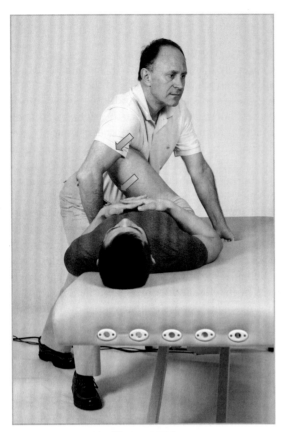

Figure 6-38A

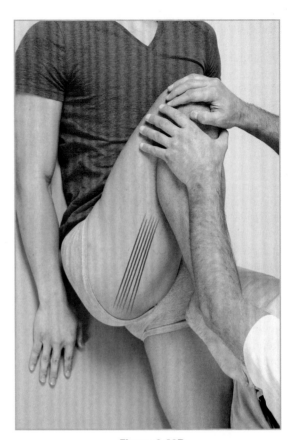

Figure 6-38B

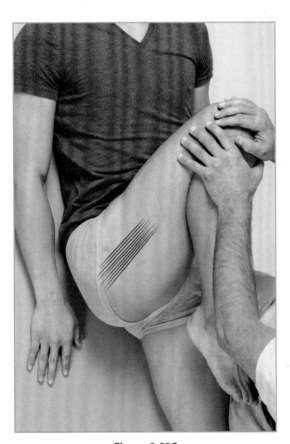

Figure 6-38C

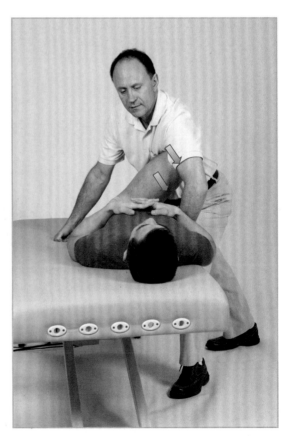

Figure 6-38D

Deep Lateral Rotator Stretch and Groin Pain

The direction that you move the client's thigh during the deep lateral rotator horizontal adduction stretch is extremely important. If the direction is too horizontal (parallel with the table), the client's pelvis will no longer be stabilized and will lift from the table, causing the stretch to travel into the LSp and be lost to the target musculature of the pelvis. However, if you press the client's thigh too downward, it may compress the anterior hip joint region (groin) and cause discomfort or pain for the client. The ideal direction to press the thigh is as downward into the chest as possible without causing pain, or conversely, it could be looked at as being as horizontal as possible without

allowing the pelvis to lift from the table. The exact degree of this ideal direction will vary from client to client. If it is impossible to find an angle that both stabilizes the client's pelvis and keeps the client pain-free, then you can use your hands to grasp the client's proximal femur and soft tissue of the proximal thigh and traction the thigh away from the pelvis (**Fig. A**). This often removes the pinching discomfort/pain that clients experience. If the client is being instructed to do this stretch as part of self-care, then it can be beneficial to place a small cushion or towel in the crease of the pelvis/thigh to make space in this area to decrease the pinching discomfort/pain (**Fig. B**).

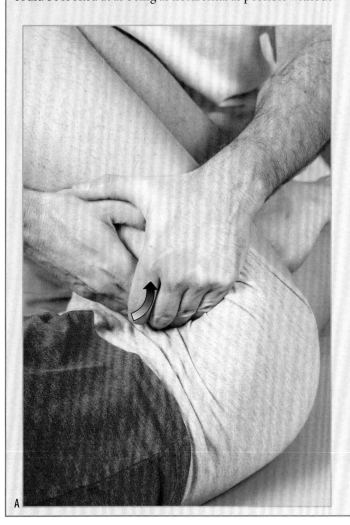 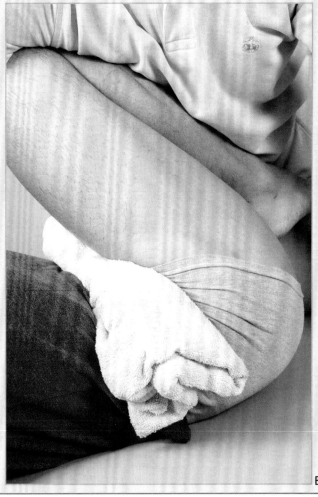

 As previously mentioned, placing pressure through an unhealthy knee joint can be difficult and painful for the client. However, the stretch can be modified to obviate pressure to the knee joint by instead placing and resting the client's leg on your shoulder.

Stretch #2: Figure 4

- Have the client supine toward the right side of the table.
- Position yourself at the right side of the table.
- Flex and laterally rotate the client's right hip joint and flex his right knee joint and place his distal right leg on his flexed left thigh. This forms the Figure 4 position for which the stretch is named.
- Both of your hands are treatment hands. Place your left hand on the posterior surface of his distal right thigh, and place your right hand on the posterior surface of his distal left thigh (Fig. 6-39A).

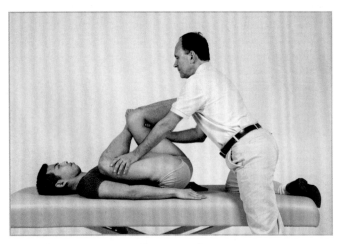

Figure 6-39A

- No stabilization hand is necessary; the client's body weight and contact with the table stabilize his pelvis.
- Using core body weight, gently lean forward into the client, pressing equally with both hands and bringing his laterally rotated right thigh farther into flexion, in other words, down toward his chest (Fig. 6-39B). Be sure that the direction of your pressure is such that the client's pelvis remains stabilized down onto the table.

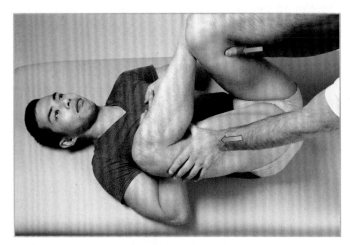

Figure 6-39B

- After performing the appropriate stretches as indicated for the right side, switch to the left side of the client's body and perform these stretches there (Fig. 6-39C).

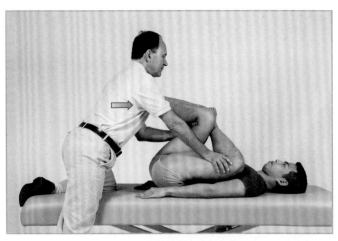

Figure 6-39C

CHAPTER SUMMARY

Stretching is an invaluable treatment tool when working with clients who have tight muscles and other taut soft tissues. However, a typical stretch often creates a line of tension that spreads across an entire functional group of muscles. Multiplane stretching is a technique that allows the therapist to focus a stretch specifically on the desired target muscle. It also optimizes the effectiveness of the stretch of the target muscle by stretching it across all its planes of action. Performing multiplane stretching for a target muscle is easy and straightforward because it involves simply stretching the client's LSp or pelvis into the opposite action of each and every one of the mover actions of the target muscle being stretched.

CASE STUDY

FELIX

■ History and Physical Assessment

A new client, Felix Madison, age 53 years, comes to your office complaining of pain and stiffness in his right hip and tightness across his low back. He tells you that he has been experiencing pain and stiffness for 3 weeks. Because he is a nurse, his hip and low back pain has made it difficult to work. He was referred to you by his fitness trainer because the trainer heard that you are skilled at working with low back problems and stretching techniques.

You perform a thorough client history, which reveals that he has had multiple low back sports injuries when he was younger and played lacrosse in high school. Since high school, he has had occasional episodes of hip tightness and pain as well as low back tightness, but these episodes have never lasted more than a few days. His present episode is more intense and is not going away. It began during a vacation in which he was walking many hours each day.

Felix has seen his massage therapist twice now. In the past, massage has always helped to loosen his hip and low back and eliminate the pain and stiffness, but this time, the relief has only been temporary. Felix also has a regular stretching routine that he does whenever his low back and hip act up. These stretches also usually help, but this time they have not. At this point, his current episode of stiffness and pain has not improved, and he is very discouraged.

Postural examination shows that Felix has a mildly excessive anterior tilt of his pelvis with a concomitantly increased lumbar lordosis. Your LSp range of motion assessment shows that left lateral flexion is decreased by 10 degrees, and flexion is decreased by 15 degrees. His right hip joint range of motion assessment shows that extension and adduction are decreased on the right side compared to the left side and also cause mild pain in the front of his right hip. Manual resistance to right hip joint flexion and abduction reproduces the characteristic pain that he has been experiencing in the front of the right hip. You perform active and passive straight leg raise, Nachlas', and Yeoman's tests and ask the client to perform the cough test and Valsalva maneuver, all of which produce negative results (for a review of assessment procedures, see Chapter 3).

Palpatory examination reveals that his hip flexors on the right side are all mildly tight, but his TFL is markedly tight and is the source of his anterior hip pain. His adductors and hamstrings are fine. In the low back, his erector spinae musculature is moderately tight, with his right side tighter than the left side. The gluteal musculature, deep lateral rotators, and quadratus lumborum muscles bilaterally are all within normal limits of tone.

At the end of the examination, you ask him to show you the stretches that he has been doing. He demonstrates single knee-to-chest and double knee-to-chest for his low back and a lunge stretch for his hip flexors as well as stretches for his hamstrings and quadriceps femoris. You note that when he shows you the lunge stretch, his right thigh is abducted as he performs the stretch.

■ Think-It-Through Questions:

1. Should you include a multiplane stretching technique in your treatment plan for Felix? Why, or why not?
2. If multiplane stretching would be of value, is it safe to use with him? If yes, how do you know?
3. If you do perform multiplane stretching, which specific stretching routines should you do? Why?

Answers to these Think-It-Through Questions and the Treatment Strategy employed for this client are available online at thePoint.lww.com/MuscolinoLowBack

OBJECTIVES

After completing this chapter, the student should be able to:

1. Explain why contract relax (CR) stretching is also known as proprioceptive neuromuscular facilitation stretching and/or postisometric relaxation stretching.
2. Describe the mechanism of CR stretching.
3. Describe in steps an overview of the usual protocol for carrying out the CR stretching technique.
4. Describe the roles of the treatment hand and the stabilization hand.
5. Explain why the client may perform either an isometric or concentric contraction during a CR stretch.
6. Describe the usual breathing protocol for the client during the CR stretching technique.
7. Explain why stretching should never be performed too fast or too far.
8. Define each key term in this chapter and explain its relationship to the CR stretching technique.
9. Perform the CR stretching technique for each of the muscle groups presented in this chapter.

KEY TERMS

assisted CR stretching
contract relax (CR) stretching
Golgi tendon organ (GTO) reflex
lengthened active insufficiency

muscle spindle reflex
postisometric relaxation (PIR) stretching
preset the rotation

proprioceptive neuromuscular facilitation (PNF) stretching
resistance hand
stabilization hand

stretch reflex
stretching hand
treatment hand
unassisted CR stretching

INTRODUCTION

Contract relax (CR) stretching is a stretching technique in which the client first *contracts* and then *relaxes* the target muscle to be stretched, hence the name. CR stretching has classically been stated to utilize the proprioceptive neurologic reflex known as the **Golgi tendon organ (GTO) reflex** (also addressed in Chapter 9) to facilitate the stretch of the target muscle. For this reason, it is also known as **proprioceptive neuromuscular facilitation (PNF) stretching**. It is also known as **postisometric relaxation (PIR) stretching** because the client usually performs an isometric contraction of the target muscle, followed by relaxation. Because CR stretching involves a neurologic re-flex to facilitate the stretch, it is considered to be an advanced form of stretching; in addition, it is usually more effective than standard mechanical stretching alone. The beauty of CR stretching is that once a therapist is familiar and comfortable with the mechanism that underlies it, almost any stretch can be converted into a CR stretch. CR stretching is especially useful for clients whose problem is chronic and stubborn and does not respond well to standard stretching.

MECHANISM

The classically proposed physiologic mechanism that underlies CR stretching is the GTO reflex, which is a protective reflex that prevents a muscle's tendon from being torn. CR stretching is a technique that allows the therapist to make use of this reflex to facilitate stretching clients.

Note: In the Technique and Self-Care chapters of this book (Chapters 4 to 12), green arrows indicate movement, red arrows indicate stabilization, and black arrows indicate a position that is statically held.

When a muscle is contracted, the GTO reflex sends inhibitory signals to the muscle, causing it to relax. This is why the first step in the CR stretch procedure is usually to have the client isometrically contract the target muscle against the therapist's resistance. The client typically holds the isometric contraction against resistance for approximately 5 to 8 seconds. When the client relaxes the target muscle, the therapist can passively move the client's body part farther because the GTO reflex has inhibited the target muscle. This allows for a greater stretch of the target muscle than would otherwise be possible. This procedure is usually repeated three to four times. *Note*: It should be mentioned that there is controversy whether the GTO reflex is the operative mechanism of CR stretching.

CR stretching is usually performed with the client isometrically contracting the target muscle because this creates maximal tension in the muscle to trigger the GTO reflex. However, the client can concentrically contract the target muscle instead. Both methods are effective. The choice of whether to have the client perform the contraction isometrically or concentrically is best based on the client's comfort (this book consistently demonstrates it as an isometric contraction). *Note*: Your hand that resists the client's contraction and performs the stretch of the client is known as the **treatment hand**; it is also known as the

---

BOX 7.1

Contract Relax Routines

The following CR stretching routines are presented in this chapter:
- Section 1: lumbar spine (LSp) contract relax stretches:
    - Routine 7-1—LSp extensors
    - Routine 7-2—LSp flexors
    - Routine 7-3—LSp right lateral flexors
    - Routine 7-4—LSp left lateral flexors
    - Routine 7-5—LSp right rotators—seated
    - Routine 7-6—LSp left rotators—seated
- Section 2: hip joint/pelvis contract relax stretches:
    - Routine 7-7—hip abductors
    - Routine 7-8—hip adductors
    - Routine 7-9—hip flexors
    - Routine 7-10—hip extensors: hamstrings
    - Routine 7-11—hip extensors: gluteals
    - Routine 7-12—hip deep lateral rotators
    - Routine 7-13—hip medial rotators

BOX 7.2

Golgi Tendon Organ Reflex

The GTO reflex is a proprioceptive neurologic reflex that protects the tendons of a muscle from tearing. The force of the contraction of the muscle belly is transmitted to its bony attachments by pulling on its tendons. If this contraction is too great, the pulling force may tear the tendon. The GTO reflex works to prevent this by monitoring the tension (stretch) within a tendon. If the stretch is too great, the GTO reflex sends a signal into the spinal cord via a sensory neuron, which synapses with an interneuron that inhibits the (alpha) lower motor neurons (LMNs) that control that muscle. Inhibition of a muscle's LMNs results in relaxation of the muscle, thereby relieving the force on its tendon (see accompanying figure). Therapists can take advantage of the GTO reflex through CR stretching by asking the client to begin by contracting the target muscle. If the contraction is sufficiently strong, it triggers the GTO reflex so that the target muscle is inhibited and relaxed. The target muscle can then be stretched farther than it otherwise would have been.

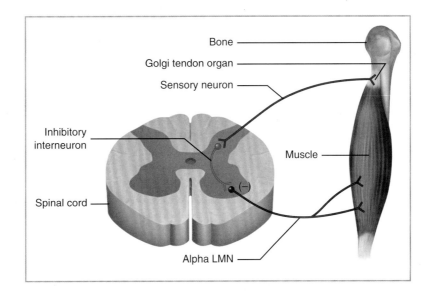

stretching hand or **resistance hand**. Your other hand is used as a **stabilization hand** to stabilize the client's pelvis and/or trunk.

OVERVIEW OF TECHNIQUE

If the GTO reflex is the scientific principle that underlies CR stretching, then the manner in which it is carried out is its art. The following is an overview of the CR stretching technique using the right hamstring muscle group as the target muscle group being stretched. The following overview of the CR stretching technique protocol describes **assisted CR stretching** in which the client is stretched with the assistance of a therapist. However, it is often possible for a client to perform **unassisted CR stretching** without the assistance of a therapist. For more on unassisted CR stretching, refer to Chapter 11 (available online at thePoint.lww.com).

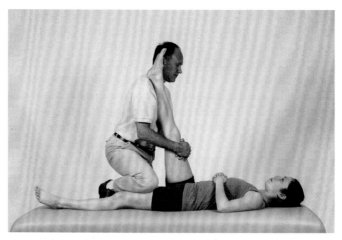

Figure 7-1 Starting position for CR stretching of the right hamstring muscle group. Note that the therapist's elbows are tucked in.

> ### 7.1   THERAPIST TIP
>
> #### Communication with the Client
>
> Because CR stretching involves a number of steps and utilizes a specific breathing pattern, it is best to practice it before working with clients. The first time you perform CR stretching on a client who has never done it before, it can also be helpful to start by giving the client a brief overview of how CR stretching is done. Explain that the client will need to press against your resistance and then relax as you perform the stretch. Tell the client approximately how long to press against your resistance and how many repetitions there will be. Describe the breathing protocol as well. This will allow the client to give informed verbal consent before you begin the technique and also will make it easier to carry out the CR protocol once you begin.

Starting Position:

- The client is supine and positioned as far to the right side of the table as possible; you are standing at the right side of the table.
- The client's right thigh is flexed at the hip joint with her right leg extended at the knee joint; her right leg is placed on your right shoulder.
- Both of your hands are treatment hands and are placed on the anterior surface of the client's distal right thigh.
- Your right knee is the stabilization contact and is placed on the anterior surface of the client's left thigh.
- Note that your elbows are tucked in front of your body so that you can use your core body weight behind your forearms and hands when pressing on the client with your treatment hands (Fig. 7-1).

Alternative Positions:

Four alternative positions are commonly used.

- The first is to instead place only one treatment hand (usually the left hand) on the anterior surface of the client's

distal right thigh; the other (right) treatment hand is placed on the posterior surface of the client's right leg. This assists in keeping the client's knee joint extended during the stretch (Fig. 7-2A).

- The second is to use your right hand instead of your right knee to stabilize her left thigh/pelvis (Fig. 7-2B).
- A third position is to place your right hand on the plantar surface of the client's right foot. This is done to increase the client's stretch by dorsiflexing the foot at the ankle joint (Fig. 7-2C). Dorsiflexing the foot will stretch the gastrocnemius musculature, which, via its myofascial attachment into the hamstrings, will increase the tension and therefore the stretch to the hamstrings.

> ### 7.2   THERAPIST TIP
>
> #### Stabilizing the Client's Pelvis
>
> When stretching musculature that crosses the client's hip joint, the thigh is moved and the pelvis must be stabilized because if the pelvis is allowed to move, the line of tension of the stretch will extend into the LSp, and the stretch across the hip joint will be lost. To stabilize the pelvis, the direction of the stabilization pressure must be opposite of how the pelvis would have moved (had it not been stabilized). When stretching the right hamstrings, as they are lengthened and pulled taut, they will exert a pull on the right side of the pelvis toward posterior tilt; this will pull the right pelvic bone and indeed the entire pelvis into posterior tilt. Therefore, to stabilize and prevent posterior tilt of the pelvis, you would need to exert a force toward anterior tilt. The problem is that with the client supine, there is no easy way to contact the pelvis to accomplish this. What can be done instead is indirectly stabilize the pelvis from posteriorly tilting by contacting the client's left thigh. Had the pelvis posteriorly tilted, the client's left thigh would have lifted off the table. By placing your knee on the client's left anterior thigh, you hold the left thigh down, which prevents the pelvis from posteriorly tilting. Therefore, the pelvis is stabilized.

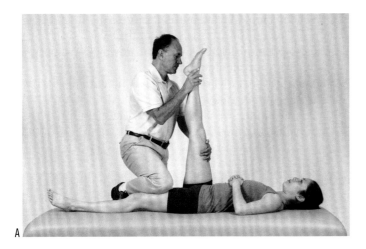
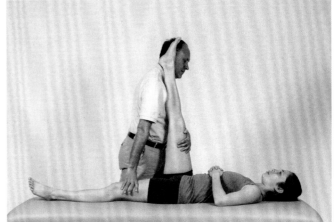
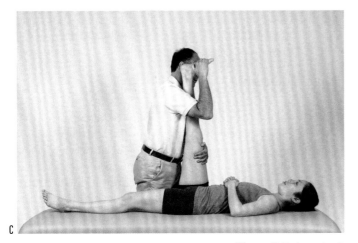
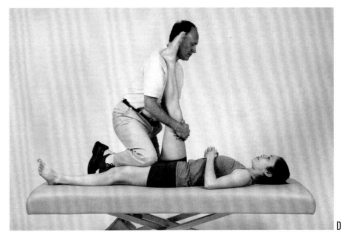

Figure 7-2 (**A–D**) Alternative starting positions.

- The fourth position is to actually climb up onto the table so that you can position your trunk/core directly in line with the force that the client will be creating. Using your core in this manner is the most efficient position for body mechanics. If this position is used, it is better to have the client supine toward the middle of the table instead of the side; this gives you more room to comfortably position your body on the table. Of course, before climbing on the table, be sure that the table can support the weight of both you and the client (Fig. 7-2D).

If when stretching the hamstrings, the client's knee joint flexes, the hamstrings will slacken, and the tension of the stretch will be lost. For this reason, the client's knee joint must remain extended during the entire stretch. However, it is important to not allow or force the client's knee joint to hyperextend.

7.3 THERAPIST TIP

Using Your Core

It may seem uncomfortable at first to tuck your elbows in front of your body. However, with a little practice, this position will become comfortable. It is well worth it because the advantage of this position is that you can use your core strength to resist the client's contraction and to stabilize the client instead of overtaxing the musculature of your shoulder. For overweight therapists and large-breasted female therapists, if it is difficult to tuck your elbows in front of your body, the closer you can place them to being in front of your core, the better. If you find that it is difficult to get both of your elbows in front, then focus on getting the one in front that requires the most effort. With some clients, this may be the treatment hand; with other clients, it may be the stabilization hand. Consciously laterally rotating your arms at the glenohumeral joints helps you to keep your elbows in. Once you have practiced this position for a little while, it will come naturally.

Placing the client's leg against your shoulder directly engages your core in the performance of this stretch and allows for even greater strength and efficiency of body mechanics.

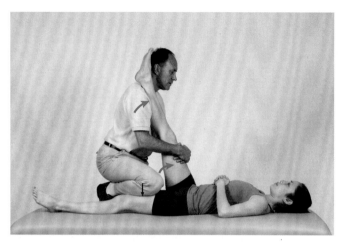

Figure 7-3 Initial stretch of the client's right thigh into flexion at the hip joint by the therapist. Note that the client's right knee remains extended.

Initial Client Stretch:

- Gently stretch the client's target (right hamstring) musculature by moving the client's thigh into flexion until you meet tissue resistance. *Note*: Make sure that the client's knee joint stays extended.
- This begins the stretch of the target hamstring muscles (Fig. 7-3).
- Note that your right knee acts as the stabilization contact, holding down and stabilizing the client's left thigh. Stabilizing the left thigh acts to stabilize the pelvis

First Repetition, Step 1: Client Contraction:

- In this position of stretch of the target muscles, ask the client to inhale and then gently isometrically contract the target muscles for approximately 5 to 8 seconds against the resistance of your treatment hands (and/or shoulder).

The client should be attempting to press the thigh down into extension toward the table against your resistance and also press the leg toward flexion down against the resistance of your shoulder.

- This engages the GTO reflex, which inhibits and therefore relaxes the target muscles.
- In this example, the client isometrically contracts the right hamstring muscle group, attempting to return the right lower extremity back to anatomic position (Fig. 7-4A).
- The breathing protocol for every repetition is to have the client either hold the breath or exhale when contracting against your resistance.

| 7.4 | **THERAPIST TIP** |

Counting Down

While the client is contracting for 5 to 8 seconds, some therapists like to encourage the client to keep contracting by gently repeating something like *resist* or *keep contracting*. Other therapists like to count down as the client contracts. This can be done by asking the client to contract and then gently counting out loud starting with the number of seconds that you want the client to contract for. For example, you might say *contract, 7, 6, 5, 4, 3, 2, 1, relax*. Or you may begin with words to encourage the client's contraction and then complete the time with the remainder of the countdown, such as *resist . . . that's it . . . keep contracting . . . 3, 2, 1, relax*. The advantage to counting down is that the client knows how long he or she will have to continue contracting.

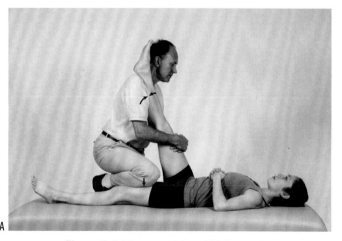
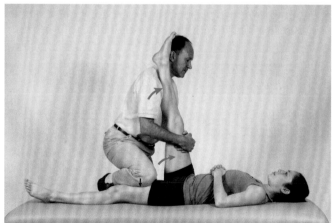

Figure 7-4 First repetition. **(A)** Step 1: Isometric contraction of the client's right hamstring musculature against the resistance of the therapist. **(B)** Step 2: After contracting, the client relaxes and is stretched farther into flexion by the therapist.

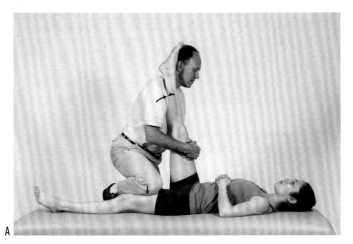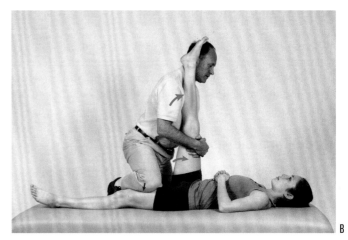

Figure 7-5 Second repetition. **(A)** Step 1: Contraction by the client. **(B)** Step 2: Further stretch of the client.

First Repetition, Step 2: Postcontraction Stretch:

- The client relaxes, and you passively stretch the target muscle group farther until you feel tissue resistance.
- Hold this position of stretch for approximately 1 to 3 seconds.
- Because of the GTO reflex, the target muscle group will be better stretched than would have been possible otherwise.
- In this example, the client's right thigh is moved farther into flexion (Fig. 7-4B).

Second Repetition:

- Beginning from the position of stretch attained at the end of the first repetition, perform a second repetition by repeating steps 1 and 2 (Fig. 7-5).
- This time, the client's isometric contraction (again held for approximately 5 to 8 seconds) can be moderately strong.
- When the client relaxes, gently increase the stretch of the client's target musculature by moving the right thigh farther into flexion until you meet tissue resistance.

Third Repetition:

- Beginning from the position of stretch attained at the end of the second repetition, perform a third repetition by repeating steps 1 and 2 (Fig. 7-6).
- This time, the client's isometric contraction (again held for approximately 5 to 8 seconds) can be as strong as is comfortable for the client.
- When the client relaxes, gently increase the stretch of the client's target musculature by moving the right thigh farther into flexion until you meet tissue resistance.
- *Note*: If desired, a fourth repetition could be performed, following the same steps.
- Once the final position of stretch is reached at the end of the last CR repetition, many therapists like to hold this position of stretch for a longer period, often 10 to 20 seconds or more.
- *Note*: It is extremely important that the client's right knee joint is never allowed to move into flexion during this entire routine. If this occurs, hamstring tension will be lost and they will not be stretched as well.

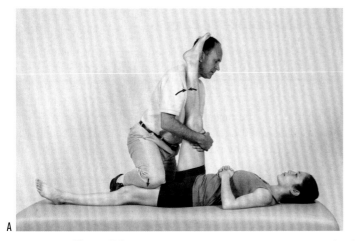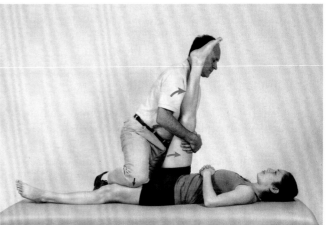

Figure 7-6 Third repetition. **(A)** Step 1: Contraction by the client. **(B)** Step 2: Further stretch of the client. Note the increased range of motion attained compared to the first two repetitions.

PERFORMING THE TECHNIQUE

When performing CR stretching, it is important to keep the following in mind: Each point addresses a specific aspect of the CR stretching technique. Understanding and applying the following guidelines will help you perform CR stretches more effectively.

7.1 Contraction: Increase Gradually

The goal for each successive CR stretch repetition is to build on the previous one so that the degree of stretch achieved gradually increases. This can be achieved by increasing the degree of the client's strength of contraction gradually. For example, if you ask the client to perform three repetitions, do the following:

- For the first repetition, ask the client to contract gently as you offer mild resistance.
- For the second repetition, ask the client to contract with moderate strength against your resistance.
- For the third (and perhaps fourth) repetition, ask the client to contract the target muscle as forcefully as is comfortable.

However, you should never ask the client to contract more forcefully than he or she is comfortable. The strength of the client's contraction against your resistance is not as important as performing the stretching protocol comfortably and smoothly.

*If the client contracts too forcefully or too suddenly, a pulled or torn muscle is possible. It may be helpful to tell the client, "Contract more forcefully, build up to it slowly so you don't hurt yourself, but contract as hard as you **comfortably** can."*

7.2 Resistance: Your Role

When you offer resistance as the client contracts isometrically, remember that it is not a contest between you and the client. It is your role to meet the client's resistance, not exceed it. Thus, you must equal whatever force the client generates so that the contraction of the client's target muscle is isometric. When you tell the client to relax, it is also important that you immediately ease off your pressure so that the client's body is not suddenly pushed into the stretch.

7.3 Position: Monitor the Client

Although it is customary to begin the resistance of each successive repetition from wherever the stretch of the previous repetition ended, it is not necessary. Sometimes, if the client's target muscle is greatly stretched and elongated, it can be difficult or uncomfortable for the client to contract the target muscle from that position. The principle of **lengthened active insufficiency** explains this difficulty. Lengthened active insufficiency is when a lengthened muscle contracts and the strength of its contraction is weakened because fewer actin–myosin crossbridges can be formed in the sarcomeres of its stretched muscle fibers than when the sarcomeres are at resting length. Asking a client to

7.5 | **THERAPIST TIP**

Bracing Your Core

If you find that the client is contracting so forcefully that you feel overpowered, perhaps because you are small and the client is large, you can usually remedy this by focusing on bringing your elbow in front of your core. This positions your body weight behind your forearm and hand. If this is still insufficient, try placing a foot behind you on the floor in the line of force so that you can engage your lower extremity muscles to brace your core. When possible, climb on the table to more directly place your core in the line of force of the stretch.

contract against your resistance under these circumstances might actually reduce the effectiveness of the GTO reflex and minimize the benefit of the stretch. It is often better to bring the client's thigh back to a more neutral (closer to anatomic) position to begin the client's contraction for the next repetition.

Even when you begin a new repetition with the client's thigh in the position of stretch attained in the previous repetition, if you allow the client to perform a concentric contraction instead of an isometric one, then the position of stretch attained in the previous repetition will be lessened or lost. Although this might not seem desirable, it is perfectly fine. The point of the CR stretching technique is that the client contracts the target musculature, thereby initiating the GTO reflex to inhibit and relax the target musculature so that it can then be stretched effectively. Whatever position facilitates the client being able to comfortably contract the target musculature is efficient for CR stretching. For the sake of consistency, each of the CR stretches demonstrated in this book shows each successive repetition beginning from the ending position of the previous repetition's stretch. When using this technique in your practice, this aspect of the stretch should be applied in the manner that is most comfortable and effective for your client.

7.4 Stretch: Slow and Easy

When stretching the client's target musculature, whether at the beginning of the technique or at the end of each of the repetitions, it is extremely important to perform the stretch slowly and never force it. If a target muscle is stretched too fast or too far, the **muscle spindle reflex**, also known as the **stretch reflex** may be triggered, causing a spasm of the target muscle, defeating the purpose of the stretch (for more on the muscle spindle reflex, see Chapter 2). Therefore, stretching should always be performed slowly and within the comfort zone of the client. It is important to emphasize that when you begin to feel the client's target tissues offering resistance to your stretch, stop increasing the stretch. Because three to four repetitions are performed, gaining a small incrementally increased stretch at each repetition will allow for a good degree of stretch at the end of the CR stretching technique.

7.5 Hand Placement: Treatment and Stabilization Hands

When performing CR stretching technique, it is important to place the treatment hand in a comfortable manner for the client. To do this, offer as broad a contact with your hand as possible so that the pressure of your hand against the client's body is distributed as evenly as possible when the client contracts. This is especially true if the stabilization contact is against a prominent bony landmark such as the anterior superior iliac spine (ASIS) or iliac crest of the pelvis (see Routines 7-7, 7-8, and 7-9).

The position of the stabilization contact is also critical. Without proper positioning, the client's pelvis will often move in such a manner as to lose the stretch of the target hip joint musculature. Placement of your stabilization hand should also be comfortable for the client and offer as broad a contact as possible.

The placement of the treatment and stabilization hands may place your wrist joints in an extended position. For the health of your wrists, your point of contact through which pressure is transmitted into the client should be the heel of your hand (the carpal region). If you direct the pressure through your palm or fingers, you will hyperextend and likely injure your wrist. Given how vulnerable the wrist joint can be, proper biomechanical positioning of the hand/wrist is crucially important.

7.6 Breathing

When performing CR stretching, it is customary for the client to inhale deeply before contracting isometrically in step 1 of the technique. During the isometric contraction, the client can either hold the breath or exhale. If the client holds the breath while contracting isometrically, then the client should exhale it when you perform the stretch in step 2. If the client exhales during the isometric contraction, then the client should continue to exhale when you perform the stretch in step 2 (if the client does not have sufficient breath to continuously breathe out while contracting and then being stretched, you can pause after the contraction for a second or two so that the client can take in another breath, which is then exhaled while being stretched). Either way, the client must then inhale again just before the beginning of the isometric contraction of the next repetition. It is generally considered better for the client to exhale instead of holding in the breath when contracting isometrically in step 2 because continuous breathing ensures better circulation of oxygenated blood to the tissues. *Note*: If CR stretching is combined with agonist contract (AC) stretching to perform contract relax agonist contract (CRAC) stretching (see Chapter 9), the client must hold the breath during the CR aspect of the protocol when isometrically contracting.

Choosing the Breathing Protocol

Given that there are two choices for how the client can breathe during the CR stretch technique, how do you decide which one to have the client do? Generally, it is considered best to have the client breathe out when pressing against your resistance. However, if you anticipate also performing CRAC stretching with that client, whether it is during that treatment session or in the future, then it may be best to instruct the client to hold his or her breath when resisting you. Otherwise, the client will need to relearn the breathing pattern for the CR component of CRAC stretching. Following one breathing pattern for CR stretching and another pattern for the CR component of CRAC stretching might be confusing.

7.7 Direction of Resistance

You can offer resistance either in a cardinal plane or in an oblique plane. The three cardinal planes are the sagittal, frontal, and transverse planes; an oblique plane is any plane that is not perfectly sagittal, frontal, or transverse (in other words, it has a component of two or three cardinal planes). Figure 1-8 in Chapter 1 provides a review of planes. When the client performs an oblique plane contraction, it is usually a "diagonal" motion that combines flexion or extension in the sagittal plane with either abduction or adduction of the thigh or right or left lateral flexion of the trunk in the frontal plane. Transverse plane rotation is usually not coupled with motion in another plane when doing CR stretching. It can be confusing to the client to ask him or her to rotate in the transverse plane while moving in another cardinal plane or oblique plane. It can also be difficult for you to resist transverse plane rotation because the twisting motion is harder to resist with your hand. In addition, if the rotation motion is not well resisted, it will pull on the client's skin in an uncomfortable way. Therefore, whenever rotation is involved with a multiplane stretch, it is best to **preset the rotation** during the starting position. This way, the client does not have to try to isometrically contract toward rotation in addition to the sagittal and/or frontal plane directions.

Adding transverse plane rotation into oblique plane stretches when performing CR stretching with your clients requires practice. It is best to practice the CR stretching routines presented in this chapter before adding in multiplane rotation components.

7.8 Electric Lift Table

As discussed in Chapter 6, when stretching the low back and pelvis/hip joint, the value of an electric lift table for optimal body mechanics cannot be overstated. Some routines require the table to be low and others require it to be high. For this reason, having an electric lift table so that table height can be easily adjusted is essential for clinical orthopedic work.

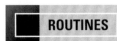

ROUTINES

CONTRACT RELAX ROUTINES

The routines that follow demonstrate 13 different applications of CR stretching to the LSp and to the muscle groups of the pelvis that cross the hip joint. They are organized according to the functional groups of muscles being stretched. The routine for the hamstring hip joint extensors has already been shown in the "Overview of Technique" section. For all the other routines, the following steps are explained and illustrated: starting position, initial client stretch, first repetition, and second repetition. An explanation is then given on how to perform the third and possibly fourth repetitions.

Because many of these stretches are identical or similar in positioning to stretches presented in Chapter 6, the reader is recommended to consult first that chapter for additional information, including alternate positioning and cautions, before reading and practicing the stretches presented in this chapter.

7.1　**PRACTICAL APPLICATION**

Lumbar Spine and Pelvis/Hip Joint Contract Relax Multiplane Stretching Routines

This chapter explains how to perform the CR stretching technique and then presents this technique applied to each of the major functional groups of muscles of the LSp and pelvis/hip joint. However, the CR technique can be applied to any stretch, including the multiplane stretches presented in Chapter 6. A number of multiplane stretches for the CR routines of this chapter are presented in Practical Application boxes that follow the CR stretching routine steps. Keep in mind that any stretch, including multiplane stretches, can be done with the CR protocol. All that is necessary to transition a stretch into a CR stretch is to add in client contraction against your resistance and then the postcontraction stretching.

SECTION 1: LUMBAR SPINE CONTRACT RELAX STRETCHES

CR stretches of the LSp can be performed in two ways. One way is to stabilize the client's pelvis and move his or her upper trunk downward toward the pelvis. This method begins the stretch of the LSp superiorly, and as the stretching force is increased and the LSp is increasingly moved downward, the stretch moves into the lower LSp. The second way is to stabilize the client's upper trunk and move his or her pelvis and lower LSp upward toward the thoracic trunk. This method begins the stretch of the LSp inferiorly, and as the stretching force is increased and the pelvis and lower spine are increasingly moved upward, the stretch moves into the upper LSp.

The following CR stretching routines for the LSp are presented in this chapter:

- Routine 7-1—LSp extensors
- Routine 7-2—LSp flexors
- Routine 7-3—LSp right lateral flexors
- Routine 7-4—LSp left lateral flexors
- Routine 7-5—LSp right rotators—seated
- Routine 7-6 —LSp left rotators—seated

7.7　**THERAPIST TIP**

Transitioning to the Thoracic Spine

Every one of the stretches presented for the LSp can be transitioned to become a stretch of the thoracic spine if the movement and/or stabilization are changed so that the line of tension of the stretch enters the thoracic region.

ROUTINE 7-1: LUMBAR SPINE EXTENSORS

Figure 7-7 shows the functional group of muscles that extend the LSp. These muscles are located on the posterior side of the trunk in the lumbar region. The CR stretching routine presented here is essentially the double knee-to-chest stretch that is presented in Chapter 11 (Self-Care Routine 11-6; available online at thePoint.lww.com), with the CR stretching protocol added.

The Lumbar Spine Extensor Functional Group
This functional group comprises the following muscles bilaterally:
Erector spinae group
Transversospinalis group
Quadratus lumborum

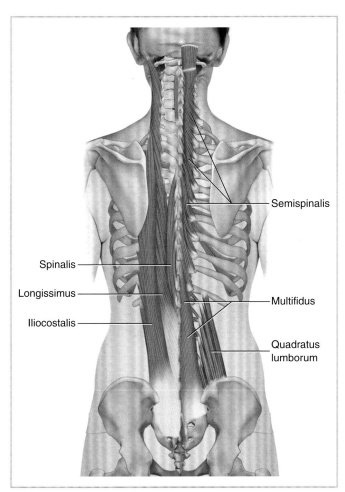

Figure 7-7

Starting Position:

- The client is supine with his hip and knee joints flexed. If you are standing on the right side of the table (as shown in Fig. 7-8A), his feet are on your right clavicle. Your left foot is on the floor; your right lower extremity is positioned on the table to be in line with the force of the stroke.

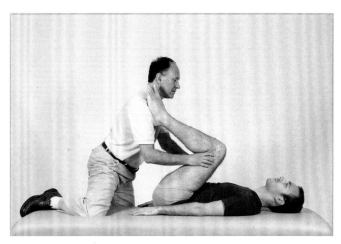

Figure 7-8A

- *Note*: This stretching routine could also be performed from the other (left) side of the table. Simply reverse the positioning of your lower extremities and on which clavicle the client places his feet.
- Both of your hands are treatment hands and are placed on the distal posterior surface of the client's thighs.
- The client's upper trunk is stabilized by body weight and contact with the table. (*Note*: The upper trunk is also stabilized by the direction in which you push on the client's thighs when performing the stretch; see Practical Application Box 6.2 in Chapter 6).
- An alternative position is to not have his feet placed on your clavicle (Fig. 7-8B).

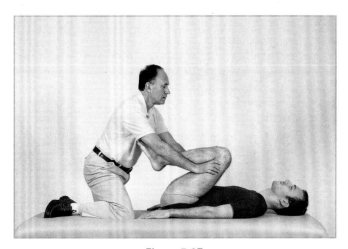

Figure 7-8B

Initial Client Stretch:

■ Begin by gently stretching the client's target (lumbar extensor) musculature by moving the client's pelvis and trunk into posterior tilt and flexion (the pelvis moves into posterior tilt, and the LSp moves into flexion) until you meet tissue resistance, beginning the stretch of the target lumbar extensor muscles (Fig. 7-9).

■ When you are supporting and holding the client's thighs, it is important for you to have a gentle and broad grasp that is comfortable for the client.

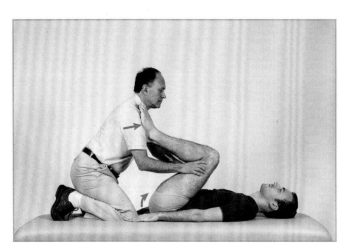

Figure 7-9

First Repetition: Client Contraction:

■ With the client in the initial stretch position, ask the client to perform a gentle isometric contraction of the target muscles for approximately 5 to 8 seconds (in an attempt to extend the trunk back down toward the table) against your resistance (Fig. 7-10A).

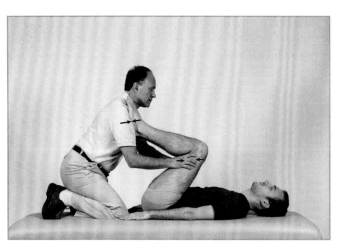

Figure 7-10A

■ Ask the client to relax.

■ Note that the breathing protocol for every repetition is to have the client either hold the breath or exhale when contracting against your resistance.

First Repetition: Postcontraction Stretch:

■ As soon as the client relaxes, gently increase the stretch of the client's target musculature by moving the client's trunk farther into flexion until you meet tissue resistance (Fig. 7-10B).

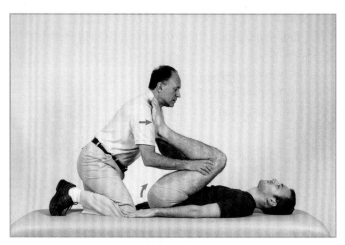

Figure 7-10B

■ Hold this position of stretch for approximately 1 to 3 seconds.

■ *Note*: To maintain stabilization of the client's trunk on the table, be sure to not press the client's thighs too horizontally and parallel with table because this would cause his trunk to excessively lift from the table, moving the stretch into the thoracic stretch, thereby losing the stretch in the lumbar region. It is important to press his thighs somewhat downward toward his chest.

Second Repetition: Client Contraction:

- Beginning from the position of stretch reached at the end of the first repetition, have the client again contract the target musculature isometrically for approximately 5 to 8 seconds against your resistance (Fig. 7-11A).
- This time, ask the client to contract against your resistance with moderate force.

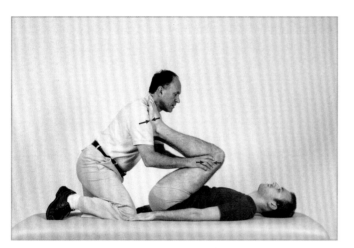

Figure 7-11A

Second Repetition: Postcontraction Stretch:

- As soon as the client relaxes, gently increase the stretch of the client's target musculature by moving the trunk farther into flexion until you meet tissue resistance (Fig. 7-11B).
- Hold this position of stretch for approximately 1 to 3 seconds.

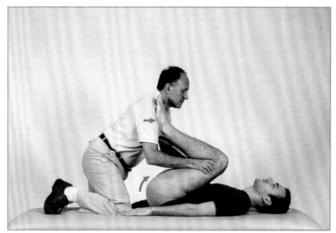

Figure 7-11B

Third Repetition:

- Beginning from the position of stretch reached at the end of the second repetition, have the client again contract the target musculature isometrically for approximately 5 to 8 seconds against your resistance, this time with as much force as is comfortable for the client.
- As soon as the client relaxes, gently increase the stretch of the client's target musculature by moving the trunk farther into flexion until you meet tissue resistance.
- If desired, a fourth repetition can be done.
- Hold the position of stretch of the last repetition for approximately 10 seconds or more.

Transitioning to Multiplane Contract Relax Stretching: Lumbar Spine Extensor Functional Group

Transitioning the CR stretching protocol for the LSp extensor functional group into a multiplane stretch that incorporates other planes of motion can be easily done by altering the direction of the movement of the client's pelvis and LSp. **Figure A** demonstrates frontal plane LSp right left lateral flexion being added into the sagittal plane lumbar flexion. This increases the stretch to the left-side extensor functional group muscles that also do left lateral flexion. **Figure B** demonstrates transverse plane left rotation of the pelvis and lower LSp (equivalent to right rotation of the upper LSp) being added into the sagittal plane lumbar flexion. This increases the stretch to the LSp extensors that are also left rotators (right-sided transversospinalis and left-sided erector spinae musculature). Of course, both frontal and transverse plane components can be added to the sagittal plane flexion when performing a CR multiplane stretch of the LSp extensor functional group.

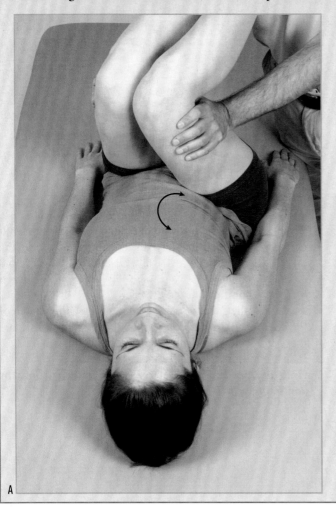

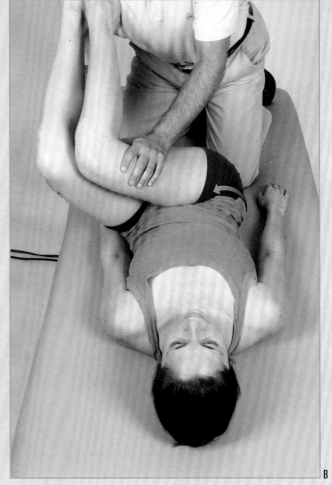

A

B

ROUTINE 7-2: LUMBAR SPINE FLEXORS

Figure 7-12 shows the functional group of muscles that flex the LSp. These muscles are often described as muscles of the anterior abdominal wall and are located on the anterior side of the trunk in the lumbar region. The following CR stretch involves the therapist climbing onto the table. For more on stretching the LSp flexor group, including alternative positioning, see Routine 6-4.

The Lumbar Spine Flexor Functional Group

This functional group comprises the following muscles bilaterally:

Rectus abdominis
External abdominal oblique
Internal abdominal oblique
Psoas major
Psoas minor

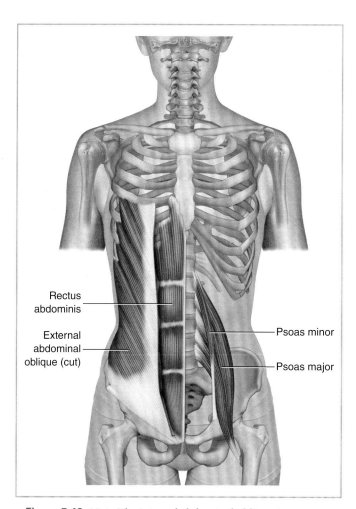

Figure 7-12 *Note*: The internal abdominal oblique is not seen.

Starting Position:

■ The client is prone with his hands clasped behind his head. You are seated on the client's buttocks and grasping the client's arms. Note the placement of the cushion for client and therapist modesty and comfort (Fig. 7-13A).

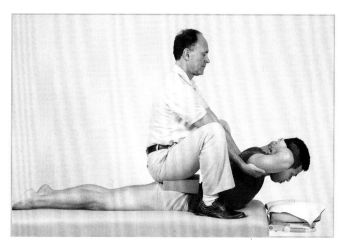

Figure 7-13A

■ Both of your hands are treatment hands.
■ The client's pelvis is stabilized by your body weight.
■ An alternative position that does not involve sitting on the client's buttocks is shown in Figure 7-13B.

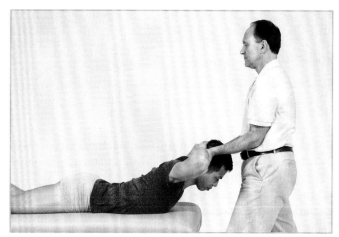

Figure 7-13B

Caution must be exercised when performing these stretches for the anterior abdominal wall.
- Bringing the client's LSp into extension approximates the facet joints and decreases the size of the intervertebral foramina and is therefore contraindicated if the client has facet syndrome or a space-occupying lesion, such as pathologic disc or a large bone spur.
- The client's glenohumeral joints must be healthy enough to reach behind him or her and have a stretching force placed through them.
- Positioning your body weight on the client's buttocks in this routine is important. If you sit too far superiorly on the pelvis, it can push it into anterior tilt, increasing the client's lumbar lordosis. If you sit too far inferiorly, the pelvis will not be adequately stabilized.

Initial Client Stretch:
- Begin by gently stretching the client's target (lumbar flexor) musculature by moving the client's trunk into extension by leaning back with core body weight until you meet tissue resistance, beginning the stretch of the target lumbar flexor muscles (Fig. 7-14).

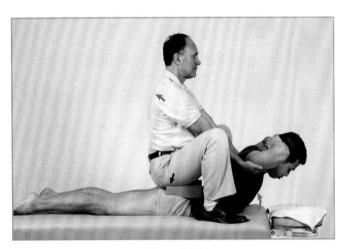

Figure 7-14

- When you are supporting and holding the client's arms, it is important for you to have a gentle and broad grasp that is comfortable for the client.
- The client has the choice of allowing the head and neck to relax into flexion or to extend the head and neck as the stretch is done. The advantage of relaxing into flexion is that it is less stressful for the posterior extensor musculature of the neck. The advantage of extending is that it can add to the effectiveness of the stretch of the anterior abdominal wall via fascial pull through the anterior thoracic region.

First Repetition: Client Contraction:
- With the client in the initial stretch position, ask the client to perform a gentle isometric contraction of the target muscles for approximately 5 to 8 seconds (in an attempt to flex the trunk back down toward the table) against your resistance (Fig. 7-15A).

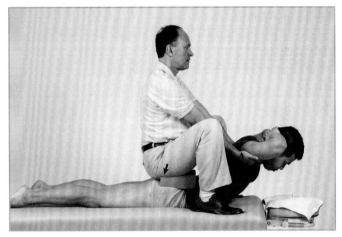

Figure 7-15A

- Ask the client to relax.
- Note that the breathing protocol for every repetition is to have the client either hold the breath or exhale when contracting against your resistance.

First Repetition: Postcontraction Stretch:
- As soon as the client relaxes, gently increase the stretch of the client's target musculature by moving the client's trunk farther into extension until you meet tissue resistance (Fig. 7-15B).
- Hold this position of stretch for approximately 1 to 3 seconds.

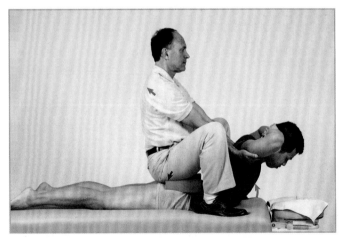

Figure 7-15B

Second Repetition: Client contraction:
- Beginning from the position of stretch reached at the end of the first repetition, have the client again contract the target musculature isometrically for approximately 5 to 8 seconds against your resistance (Fig. 7-16A).
- This time, ask the client to contract against your resistance with moderate force.

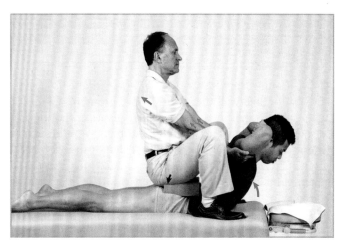

Figure 7-16B

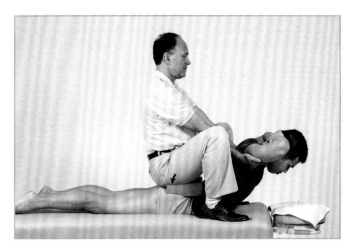

Figure 7-16A

Second Repetition: Postcontraction Stretch:
- As soon as the client relaxes, gently increase the stretch of the client's target musculature by moving the trunk farther into extension until you meet tissue resistance (Fig. 7-16B).
- Hold this position of stretch for approximately 1 to 3 seconds.

Third Repetition:
- Beginning from the position of stretch reached at the end of the second repetition, have the client again contract the target musculature isometrically for approximately 5 to 8 seconds against your resistance, this time, with as much force as is comfortable for the client.
- As soon as the client relaxes, gently increase the stretch of the client's target musculature by moving the trunk farther into extension until you meet tissue resistance.
- If desired, a fourth repetition can be done.
- Hold the position of stretch of the last repetition for approximately 10 seconds or more.

7.3   **PRACTICAL APPLICATION**

Transitioning to Multiplane Contract Relax Stretching: Lumbar Spine Flexor Functional Group

Transitioning the CR stretching protocol for the LSp (anterior abdominal wall) flexor functional group into a multiplane stretch that incorporates other planes of motion can also be easily done by altering the direction of the movement of the client's LSp. **Figure A** demonstrates frontal plane LSp right lateral flexion being added into the sagittal plane lumbar extension. This increases the stretch to the left-sided flexor functional group muscles that also do left lateral flexion (left-sided external and internal abdominal obliques). **Figure B** demonstrates frontal plane right lateral flexion and transverse plane right rotation being added into the sagittal plane lumbar extension. This focuses the stretch specifically to the left-sided left internal abdominal oblique muscle (because it does left lateral flexion and left rotation).

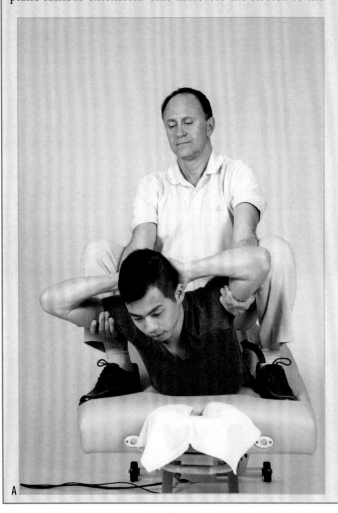

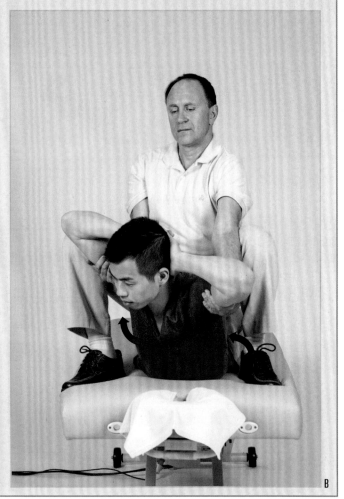

A

B

ROUTINE 7-3: LUMBAR SPINE RIGHT LATERAL FLEXORS

Figure 7-17 shows the functional group of muscles that right laterally flexes the LSp. These muscles are located on the right side of the trunk in the lumbar region.

The Lumbar Spine Right Lateral Flexor Functional Group
This functional group comprises the following right-sided muscles:
Erector spinae group
Transversospinalis group
Quadratus lumborum
Rectus abdominis
External abdominal oblique
Internal abdominal oblique
Psoas major
Psoas minor

Starting Position:

- Have the client side-lying on her left side with her bottom as close to the near (your) side of the table as possible and her left shoulder as far to the opposite side of the table as possible. This positions the client diagonally on the table so that her right thigh can be dropped off the side of the table into adduction without its path being obstructed by the table.
- Stand behind the client.
- Your right hand is the treatment hand and is placed on the lateral surface of the client's distal right thigh.
- Your left hand is the stabilization hand and is placed on the client's rib cage. It is important to press on the rib cage in a cephalad/cranial direction. Note placement of a cushion to spread out the stabilization force on the rib cage (Fig. 7-18).
- Bring the client's right thigh down into adduction off the side of the table. As the client's thigh adducts, the client's right-side pelvis will drop down into depression, thereby stretching the right lateral flexor musculature of the trunk.

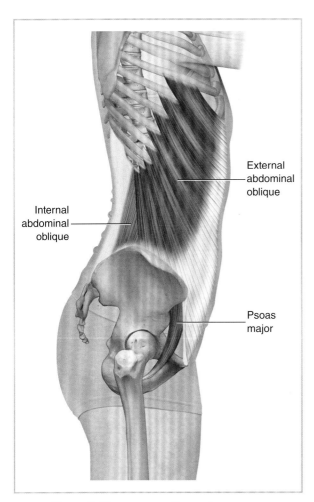

Internal abdominal oblique

External abdominal oblique

Psoas major

Figure 7-17 *Note*: Not all muscles are seen.

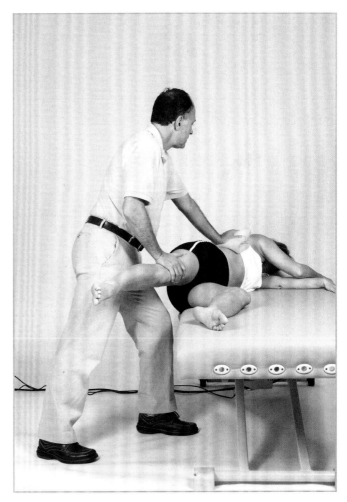

Figure 7-18

■ *It is extremely important to use a cushion to spread out the stabilization force on the client's rib cage. Too much pressure on one of the client's ribs could cause it to "release/pop" at its costospinal joints, possibly spraining the ligaments of the joint.*

■ *This stretch requires the client to be positioned far to the side of the table, so it is important to reassure the client before the stretch begins that he or she will not fall off the table. To be sure that he or she cannot fall off the table, it can be helpful to have a strong and stable lower body posture with pressure of your lower extremity against the table so that the client would have to fall through you to fall off the table.*

Initial Client Stretch:

■ Begin by gently stretching the client's target (lumbar right lateral flexor) musculature by moving the client's thigh and pelvis down toward the floor by dropping down with your core body weight until you meet tissue resistance, beginning the stretch of the target lumbar right lateral flexor muscles (Fig. 7-19).

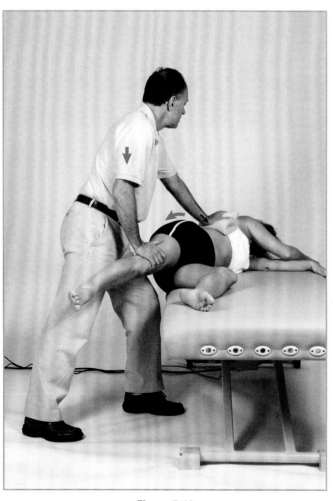

Figure 7-19

First Repetition: Client Contraction:

■ With the client in the initial stretch position, ask the client to perform a gentle isometric contraction of the target muscles for approximately 5 to 8 seconds (in an attempt to abduct the thigh back up toward the table and elevate the pelvis) against your resistance (Fig. 7-20A). It can be helpful to cue the client to engage her right lateral flexor lumbar musculature during the contraction; this can be done by touching her lateral lumbar musculature and asking her to contract from there.

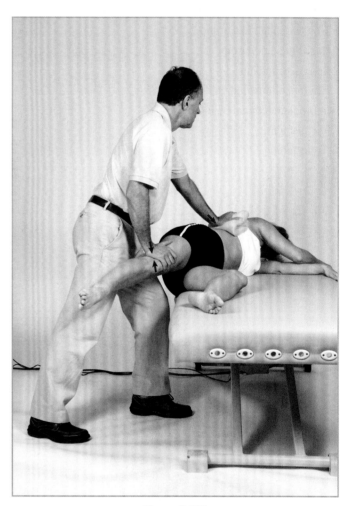

Figure 7-20A

■ Ask the client to relax.
■ Note that the breathing protocol for every repetition is to have the client either hold the breath or exhale when contracting against your resistance.

The client must attempt to isometrically contract upward against both your resistance and gravity. Therefore, it is important to ask for only a gentle contraction on the part of the client. This is especially true if the client's thigh and pelvis are stretched far toward the floor and therefore biomechanically weaker and less able to contract with much force. Further, because gravity is assisting your stretching force, it is important that you use extra caution when adding to the force of the postcontraction stretch.

Note: When the stretching routine is completed, be sure to ask the client to completely relax the thigh as you passively return it to the table.

First Repetition: Postcontraction Stretch:

■ As soon as the client relaxes, gently increase the stretch of the client's target musculature by moving the client's thigh farther toward the floor, further depressing the pelvis, until you meet tissue resistance (Fig. 7-20B).

■ Hold this position of stretch for approximately 1 to 3 seconds.

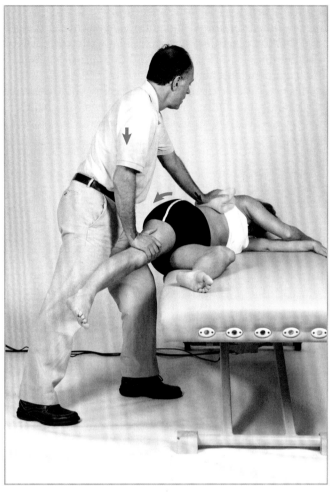

Figure 7-20B

Second Repetition: Client Contraction:

■ Beginning from the position of stretch reached at the end of the first repetition, have the client again contract the target musculature isometrically for approximately 5 to 8 seconds against your resistance (Fig. 7-21A).

■ This time, ask the client to contract against your resistance with moderate force, if it is comfortable for the client.

Second Repetition: Postcontraction Stretch:

■ As soon as the client relaxes, gently increase the stretch of the client's target musculature by moving the thigh and pelvis farther down into the stretch until you meet tissue resistance (Fig. 7-21B).

■ Hold this position of stretch for approximately 1 to 3 seconds.

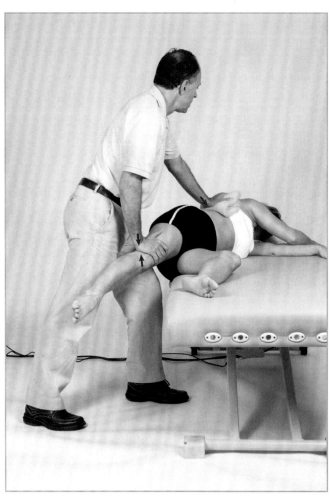

Figure 7-21A

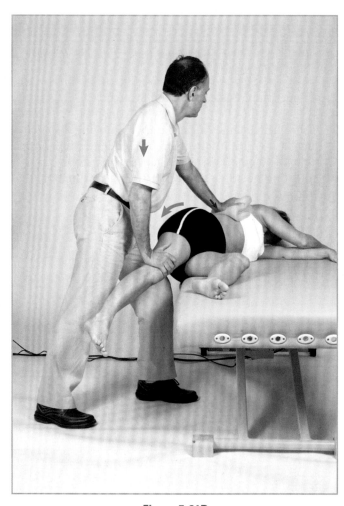

Figure 7-21B

Third Repetition:

- Beginning from the position of stretch reached at the end of the second repetition, have the client again contract the target musculature isometrically for approximately 5 to 8 seconds against your resistance, this time, with as much force as is comfortable for the client.
- As soon as the client relaxes, gently increase the stretch of the client's target musculature by moving the thigh and pelvis farther into the stretch until you meet tissue resistance.
- If desired, a fourth repetition can be done.
- Hold the position of stretch of the last repetition for approximately 10 seconds or more.
- When the stretching routine is complete, ask the client to completely relax the thigh as you passively return it to the table.

7.4   PRACTICAL APPLICATION

Contract Relax Stretching of the Lumbar Spine Right Lateral Flexors with the Client Seated

It is also possible to perform CR stretching of the LSp right lateral flexor musculature with the client seated at the end of the table. For this option, you would be standing to the right side of the client. Your right hand is the treatment hand and is placed on right side of the client's trunk. Your left hand is the stabilization hand and functions to stabilize the client's pelvis. It is placed across the top of the client's right iliac crest (**Fig. A**); if it is not possible to grasp the client's iliac crest, the stabilization hand can be placed on the proximal anterior surface of the client's right thigh (**Fig. B**). In either case, your stabilization hand contact should be broad in contact so it is both firm and comfortable for the client; if desired, a cushion can be used. The advantage of the seated position is that the client's hip joint is not involved with the stretch. The disadvantage is that it can be challenging to adequately stabilize the client's pelvis and to control the motion of the client's trunk.

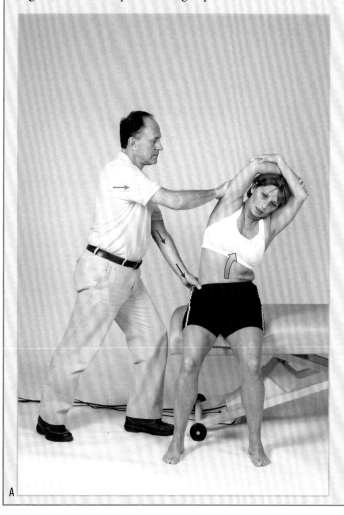
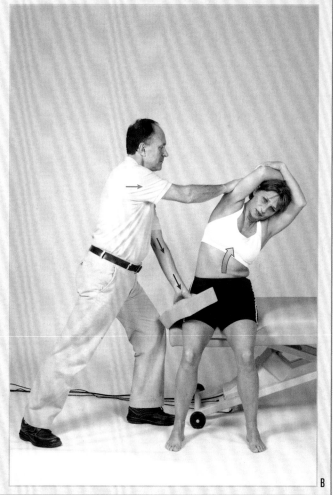

ROUTINE 7-4: LUMBAR SPINE LEFT LATERAL FLEXORS

Figure 7-22 shows the functional group of muscles that left laterally flex the LSp. These muscles are located on the left side of the trunk in the lumbar region. To use CR stretching to stretch this functional group of muscles, follow the directions given in Figures 7-18 through 7-21 to stretch the right lateral flexor group but switch for the left side of the body.

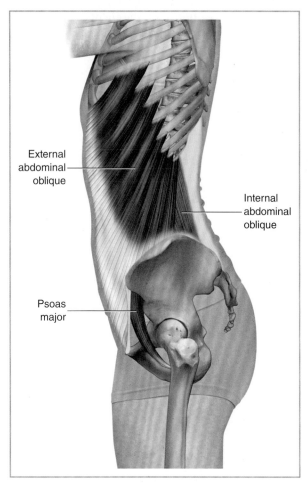

External abdominal oblique

Internal abdominal oblique

Psoas major

Figure 7-22 *Note*: Not all muscles are seen.

ROUTINE 7-5: LUMBAR SPINE RIGHT ROTATORS—SEATED

Figure 7-23 shows the functional group of muscles that right rotate the LSp. These muscles are located both anteriorly and posteriorly and on both the right and left sides of the trunk in the lumbar region.

The Lumbar Spine Right Rotator Functional Group
This functional group comprises the following muscles:
Left transversospinalis group
Right erector spinae group
Left external abdominal oblique
Right internal abdominal oblique

Starting Position:

■ Have the client seated at the right end of the table with her arms crossed so that her hands are on the opposite shoulders, but her arms should be adducted at the glenohumeral joints so that her elbows meet at the center of the body.

■ Stand to the right side of the client.

■ Your right hand is the treatment hand and is placed on the client's elbows.

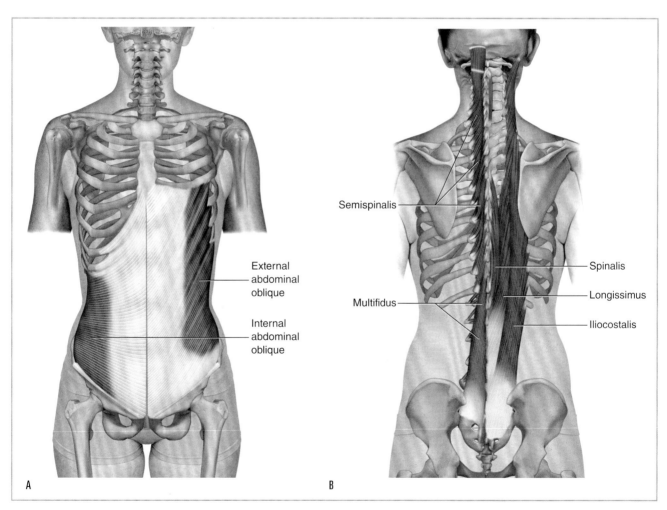

Figure 7-23 (**A**) Anterior view. (**B**) Posterior view.

■ Your left hand is the stabilization hand and functions to stabilize the client's pelvis. It is placed across the top of the client's right iliac crest (Fig. 7-24); if it is not possible to grasp the client's iliac crest, the stabilization hand can be placed on the proximal anterior surface of the client's right thigh; if desired, a cushion can be used for comfort to broaden the stabilization contact as described in Practical Application Box 7.4.

Initial Client Stretch:

■ Begin by gently stretching the client's target (lumbar right rotator) musculature by moving the client's trunk into left rotation until you meet tissue resistance, beginning the stretch of the target lumbar right rotator muscles (Fig. 7-25).

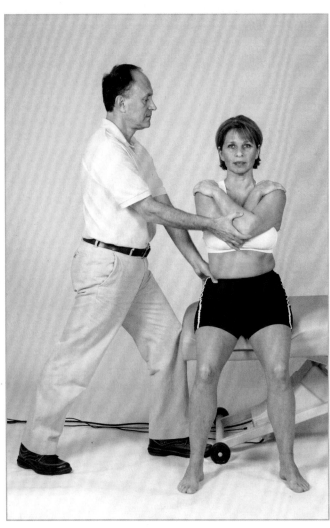

Figure 7-24

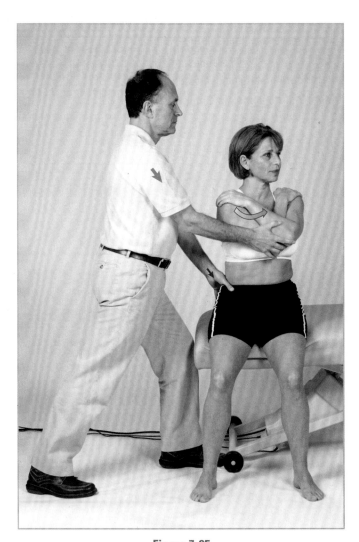

Figure 7-25

First Repetition: Client Contraction:
- With the client in the initial stretch position, ask the client to perform a gentle isometric contraction of the target muscles for approximately 5 to 8 seconds (in an attempt to right rotate the trunk against your resistance) (Fig. 7-26A).

First Repetition: Postcontraction Stretch:
- As soon as the client relaxes, gently increase the stretch of the client's target musculature by moving the client's trunk farther into left rotation until you meet tissue resistance (Fig. 7-26B).
- Hold this position of stretch for approximately 1 to 3 seconds.

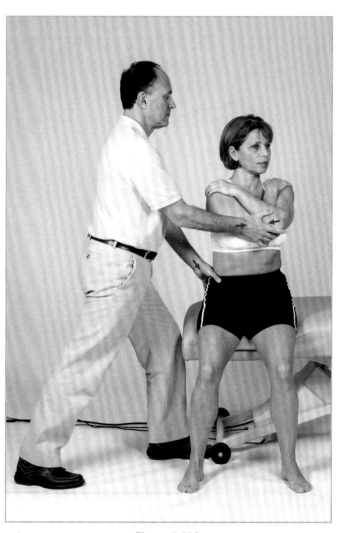

Figure 7-26A

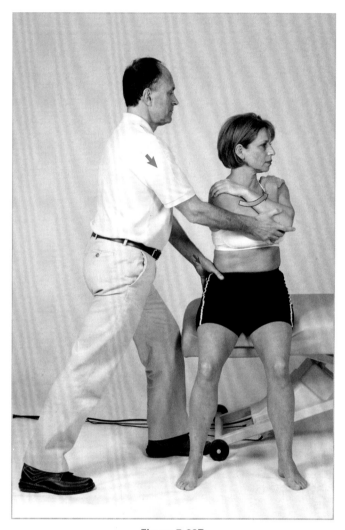

Figure 7-26B

- It can be helpful to cue the client to engage this motion from her lumbar musculature and not her thoracic musculature; this can be done by touching her lumbar (low back and anterior abdominal wall) musculature and asking her to contract from there.
- Ask the client to relax.
- Note that the breathing protocol for every repetition is to have the client either hold the breath or exhale when contracting against your resistance.

Second Repetition: Client Contraction:

- Beginning from the position of stretch reached at the end of the first repetition, have the client again contract the target musculature isometrically for approximately 5 to 8 seconds against your resistance (Fig. 7-27A).
- This time, ask the client to contract against your resistance with moderate force, if it is comfortable for the client.

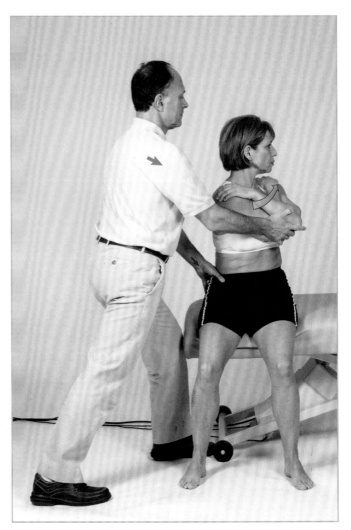

Figure 7-27B

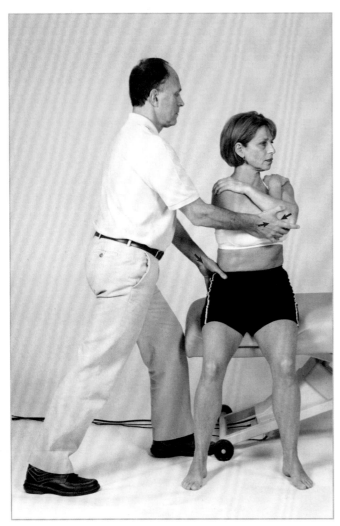

Figure 7-27A

Second Repetition: Postcontraction Stretch:

- As soon as the client relaxes, gently increase the stretch of the client's target musculature by moving the trunk farther into left rotation until you meet tissue resistance (Fig. 7-27B).
- Hold this position of stretch for approximately 1 to 3 seconds.

Third Repetition:

- Beginning from the position of stretch reached at the end of the second repetition, have the client again contract the target musculature isometrically for approximately 5 to 8 seconds against your resistance, this time, with as much force as is comfortable for the client.
- As soon as the client relaxes, gently increase the stretch of the client's target musculature by moving the trunk farther into left rotation until you meet tissue resistance.
- If desired, a fourth repetition can be done.
- Hold the position of stretch of the last repetition for approximately 10 seconds or more.

ROUTINE 7-6: LUMBAR SPINE LEFT ROTATORS—SEATED

Figure 7-28 shows the functional group of muscles that left rotate the LSp. These muscles are located both anteriorly and posteriorly and on both the left and right sides of the trunk in the lumbar region. To use CR stretching to stretch this functional group of muscles, follow the directions given in Figures 7-24 through 7-27 to stretch the right rotator group but switch for the left side of the body.

The Lumbar Spine Left Rotator Functional Group
This functional group comprises the following muscles:
Right transversospinalis group
Left erector spinae group
Right external abdominal oblique
Left internal abdominal oblique

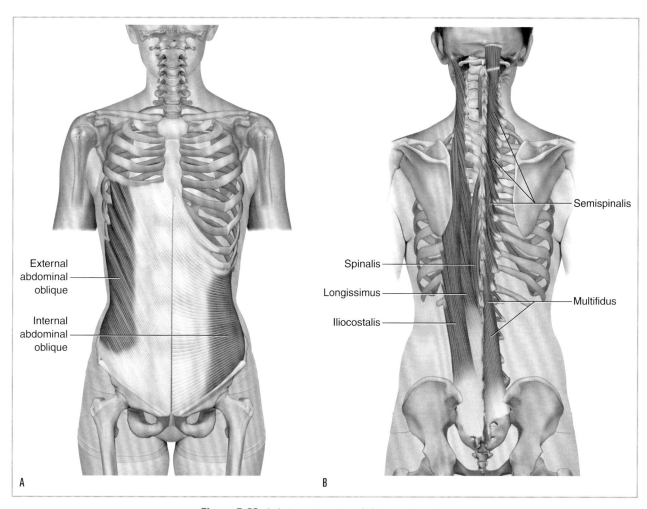

Figure 7-28 (**A**) Anterior view. (**B**) Posterior view.

SECTION 2: HIP JOINT/PELVIS CONTRACT RELAX STRETCHES

As a rule, CR stretches to the muscles of the pelvis that cross the hip joint are performed by stabilizing the client's pelvis and moving his or her thigh to create the stretch. For the stretch to be effective, it is extremely important that the pelvis is well stabilized. Otherwise, the stretching force will enter the LSp. This will not only dissipate the stretching force at the hip joint causing it to lose its effectiveness but it might also place a torque force into the LSp that can cause pain or injury.

The following CR stretching routines for muscles of the pelvis that cross the hip joint are presented in this chapter:

- Routine 7-7—hip abductors
- Routine 7-8—hip adductors
- Routine 7-9—hip flexors
- Routine 7-10—hip extensors: hamstrings
- Routine 7-11—hip extensors: gluteals
- Routine 7-12—hip deep lateral rotators
- Routine 7-13—hip medial rotators

ROUTINE 7-7: HIP ABDUCTORS

Figure 7-29 shows the functional group of muscles that abduct the right thigh at the hip joint. These muscles are located on the lateral side of the pelvis and thigh, crossing the hip joint between them. The CR stretching routine presented here for the hip abductor functional group is similar to the CR stretching routine presented for the lateral flexor functional group of the LSp (see Routines 7-3 and 7-4). The difference is that the pelvis (instead of the rib cage) is stabilized when performing this CR stretch for the hip joint. Following is the CR stretching routine shown for the hip abductor functional group on the right side of the body.

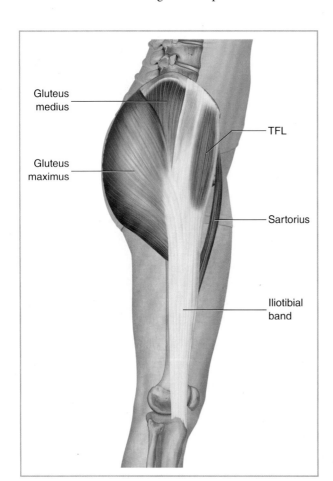

Gluteus medius

Gluteus maximus

TFL

Sartorius

Iliotibial band

Figure 7-29 *Note*: The gluteus minimus is not seen.

The Pelvis/Hip Joint Abductor Functional Group
This functional group comprises the following muscles:
Gluteus medius
Gluteus minimus
Gluteus maximus (upper fibers)
Tensor fasciae latae (TFL)
Sartorius

Starting Position:

■ Have the client side-lying on her left side with her bottom as close to the back of the table (where you are standing) as possible and her left shoulder as far to the opposite side of the table as possible. This positions the client diagonally on the table so that her right thigh can be dropped off the back side of the table into adduction without its path being obstructed by the table.

■ Stand behind the client.

■ Your right hand is the treatment hand and is placed on the lateral surface of the client's distal right thigh.

■ Your left hand is the stabilization hand and is placed on the client's pelvis, just inferior to the iliac crest. It is important to press on the iliac crest with your force directed toward elevation of the pelvis on that side. Otherwise, the right-side pelvic bone will depress and the stretch at the hip joint will be lost. Note placement of a cushion to spread out the stabilization force on the iliac crest (Fig. 7-30).

■ Bring the client's right thigh down into adduction off the side of the table. As the client's thigh adducts, be sure to stabilize the pelvis by preventing it from depressing.

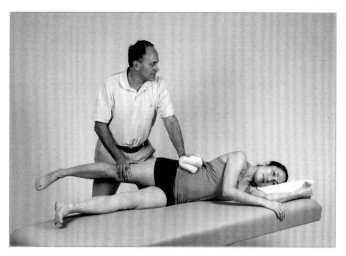

Figure 7-30

This stretch requires the client to be positioned far to the side of the table so it is important to reassure the client before the stretch begins that he or she will not fall off the table. To be sure that he or she cannot fall off the table, have a strong and stable lower body posture with pressure of your lower extremity against the table so that the client would have to fall through you to fall off the table.

Initial Client Stretch:

■ Begin by gently stretching the client's target (hip abductor) musculature by moving the client's thigh down toward the floor into adduction by dropping down with your core body weight until you meet tissue resistance, beginning the stretch of the target hip abductor muscles (Fig. 7-31).

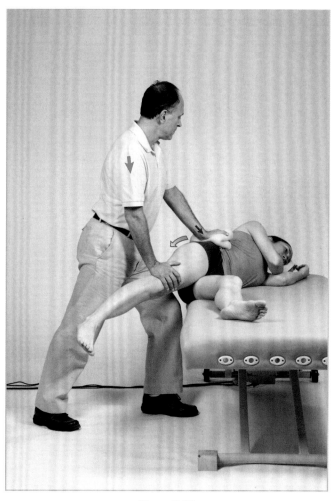

Figure 7-31

First Repetition: Client Contraction:

■ With the client in the initial stretch position, ask the client to perform a gentle isometric contraction of the target muscles for approximately 5 to 8 seconds (in an attempt to abduct the thigh back up toward the table) against your resistance (Fig. 7-32A).

■ Ask the client to relax.

■ Note that the breathing protocol for every repetition is to have the client either hold the breath or exhale when contracting against your resistance.

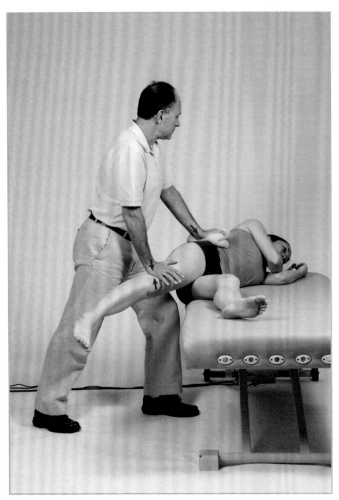

Figure 7-32A

🚦 ■ *The client must attempt to isometrically contract upward against both your resistance and gravity. Therefore, it is important to ask for only a gentle contraction on the part of the client. This is especially true if the client's thigh is stretched far toward the floor and therefore biomechanically weaker and less able to contract with much force.*

■ *Further, because gravity is assisting your stretching force, it is important that you use extra caution when adding to the force of the postcontraction stretch.*

■ *Caution should always be employed with stretches of the hip joint with clients who have hip replacements and or marked degenerative changes to the hip joint. Extra caution should be employed with stretches into adduction and medial rotation.*

■ *Note: When the stretching routine is completed, be sure to ask the client to completely relax the thigh as you passively return it to the table.*

First Repetition: Postcontraction Stretch:

■ As soon as the client relaxes, gently increase the stretch of the client's target musculature by moving the client's thigh farther into adduction toward the floor until you meet tissue resistance (Fig. 7-32B).

■ Hold this position of stretch for approximately 1 to 3 seconds.

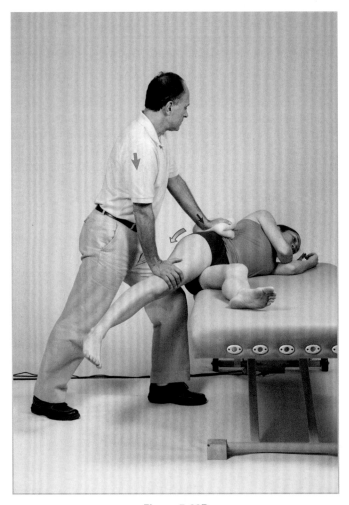

Figure 7-32B

Second Repetition: Client Contraction:

- Beginning from the position of stretch reached at the end of the first repetition, have the client again contract the target musculature isometrically for approximately 5 to 8 seconds against your resistance (Fig. 7-33A).
- This time, ask the client to contract against your resistance with moderate force, if it is comfortable for the client.

Second Repetition: Postcontraction Stretch:

- As soon as the client relaxes, gently increase the stretch of the client's target musculature by moving the thigh farther into adduction until you meet tissue resistance (Fig. 7-33B).
- Hold this position of stretch for approximately 1 to 3 seconds.

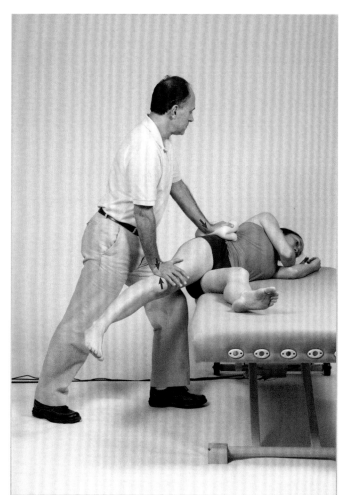

Figure 7-33A

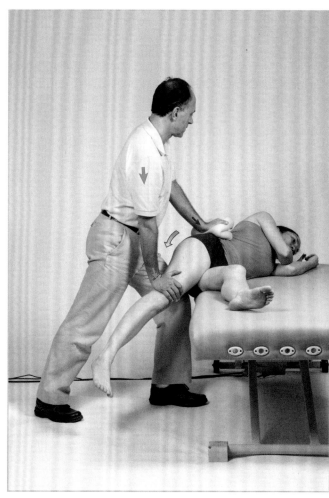

Figure 7-33B

Third Repetition:

■ Beginning from the position of stretch reached at the end of the second repetition, have the client again contract the target musculature isometrically for approximately 5 to 8 seconds against your resistance, this time with as much force as is comfortable for the client.

■ As soon as the client relaxes, gently increase the stretch of the client's target musculature by moving the thigh farther into adduction until you meet tissue resistance.

■ If desired, a fourth repetition can be done.

■ Hold the position of stretch of the last repetition for approximately 10 seconds or more.

■ When the stretching routine is complete, ask the client to completely relax the thigh as you passively return it to the table.

Left-Side Abductor Group:

■ Repeat for the pelvis/hip joint abductor functional group on the left side of the body (Fig. 7-34).

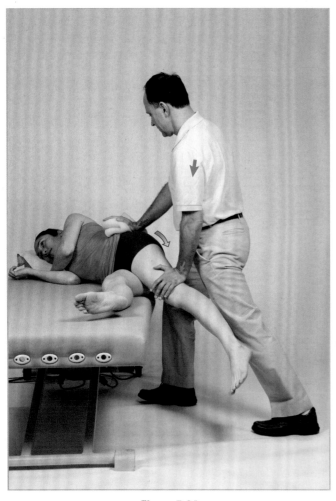

Figure 7-34

7.5	**PRACTICAL APPLICATION**

Transitioning to Multiplane Contract Relax Stretching: Hip Joint Abductor Functional Group

Transitioning the CR stretching protocol for the hip joint abductor functional group into a multiplane stretch that incorporates another plane of motion can be done by altering the position and/or direction of movement of the client's thigh. The accompanying figure demonstrates transverse plane lateral rotation added into the frontal plane adduction of the thigh; this is accomplished by presetting the lateral rotation of the thigh and then stretching it down into adduction. This multiplane stretch focuses the stretch toward the abductor musculature that also does medial rotation, such as the TFL and anterior fibers of the gluteus medius and minimus. Differing degrees of sagittal plane flexion/extension can also be combined with the frontal plane stretch into adduction.

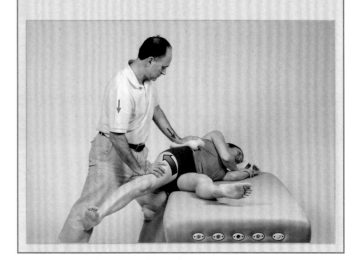

ROUTINE 7-8: HIP ADDUCTORS

Figure 7-35 shows the functional group of muscles that adduct the right thigh at the hip joint. These muscles are located on the medial side of the pelvis and thigh, crossing the hip joint between them. As with all stretches for hip joint musculature, it is extremely important that the pelvis is completely stabilized. Following is the CR stretching routine shown for the hip adductor functional group on the right side of the body.

The Pelvis/Hip Joint Adductor Functional Group
This functional group comprises the following muscles:
Pectineus
Adductor longus
Adductor brevis
Gracilis
Adductor magnus
Gluteus maximus (lower fibers)
Quadratus femoris

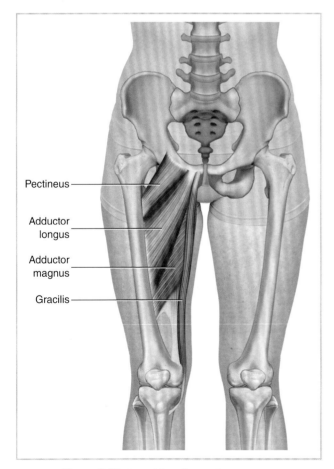

Figure 7-35 *Note*: Not all muscles are seen.

Starting Position:

- Have the client supine toward the right side of the table. Her right hip joint is abducted and laterally rotated at the hip joint, and her right leg is flexed at the knee joint; her right foot is placed on your left ASIS (Fig. 7-36). (*Note*: If the client's adductor musculature is tight, it is likely that she will need to also flex the right thigh at the hip joint to attain this position.)

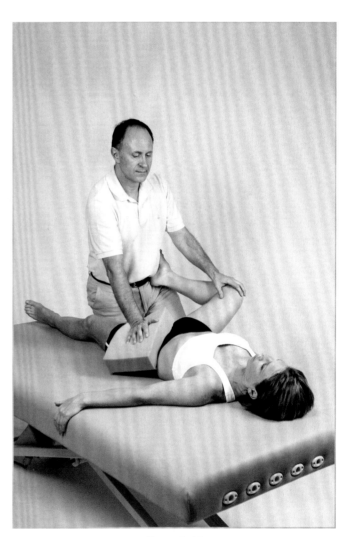

Figure 7-36

- Stand to the side of the client.
- Your left hand is the treatment hand and is placed on the medial side of the client's distal right thigh. Your left side pelvis is also a treatment contact and is placed against the client's right foot.
- Your right hand is the stabilization hand and is placed on the client's left ASIS. *Note*: A cushion is used to spread out and soften the contact pressure on the client.

Initial Client Stretch:

- First, press downward toward the floor on the client's right distal thigh by dropping with your core body weight. This motion is horizontal abduction (also known as horizontal extension) of the thigh at the hip joint and, because of the position of the client's thigh, stretches the more anteriorly placed fibers of the adductor group. During this stretch, the pelvis will tend to rotate to the right, so your stabilization pressure must be oriented toward left rotation (Fig. 7-37A).

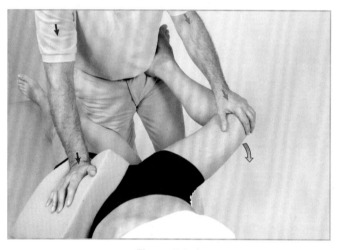

Figure 7-37A

- Now lean in with your pelvis against the client's foot, further stretching the client's thigh into abduction. Because of the position of the client's thigh, this focuses the stretch to the more posteriorly oriented fibers of the adductor group. During this stretch, the pelvis will tend to depress on the left side (and elevate on the right side), so your stabilization pressure must be oriented toward elevation of the left side of the pelvis (Fig. 7-37B).

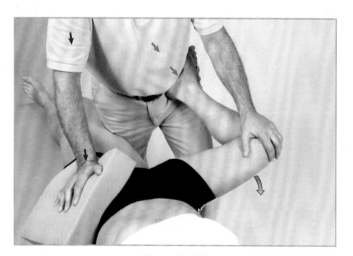

Figure 7-37B

First Repetition: Client Contraction:

- With the client in the initial stretch position, ask the client to perform a gentle isometric contraction of the target muscles for approximately 5 to 8 seconds by pressing her thigh up against the resistance of your hand (Fig. 7-38A).
- Ask the client to relax.
- Note that the breathing protocol for every repetition is to have the client either hold the breath or exhale when contracting against your resistance.

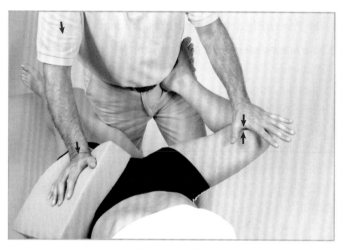

Figure 7-38A

The client must attempt to isometrically contract upward against both your resistance and gravity. Therefore, it is important to ask for only a gentle contraction on the part of the client. Further, because gravity is assisting your stretching force, it is important that you use extra caution when adding to the force of the postcontraction stretch.

First Repetition: Postcontraction Stretch:

■ As soon as the client relaxes, gently increase the stretch of the client's target musculature by moving the client's thigh farther into horizontal abduction (horizontal extension) down toward the floor until you meet tissue resistance (Fig. 7-38B).

■ Hold this position of stretch for approximately 1 to 3 seconds.

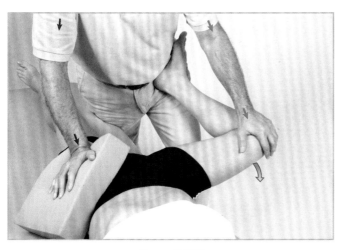

Figure 7-38B

Second Repetition: Client Contraction:

■ Beginning from the position of stretch reached at the end of the first repetition, now have the client contract the target musculature isometrically for approximately 5 to 8 seconds, this time, gently pressing her foot against the resistance of your pelvis (Fig. 7-39A).

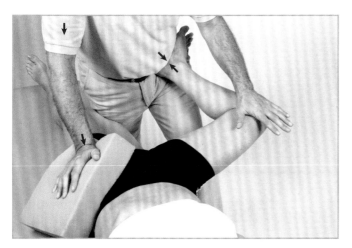

Figure 7-39A

Second Repetition: Postcontraction Stretch:

■ As soon as the client relaxes, increase the stretch of the client's target musculature by gently leaning in with your pelvis and moving the client's thigh farther into abduction until you meet tissue resistance (Fig. 7-39B).

■ Hold this position of stretch for approximately 1 to 3 seconds.

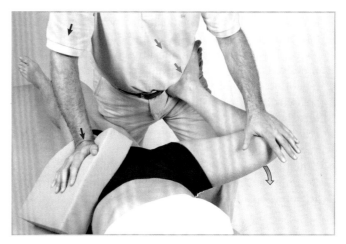

Figure 7-39B

Third Repetition:

■ Beginning from the position of stretch reached at the end of the second repetition, have the client again contract the target musculature isometrically for approximately 5 to 8 seconds, this time, pressing both her thigh against the resistance of your hand and her foot against the resistance of your pelvis (Fig. 7-40). The client can isometrically contract with moderate force this time.

■ As soon as the client relaxes, gently increase the stretch of the client's target musculature by using your left hand to move the client's thigh farther into horizontal abduction and leaning in with your pelvis to further abduct her thigh until you meet tissue resistance.

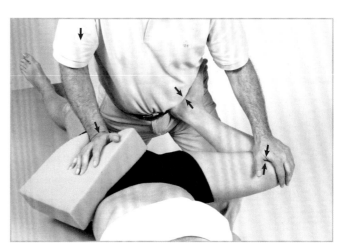

Figure 7-40

Fourth Repetition:

- Beginning from the position of stretch reached at the end of the third repetition, have the client again contract the target musculature isometrically for approximately 5 to 8 seconds, pressing against the resistance of both your hand and your pelvis, this time, with as much force as is comfortable for the client.
- As soon as the client relaxes, gently increase the stretch of the client's target musculature by again using your left hand to move the client's thigh farther into horizontal abduction and leaning in with your pelvis to further abduct her thigh until you meet tissue resistance.
- If desired, a fifth repetition can be done. *Note:* An extra repetition is usually done with this routine because there are two different aspects of the client's adductor musculature that are being stretched.
- Hold the position of stretch of the last repetition for approximately 10 seconds or more.
- When the stretching routine is complete, ask the client to completely relax the thigh as you passively return it to anatomic position on the table.

Left-Side Adductor Group:

- Repeat for the pelvis/hip joint adductor functional group on the left side of the body (Fig. 7-41).

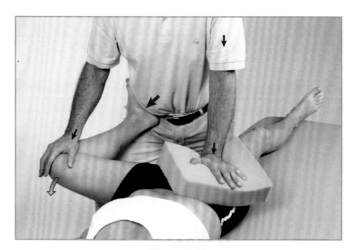

Figure 7-41

ROUTINE 7-9: HIP FLEXORS

Figure 7-42 shows the functional group of muscles that flex the right thigh at the hip joint. These muscles are located on the anterior side of the pelvis and thigh, crossing the hip joint between them. With all CR stretches to the hip joint, it is important to stabilize the pelvis. With this stretch, it is especially important because if the pelvis is not well stabilized, it will anteriorly tilt, causing increased lordosis of the LSp. Following is the CR stretching routine shown for the hip flexor functional group on the right side of the body.

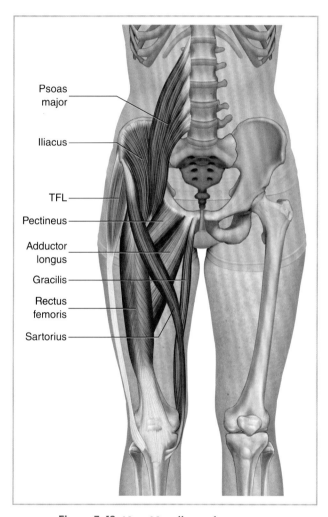

Figure 7-42 *Note*: Not all muscles are seen.

The Pelvis/Hip Joint Flexor Functional Group
This functional group comprises the following muscles:
Gluteus medius (anterior fibers)
Gluteus minimus (anterior fibers)
TFL
Rectus femoris
Sartorius
Iliacus
Psoas major
Pectineus
Adductor longus
Adductor brevis
Gracilis

7.8   THERAPIST TIP

Gaenslen's Test

The position of this stretching routine not only places a stretching tension force into the flexor musculature of the hip joint but also places a force into the same-side (and possibly the opposite-side) sacroiliac joint. In fact, this position is also known as Gaenslen's test and is used to assess the sacroiliac joint. For more on assessment tests, see Chapter 3.

Starting Position:

■ Have the client supine as far to the right side of the table as possible.

■ Stand to the right side of the client.

■ Your right hand is the treatment hand and will be placed on the anterior surface of the client's distal right thigh. Initially, to bring her thigh over and off the side of the table, your right hand will need to be under (on the posterior side of the thigh).

■ Your left hand is the stabilization hand and is placed on the client's left ASIS. *Note*: A cushion is used to spread out and soften the contact pressure on the client (Fig. 7-43).

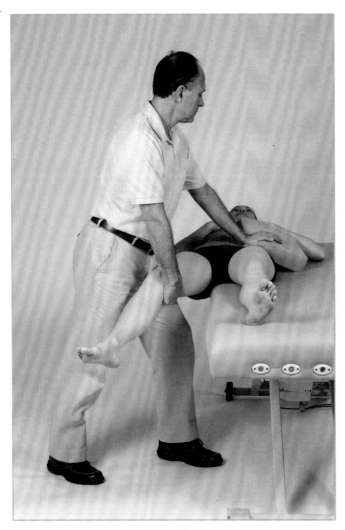

Figure 7-43

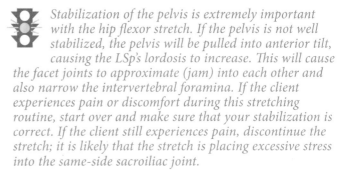

Stabilization of the pelvis is extremely important with the hip flexor stretch. If the pelvis is not well stabilized, the pelvis will be pulled into anterior tilt, causing the LSp's lordosis to increase. This will cause the facet joints to approximate (jam) into each other and also narrow the intervertebral foramina. If the client experiences pain or discomfort during this stretching routine, start over and make sure that your stabilization is correct. If the client still experiences pain, discontinue the stretch; it is likely that the stretch is placing excessive stress into the same-side sacroiliac joint.

Initial Client Stretch:

■ Begin by gently stretching the client's target (hip flexor) musculature by moving the client's thigh down toward the floor into extension until you meet tissue resistance, beginning the stretch of the target hip flexor muscles (Fig. 7-44).

■ *Note*: The client needs to be positioned far enough to the right side so that her right thigh can be slightly abducted off the table and then dropped down into extension without the table obstructing its path. The table must also be set high enough so that the excursion of the client's thigh is not blocked by her foot hitting the floor.

■ Gently press the client's right thigh farther downward into extension (toward the floor) by dropping with your core body weight. During this stretch, the pelvis will tend to anteriorly tilt and rotate to the right, so your stabilization pressure must be oriented toward posterior tilt and left rotation.

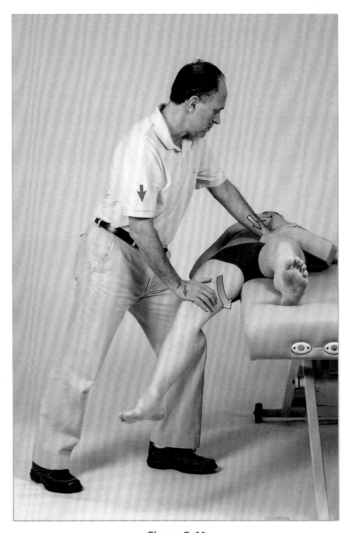

Figure 7-44

First Repetition: Client Contraction:

- With the client in the initial stretch position, ask the client to perform a gentle isometric contraction of the target muscles for approximately 5 to 8 seconds (in an attempt to flex the thigh back up toward the table) against your resistance (Fig. 7-45A).
- Ask the client to relax.
- Note that the breathing protocol for every repetition is to have the client either hold the breath or exhale when contracting against your resistance.

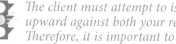

The client must attempt to isometrically contract upward against both your resistance and gravity. Therefore, it is important to ask for only a gentle contraction on the part of the client. This is especially true if the client's thigh is stretched far toward the floor into extension and therefore biomechanically weaker and less able to contract with much force. Further, because gravity is assisting your stretching force, it is important that you use extra caution when adding to the force of the postcontraction stretch.

Note: When the stretching routine is completed, be sure to ask the client to completely relax the thigh as you passively return it to the table.

First Repetition: Postcontraction Stretch:

- As soon as the client relaxes, gently increase the stretch of the client's target musculature by moving the client's thigh farther into extension toward the floor until you meet tissue resistance (Fig. 7-45B).
- Hold this position of stretch for approximately 1 to 3 seconds.

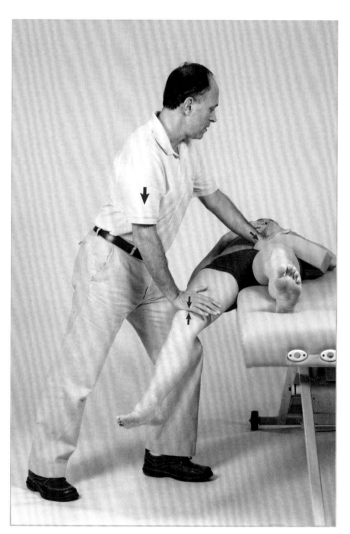

Figure 7-45A

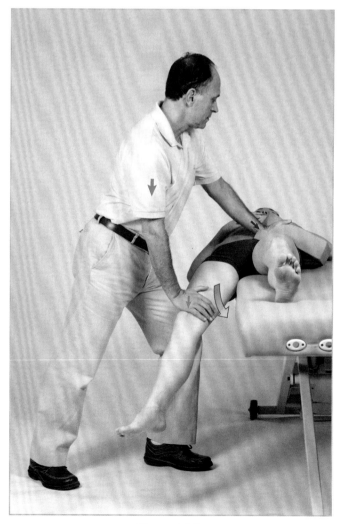

Figure 7-45B

Second Repetition: Client Contraction:

■ Beginning from the position of stretch reached at the end of the first repetition, have the client again contract the target musculature isometrically for approximately 5 to 8 seconds against your resistance (Fig. 7-46A).

■ This time, ask the client to contract against your resistance with moderate force, if it is comfortable for the client.

Second Repetition: Postcontraction Stretch:

■ As soon as the client relaxes, gently increase the stretch of the client's target musculature by moving the thigh farther into extension until you meet tissue resistance (Fig. 7-46B).

■ Hold this position of stretch for approximately 1 to 3 seconds.

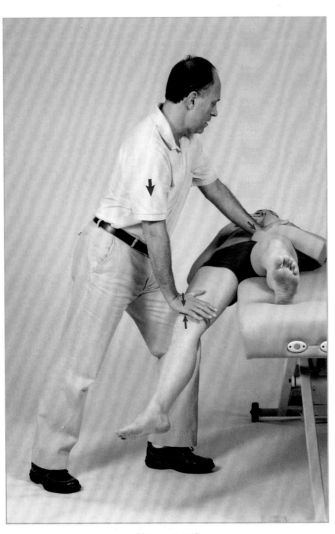

Figure 7-46A

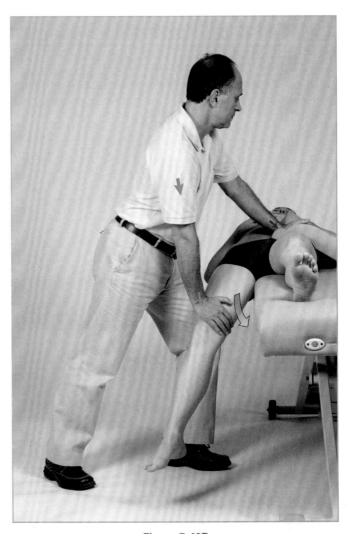

Figure 7-46B

Third Repetition:

- Beginning from the position of stretch reached at the end of the second repetition, have the client again contract the target musculature isometrically for approximately 5 to 8 seconds against your resistance, again with moderate force if it is comfortable for the client.
- As soon as the client relaxes, gently increase the stretch of the client's target musculature by moving the thigh farther into extension until you meet tissue resistance.
- If desired, a fourth repetition can be done.
- Hold the position of stretch of the last repetition for approximately 10 seconds or more.
- When the stretching routine is complete, ask the client to completely relax the thigh as you passively return it to the table.

Left-Side Flexor Group:

- Repeat for the pelvis/hip joint flexor functional group on the left side of the body (Fig. 7-47).

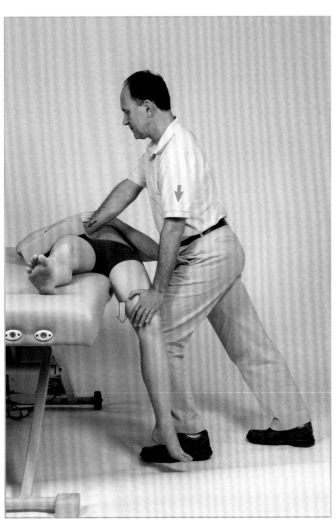

Figure 7-47

7.6 PRACTICAL APPLICATION

Transitioning to Multiplane Contract Relax Stretching: Hip Joint Flexor Functional Group

Transitioning the CR stretching protocol for the hip joint flexor functional group into a multiplane stretch that incorporates other planes of motion can be done by altering the position and/or direction of movement of the client's thigh. The accompanying figure demonstrates frontal plane abduction and transverse plane lateral rotation added into the sagittal plane extension of the thigh. This focuses the stretch toward the flexors that are also adductors and medial rotators, such as the pectineus and adductors longus and brevis. This is accomplished by presetting the abduction and lateral rotation of the thigh and then stretching it down into extension. This stretch can also be considered a multijoint stretch if the knee joint is involved. If the client's leg at the knee joint is flexed while the thigh is extended at the hip joint, multiple joints are involved, and the stretch is focused toward the rectus femoris muscle.

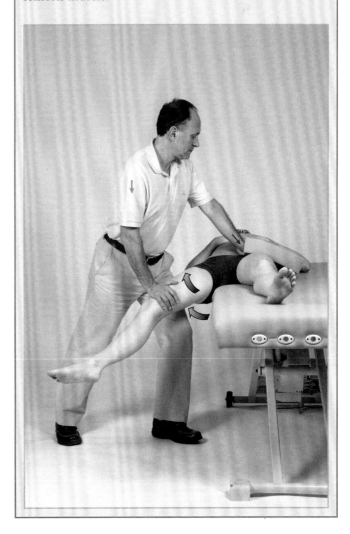

| 7.7 | **PRACTICAL APPLICATION** |

Contract Relax Stretching of the Hip Flexors at the End of the Table

It is also possible to perform CR stretching of the hip flexor functional group with the client at the end of the table. Following is the protocol for the hip flexor group on the right side of the body. Ask the client to stand facing away from the end of the table, place her tailbone (coccyx) at the top of the table, and lean back onto the table to lie supine, hugging her left thigh into her chest. You stand facing the client at the end of the table, placing your right hand on her distal posterior left thigh to assist in stabilizing her body; her left foot can be placed on your right clavicle to further assist stabilization. Your left hand is placed on her distal anterior right thigh. To perform the stretch, gently drop down with body weight, pushing her right thigh into extension. The CR protocol of client isometric contraction and postcontraction stretch would then be performed from this position. Similar to the side of table hip flexor stretch, use caution because the client must contract against both your resistance and gravity. This protocol can then be repeated for the client's left side.

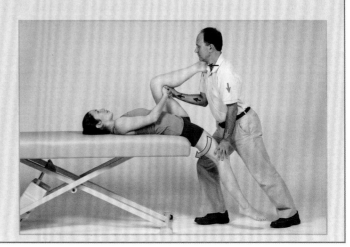

ROUTINE 7-10: HIP EXTENSORS: HAMSTRINGS

 View the video "Contract Relax Stretching of the Hamstring Group" online on thePoint.lww.com

Figure 7-48 shows the hamstring muscles on the right side. They are located in the posterior thigh, crossing from the pelvis to the proximal leg. The hamstrings are hip extensor muscles because they cross the hip joint posteriorly with a vertical orientation to their fibers. However, unlike the gluteal muscles, which also cross the hip joint posteriorly with somewhat of a vertical orientation to their fibers, the hamstrings also cross the knee joint posteriorly; therefore, they also flex the knee joint. This is important to know when stretching them. CR stretching routine of the hamstring group was demonstrated in the "Overview of Technique" section, Figures 7-1 through 7-6.

The Hamstring Group
This group comprises the following muscles:
Biceps femoris
Semitendinosus
Semimembranosus

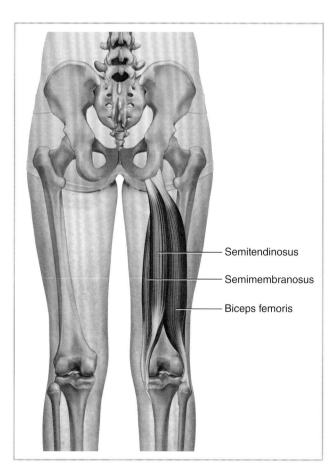

Semitendinosus

Semimembranosus

Biceps femoris

Figure 7-48

7.8 PRACTICAL APPLICATION

Transitioning to Multiplane Contract Relax Stretching: Hip Joint Extensor—Hamstring Group

Transitioning the CR stretching protocol for the hamstring group into a multiplane stretch that incorporates other planes of motion can be done by altering the position and/or direction of movement of the client's thigh. The accompanying figure demonstrates frontal plane adduction and transverse plane lateral rotation added into the sagittal plane flexion of the thigh; this is accomplished by presetting the lateral rotation of the thigh and then stretching it into flexion and adduction. As discussed with other multiplane CR stretches, multiplane stretching can involve motion in all three cardinal planes, so both frontal and transverse plane motion can be added to the sagittal plane flexion of the thigh. Each cardinal plane component that is involved focuses the stretch toward specific aspects of the hamstring musculature. *Note*: Whenever stretching the hamstring group across the hip joint, whether it is purely into sagittal plane flexion or a multiplane stretch that involves other planes of motion, the knee joint must be kept extension.

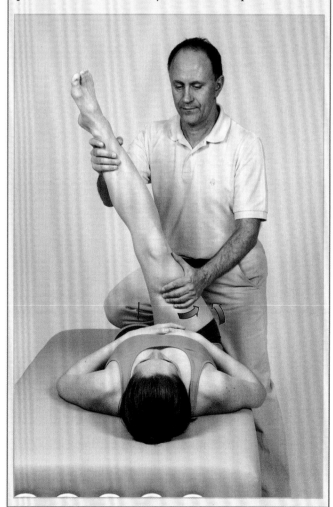

ROUTINE 7-11: HIP EXTENSORS: GLUTEALS

Figure 7-49 shows the functional group of gluteal muscles on the right side of the body. These muscles are located in the posterior pelvis in the buttock region and cross the hip joint between the pelvis and thigh. The gluteal muscles are extensors of the hip joint as are the hamstrings (see Routine 7-10). The difference is that the hamstrings cross the knee joint posteriorly, whereas the gluteals do not cross the knee joint. So to most efficiently stretch the gluteals, the knee joint is flexed to slacken and knock the hamstrings out of the stretch.

Following is the CR stretching routine shown for the gluteal group on the right side of the body. *Note*: The gluteus medius and minimus also have middle and anterior fibers that are located laterally and anteriorly in the pelvis/thigh region. These fibers are stretched with Routines 7-7 and 7-9, respectively. Routine 7-11 presented here stretches the posterior fibers of the gluteal group.

The Gluteal Group
This functional group comprises the following muscles:
Gluteus maximus
Gluteus medius
Gluteus minimus

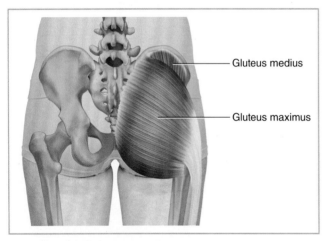

Figure 7-49 *Note*: The gluteus minimus is not seen.

Starting Position:

■ Have the client supine toward the right side of the table with her right hip and knee joints in flexion.

■ Position yourself at the right side of the table.

■ Both of your hands are treatment hands, grasping the client's distal posterior right thigh.

■ Your right leg/knee is the stabilization contact and is placed on the client's left anterior thigh to stabilize her pelvis (Fig. 7-50A).

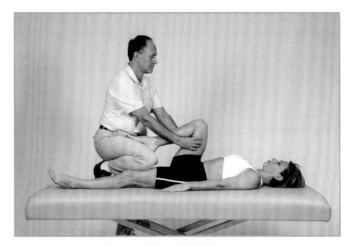

Figure 7-50A

■ An alternate position to contact the client's right lower extremity is to place the client's right foot on your right clavicle (Fig. 7-50B).

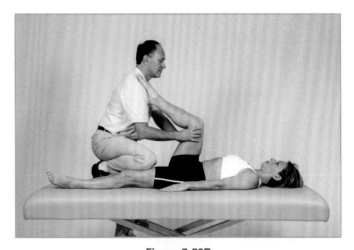

Figure 7-50B

Initial Client Stretch:

■ Begin by gently stretching the client's target (gluteal) musculature by moving the client's thigh toward her chest into flexion until you meet tissue resistance, beginning the stretch of the target gluteal muscles (Fig. 7-51).

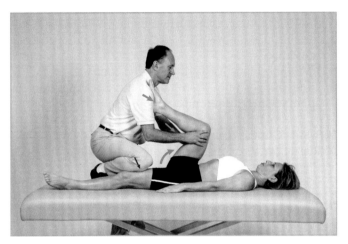

Figure 7-51

Protecting the Knee Joint

Pressing the knee toward the chest can be uncomfortable for the client if she has an unhealthy knee joint. However, if you perform this stretch with the knee joint fully extended, the hamstrings will be pulled taut and not allow the stretch to be experienced by the gluteal muscles. For clients with an unhealthy knee joint, allow the knee to partially extend. If needed, to further remove stress from the knee joint, the client's leg can even be supported on your shoulder.

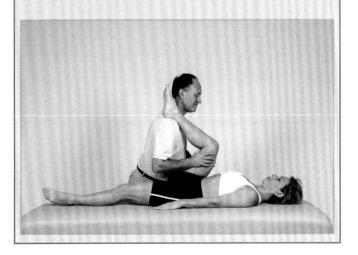

First Repetition: Client Contraction:

■ With the client in the initial stretch position, ask the client to perform a gentle isometric contraction of the target muscles for approximately 5 to 8 seconds (in an attempt to extend the thigh back down toward the table) against your resistance (Fig. 7-52A).

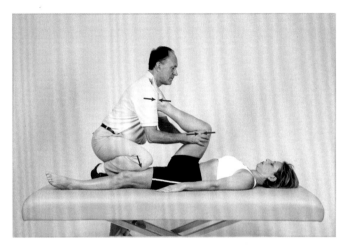

Figure 7-52A

■ Ask the client to relax.

■ Note that the breathing protocol for every repetition is to have the client either hold the breath or exhale when contracting against your resistance.

First Repetition: Postcontraction Stretch:

■ As soon as the client relaxes, gently increase the stretch of the client's target musculature by moving the client's thigh farther into flexion toward her chest until you meet tissue resistance (Fig. 7-52B).

■ Hold this position of stretch for approximately 1 to 3 seconds.

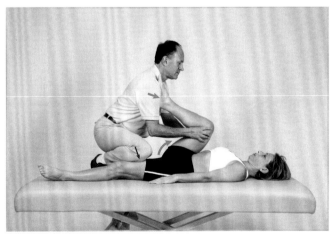

Figure 7-52B

Second Repetition: Client Contraction:

■ Beginning from the position of stretch reached at the end of the first repetition, have the client again contract the target musculature isometrically for approximately 5 to 8 seconds against your resistance (Fig. 7-53A).

■ This time, ask the client to contract against your resistance with moderate force, if it is comfortable for the client.

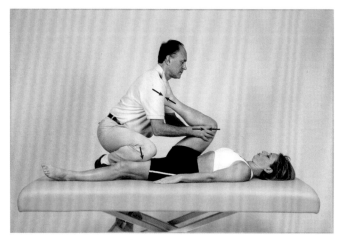

Figure 7-53A

Second Repetition: Postcontraction Stretch:

■ As soon as the client relaxes, gently increase the stretch of the client's target musculature by moving the thigh farther into flexion toward her chest until you meet tissue resistance (Fig. 7-53B).

■ Hold this position of stretch for approximately 1 to 3 seconds.

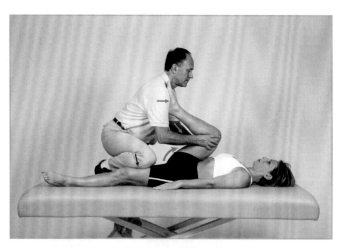

Figure 7-53B

Third Repetition:

■ Beginning from the position of stretch reached at the end of the second repetition, have the client again contract the target musculature isometrically for approximately 5 to 8 seconds against your resistance, this time, with as much force as is comfortable for the client.

■ As soon as the client relaxes, gently increase the stretch of the client's target musculature by moving the thigh farther into flexion toward her chest until you meet tissue resistance.

■ If desired, a fourth repetition can be done.

■ Hold the position of stretch of the last repetition for approximately 10 seconds or more.

Left-Side Gluteal Group:

■ Repeat for the gluteal group on the left side of the body (Fig. 7-54).

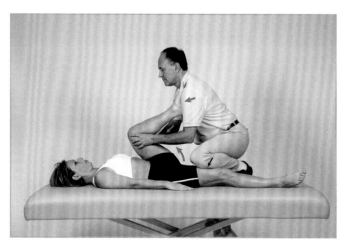

Figure 7-54

ROUTINE 7-12: HIP DEEP LATERAL ROTATORS

Figure 7-55 shows the functional group of deep lateral rotator muscles on the right side of the body. These muscles are located in the posterior pelvis in the buttock region, deep to the gluteus maximus, and cross the hip joint between the pelvis and thigh. *Note*: The posterior capsular ligament of the hip joint (ischiofemoral ligament) is stretched with medial rotation, as are the deep lateral rotator muscles. Therefore, the stretching protocol presented here for the deep lateral rotators is also very effective at stretching and loosening a taut posterior hip joint capsule. Following is the CR stretching routine shown for the deep lateral rotator group on the right side of the body.

The Deep Lateral Rotator Group
This functional group comprises the following muscles:
Piriformis
Superior gemellus
Obturator internus
Inferior gemellus
Obturator externus
Quadratus femoris

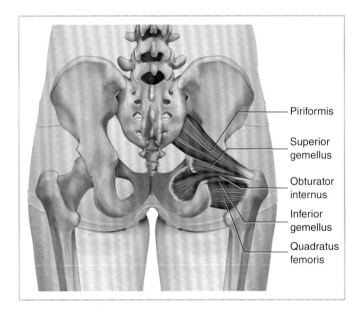

Piriformis

Superior gemellus

Obturator internus

Inferior gemellus

Quadratus femoris

Figure 7-55 *Note*: The obturator externus is not seen.

Starting Position:

- Have the client supine toward the left side of the table.
- Position yourself at the left side of the table.
- Flex the client's right hip and knee joints into flexion and then horizontally adduct the right thigh at the hip joint and trap the client's right knee between your trunk and right arm, in other words, under your right axillary region.
- No stabilization hand is necessary; the client's body weight and contact with the table, as well as the direction that you move her thigh, stabilize her pelvis (Fig. 7-56).
- Using core body weight, gently lean into the client, bringing her thigh down and across her chest, farther into horizontal adduction. Be sure that the client's pelvis remains stabilized down onto the table.

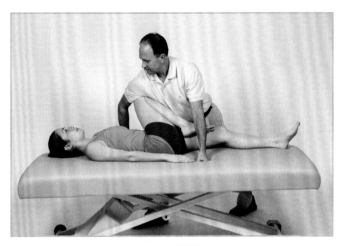

Figure 7-56

7.10 PRACTICAL APPLICATION

Deep Lateral Rotator Stretch and Groin Pain

The direction that you move the client's thigh during CR stretching of the deep lateral rotator group is extremely important. If the direction is too horizontal (parallel with the table), the client's pelvis will no longer be stabilized and will lift from the table, causing the stretch to travel into the LSp and be lost to the target musculature of the pelvis. However, if you press the client's thigh too downward into their body, it may compress the anterior hip joint region (groin) and cause discomfort or pain for the client. The ideal balance between these two directions will vary from client to client. If it is not possible to find an angle that both stabilizes the client's pelvis and keeps the client pain-free, then you can use your hands to grasp the client's proximal femur and soft tissue of the proximal thigh and traction the thigh away from the pelvis (see figure in Practical Application Box 6.6). This often removes the pinching discomfort/pain that some clients experience.

Initial Client Stretch:

- Begin by gently stretching the client's target (deep lateral rotator) musculature by moving the client's thigh down and across her chest into horizontal adduction (horizontal flexion) until you meet tissue resistance, beginning the stretch of the target deep lateral rotator muscles (Fig. 7-57).

First Repetition: Client Contraction:

- With the client in the initial stretch position, ask the client to perform a gentle isometric contraction of the target muscles for approximately 5 to 8 seconds (in an attempt to horizontally abduct the thigh back across her body) against your resistance (Fig. 7-58A).
- Ask the client to relax.
- Note that the breathing protocol for every repetition is to have the client either hold the breath or exhale when contracting against your resistance.

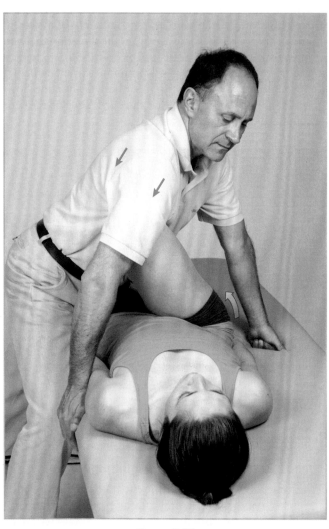

Figure 7-57

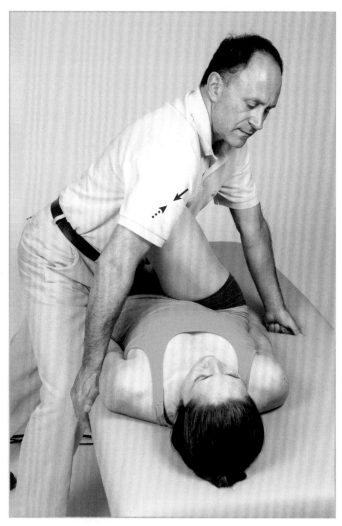

Figure 7-58A

First Repetition: Postcontraction Stretch:

■ As soon as the client relaxes, gently increase the stretch of the client's target musculature by moving the client's thigh farther into horizontal adduction across her body and toward her chest until you meet tissue resistance (Fig. 7-58B).

■ Hold this position of stretch for approximately 1 to 3 seconds.

Second Repetition: Client Contraction:

■ Beginning from the position of stretch reached at the end of the first repetition, have the client again contract the target musculature isometrically for approximately 5 to 8 seconds against your resistance (Fig. 7-59A).

■ This time, ask the client to contract against your resistance with moderate force, if it is comfortable for the client.

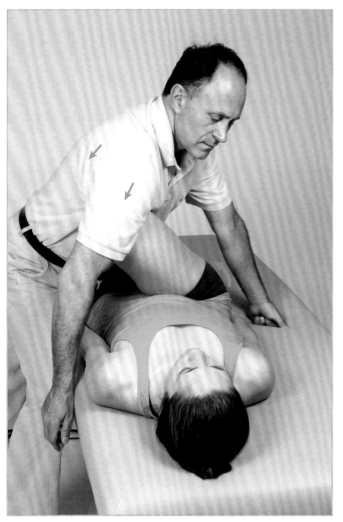

Figure 7-58B

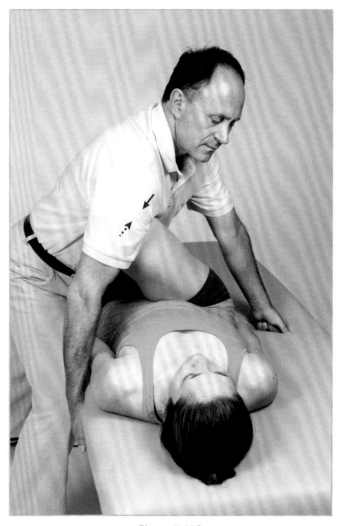

Figure 7-59A

Second Repetition: Postcontraction Stretch:
- As soon as the client relaxes, gently increase the stretch of the client's target musculature by moving the thigh farther across her body and toward her chest into horizontal adduction until you meet tissue resistance (Fig. 7-59B).
- Hold this position of stretch for approximately 1 to 3 seconds.

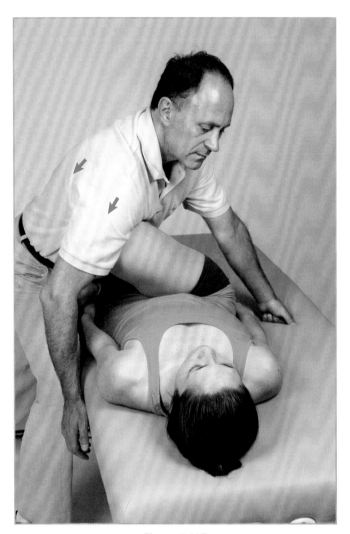

Figure 7-59B

Third Repetition:
- Beginning from the position of stretch reached at the end of the second repetition, have the client again contract the target musculature isometrically for approximately 5 to 8 seconds against your resistance, this time, with as much force as is comfortable for the client.
- As soon as the client relaxes, gently increase the stretch of the client's target musculature by moving the thigh farther across her body and toward her chest into horizontal adduction until you meet tissue resistance.
- If desired, a fourth repetition can be done.
- Hold the position of stretch of the last repetition for approximately 10 seconds or more.

Left-Side Deep Lateral Rotator Group:
- Repeat for the deep lateral rotator group on the left side of the body (Fig. 7-60).

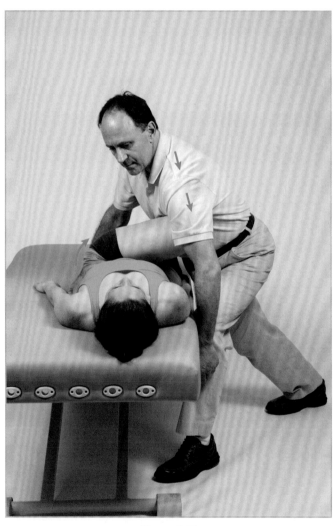

Figure 7-60

7.11   PRACTICAL APPLICATION

Contract Relax Stretching of the Deep Lateral Rotators Using the "Figure 4" Stretch

It is also possible to perform CR stretching of the deep lateral rotator functional group using the Figure 4 stretch (see Routine 6-10 in Chapter 6 for more details on this stretch). Following is the protocol for this stretch on the right side of the body.

Have the client supine toward the right side of the table and position yourself at the right side of the table. Alternately, the client can lie at the center of the table, and you can climb onto the table to be centered at the midline of the client. Flex and laterally rotate the client's right hip joint, flex her right knee joint, and place her distal right leg on her flexed left thigh (forming the Figure 4 position for which the stretch is named). Both of your hands are treatment hands: Place your left hand on the posterolateral surface of her distal right thigh and place your right hand on the posterior surface of her distal left thigh. No stabilization hand is necessary; the client's body weight and contact with the table, as well as the direction that you press, stabilize

her pelvis. Using core body weight, gently lean forward into the client, pressing equally with both hands and bringing her laterally rotated right thigh farther into flexion, in other words, down toward her chest (**Fig. A**). Be sure that the direction of your pressure is such that the client's pelvis remains stabilized down onto the table.

The CR protocol of client isometric contraction and postcontraction stretch would then be performed from this position. When the client contracts, be sure that her contraction is of the target muscles in the right posterior buttock against the resistance of your left hand; in other words, she should not be pressing against your right hand contact that is on her left posterior thigh. If desired, this protocol can be performed without the involvement of the client's left thigh, in which case, you would place both treatment hands on the client's right lower extremity (**Fig. B**). This protocol can then be repeated for the client's left side.

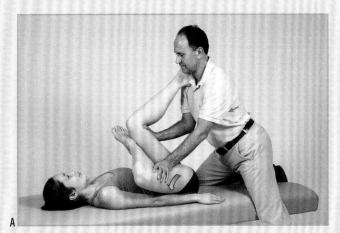

A

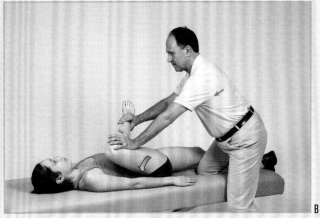

B

ROUTINE 7-13: HIP MEDIAL ROTATORS

Figure 7-61 shows the functional group of medial rotator muscles on the right side of the body. These muscles are located in the anterior pelvis and cross the hip joint between the pelvis and thigh. Following is the CR stretching routine shown for the medial rotator group on the right side of the body.

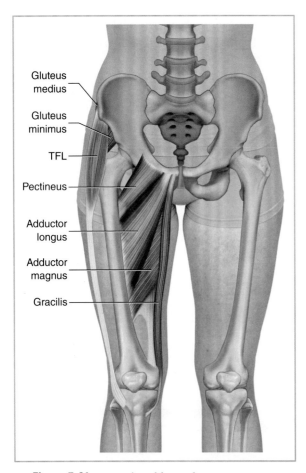

Figure 7-61 *Note:* The adductor brevis is not seen.

The Medial Rotator Group

This functional group comprises the following muscles:

TFL
Gluteus medius (anterior fibers)
Gluteus minimus (anterior fibers)
Pectineus
Adductor longus
Adductor brevis
Gracilis
Adductor magnus

Starting Position:

- Have the client prone toward the right side of the table.
- Position yourself at the right side of the table.
- Flex the client's right knee joint to 90 degrees.
- Your left hand is the treatment hand and is placed on the distal lateral surface of the client's right leg.
- Your right hand is the stabilization hand and is placed over the client's right posterior superior iliac spine (PSIS) (Fig. 7-62).

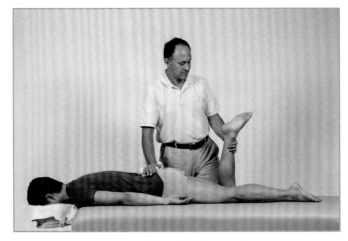

Figure 7-62

Initial Client Stretch:

- Begin by gently stretching the client's target (hip joint medial rotator) musculature by moving the client's leg medially toward the opposite side of his body until you meet tissue resistance, beginning the stretch of the target medial rotator muscles (Fig. 7-63).

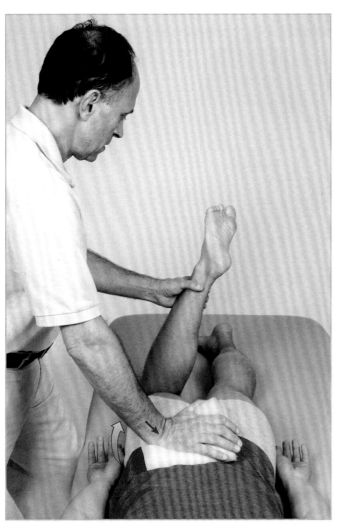

Figure 7-63

7.9	**THERAPIST TIP**

Lateral Rotation of the Thigh

Moving the client's leg medially toward the other side of the body might seem counterintuitive to create lateral rotation of the thigh at the hip joint. However, rotations are named for the orientation of the anterior surface of a body part. When the flexed leg is moved medially toward the other side of the body, the anterior surface of the thigh will be seen to orient laterally; therefore, this motion causes lateral rotation of the thigh at the hip joint and stretches the medial rotators of the thigh at the hip joint.

Using the client's leg to create lateral rotation of the hip joint to stretch the medial rotators means that force will be placed through his or her knee joint.

If the client's knee joint is unhealthy and this stretch causes pain or discomfort, this stretching protocol is contraindicated.

First Repetition: Client Contraction:

- With the client in the initial stretch position, ask the client to perform a gentle isometric contraction of the target muscles for approximately 5 to 8 seconds against your resistance. This contraction involves trying to medially rotate his thigh at the hip joint by bringing his right leg laterally toward the right side of his body (Fig. 7-64A).
- Ask the client to relax.
- Note that the breathing protocol for every repetition is to have the client either hold the breath or exhale when contracting against your resistance.

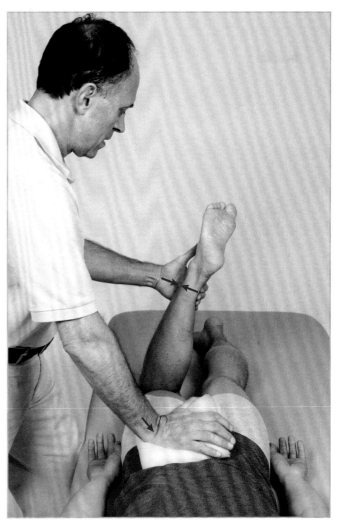

Figure 7-64A

First Repetition: Postcontraction Stretch:

■ As soon as the client relaxes, gently increase the stretch of the client's target musculature by moving the client's thigh farther into lateral rotation by moving his leg farther medially until you meet tissue resistance (Fig. 7-64B).

■ Hold this position of stretch for approximately 1 to 3 seconds.

Second Repetition: Client Contraction:

■ Beginning from the position of stretch reached at the end of the first repetition, have the client again contract the target musculature isometrically for approximately 5 to 8 seconds against your resistance (Fig. 7-65A).

■ This time, ask the client to contract against your resistance with moderate force, if it is comfortable for the client.

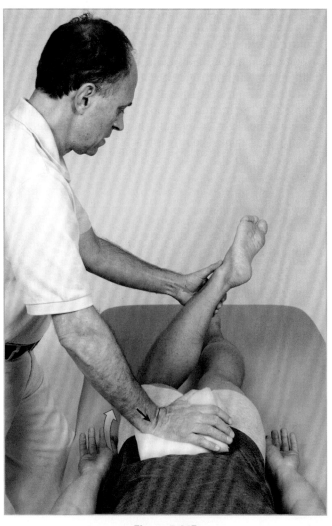

Figure 7-64B

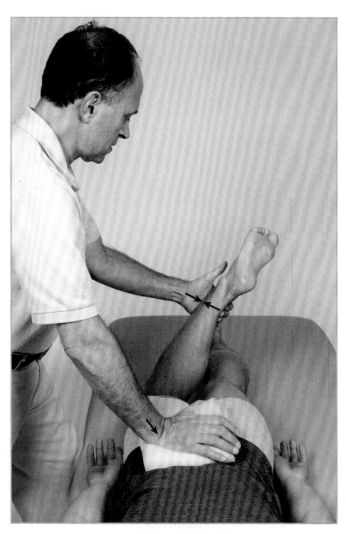

Figure 7-65A

Second Repetition: Postcontraction Stretch:

■ As soon as the client relaxes, gently increase the stretch of the client's target musculature by moving the thigh farther into lateral rotation by moving the leg farther medially until you meet tissue resistance (Fig. 7-65B).

■ Hold this position of stretch for approximately 1 to 3 seconds.

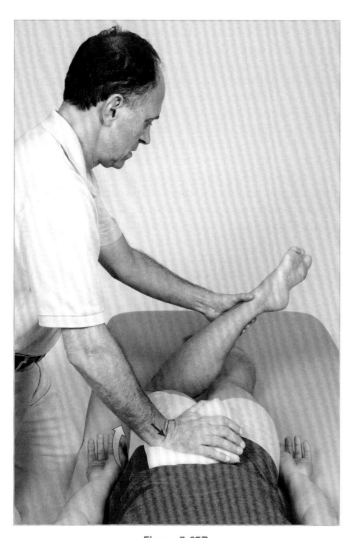

Figure 7-65B

Third Repetition:

■ Beginning from the position of stretch reached at the end of the second repetition, have the client again contract the target musculature isometrically for approximately 5 to 8 seconds against your resistance, this time, with as much force as is comfortable for the client.

■ As soon as the client relaxes, gently increase the stretch of the client's target musculature by moving the thigh farther into lateral rotation by moving his leg farther medially until you meet tissue resistance.

■ If desired, a fourth repetition can be done.

■ Hold the position of stretch of the last repetition for approximately 10 seconds or more.

Left-Side Medial Rotator Group:

■ Repeat for the medial rotator group on the left side of the body (Fig. 7-66).

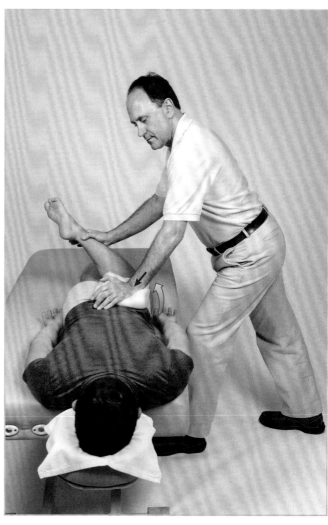

Figure 7-66

7.10 THERAPIST TIP

When Should You Use Contract Relax Stretching?

CR stretching technique is an advanced technique that can and should be employed whenever a client does not respond well to "standard" mechanical stretching techniques. Of course, it is not necessary to wait until a client stops responding to regular stretching to decide to use CR stretching. It can be incorporated into the standard care for a client. However, CR stretching does tend to require more time to perform, so you may want to be selective about when and for which areas of the client's body you use it. Another consideration is that CR stretching requires active participation on the client's part. If a client expects to come to a session and remain passive, CR stretching may not be an appropriate choice. Or, you may need to educate the client about his or her possible role during a treatment session.

A question that is often asked is, "Which advanced neural inhibition technique is the better stretching technique, CR or AC?" Although proponents of each technique may state that their method is superior to the other, the same is true here as for all treatment techniques: Each one works well for a particular subset of the client population, and neither is inherently better than the other—nor is either technique inherently superior for stretching any particular muscle or muscle group of the body. Which method a therapist chooses should be based on how well it works for each particular client, how well the client enjoys the particular technique, and/or which technique the therapist finds biomechanically easier to employ for that particular muscle/muscle group.

Having said this, because the AC technique does require more active motion on the part of the client, it is likely the better technique with regard to warming up the client's body because local fluid circulation (blood, lymph, and synovial joint fluid) would be increased. AC technique's dynamic movements would also better enforce neural patterns of movement. On the other hand, although both CR and AC stretching require the client's active participation and effort, AC stretching does tend to require more participation and effort, so for the client who is looking for a passive treatment session, CR technique might be preferred over AC technique. Also, it is generally easier to transition a stretch to CR technique than AC technique because regardless of the client position, the therapist can add the resistance needed for the CR technique, whereas AC technique usually requires the client to contract and move the body part either up against gravity or at least parallel with gravity. Therefore, the client position in relation to gravity matters with AC stretching but does not for CR stretching.

For CRAC stretching (see Chapter 9), a case probably could be made that it is more effective than either CR or AC stretching alone because it combines the effectiveness of both techniques. However, it does take twice as much time to perform, and spending more time stretching one muscle means that there is less time left to work on other areas of the client's body. Ultimately, the choice of technique is a clinical decision that will depend on the unique circumstances of each individual scenario.

7.11 THERAPIST TIP

Client Awareness of Motion

Many clients become accustomed to the limited ranges of motion of their body and learn to compensate by moving other parts of their body instead. Once a client learns this compensation pattern, it often continues in everyday life even if the client's LSp and pelvic/hip joint ranges of motion are restored through massage and stretching. Perhaps it is because the client fears that the pain will return, or perhaps, it is simply out of habit. Either way, if a client does not move the LSp and pelvis/hip joint through the increased ranges of motion created with massage and stretching, the client will lose those ranges of motion because the muscles will tighten again, and adhesions will once again build up in the tissues. As a result, the client will revert to the original limited movement pattern. For this reason, it is extremely important that a client continues to move his or her body through whatever ranges of motion are increased with treatment.

To facilitate this, it can be extremely useful at the end of a treatment session to bring the client's conscious awareness to the increased ranges of motion. This can be done in two steps. First, passively bring the client's LSp and pelvis/hip joint through the improved ranges of motion, verbally pointing out to him or her the increased motion. Second, ask the client to move the region actively through the increased ranges of motion unassisted, again as you verbally point out the improvement. Once consciously aware of the improved movements that his or her body can achieve, the client is more likely to continue moving through the restored ranges of motion. Using and moving his or her body will help to maintain its mobility, thereby increasing the likelihood that the client's condition will improve.

CHAPTER SUMMARY

CR stretching is an advanced stretching technique that can often provide the key to helping clients with tight muscles and fascial adhesions. Although the exact manner in which the technique is performed can vary, it is most commonly carried out in the following manner:

■ After the client is prestretched, the client contracts the target muscle isometrically to trigger the GTO reflex, which allows the therapist to stretch the target muscle farther afterward.

■ The client usually holds the isometric contraction for 5 to 8 seconds; three to four repetitions are typically done.

■ The client may either hold the breath or exhale when performing the isometric contraction.

Essentially, any stretch can be carried out using the CR technique. As with all stretching, CR stretching is most effective when the client's tissues have been warmed up first.

CASE STUDY

NATASHA

■ **History and Physical Assessment**

A new client, Natasha Rivera, age 24 years, comes to your office complaining of low back pain and tightness. She tells you that she was moving boxes at home the day before, and when she bent down to pick up one of the boxes, her low back went into spasm. She indicates that the pain is located bilaterally in her lumbar region but slightly more intense on the right side. There is no pain into her lower extremities. On a scale of 0 to 10, she reports that the pain is 4 to 5 when she is lying down, 6 when she stands, 7 when she sits, and a 9 if she tries to move. The client history reveals no previous incidence of low back pain or trauma in her past.

Because Natasha is so acute, you abbreviate your physical exam and eliminate range of motion assessment so as to not aggravate her condition. You perform active and passive straight leg raise tests as well as cough and Valsalva to rule out a space-occupying lesion and to determine if the injury is a strain or sprain. Active straight leg raise is positive for local lumbar pain bilaterally at approximately 45 degrees of thigh flexion. Passive straight leg raise, cough test, and Valsalva maneuver are all negative (for a review of assessment procedures, see Chapter 3). Palpation assessment reveals marked spasming of her entire lumbar paraspinal (erector spinae and transversospinalis) musculature bilaterally, with the tightness greatest on the right side, at the midlumbar region. The tone of all other trunk and pelvis musculature is within normal limits.

■ **Think-It-Through Questions:**

1. Should an advanced stretching technique such as CR stretching be included in your treatment plan for Natasha? If so, why? If not, why not?

2. If CR stretching would be of value, is it safe to use with her? If yes, how do you know? If not, why not?

3. If CR stretching is done, which specific stretching routines should be done? Why did you choose the ones you did?

Answers to these Think-It-Through Questions and the Treatment Strategy employed for this client are available online at thePoint.lww.com/MuscolinoLowBack

OBJECTIVES

After completing the chapter, the student should be able to:

1. Describe the mechanism of agonist contract (AC) stretching.
2. Describe in steps an overview of the usual protocol for carrying out the AC stretching technique.
3. Describe the roles of the treatment hand and the stabilization hand.
4. Describe the usual breathing protocol for the client during the AC stretching technique.
5. Describe the added benefits to the AC stretching technique of being a form of dynamic stretching.
6. Explain why stretching should never be performed too fast or too far.
7. Define each key term in the chapter and explain its relationship to the AC stretching technique.
8. Perform the AC stretching technique for each of the 13 groups of muscles presented in the chapter.

KEY TERMS

active isolated stretching (AIS)
agonist contract (AC) stretching
assisted AC stretching

creep
dynamic stretching
muscle spindle reflex

reciprocal inhibition (RI)
stabilization hand
stretch reflex

stretching hand
treatment hand
unassisted AC stretching

INTRODUCTION

Agonist contract (AC) stretching is another advanced stretching technique that involves a neurologic reflex to relax the target muscle that is to be stretched. Whereas contract relax (CR) stretching (covered in Chapter 7) has classically been stated as utilizing the neurologic reflex known as the *Golgi tendon organ reflex*, AC stretching utilizes the neurologic reflex known as **reciprocal inhibition (RI)**.

Note: In the Technique and Self-Care chapters of this book (Chapters 4 to 12), green arrows indicate movement, red arrows indicate stabilization, and black arrows indicate a position that is statically held.

BOX 8.1

Agonist Contract Routines

The following AC stretching routines are presented in the chapter:

- Section 1: lumbar spine (LSp) agonist contract routines:
  - Routine 8-1—LSp extensors
  - Routine 8-2—LSp flexors
  - Routine 8-3—LSp right lateral flexors
  - Routine 8-4—LSp left lateral flexors
  - Routine 8-5—LSp right rotators
  - Routine 8-6—LSp left rotators
- Section 2: hip joint/pelvis agonist contract routines:
  - Routine 8-7—hip abductors
  - Routine 8-8—hip adductors
  - Routine 8-9—hip flexors
  - Routine 8-10—hip extensors: hamstrings
  - Routine 8-11—hip extensors: gluteals
  - Routine 8-12—hip deep lateral rotators
  - Routine 8-13—hip medial rotators

BOX 8.2

Reciprocal Inhibition Reflex

The RI reflex is a proprioceptive neurologic reflex that inhibits (relaxes) the muscles that have the antagonistic action to the joint action that is occurring. For a mover muscle to contract and shorten and cause a joint action to occur, the antagonist muscles must lengthen; for the antagonist muscles to lengthen, they need to be relaxed. Therefore, whenever the nervous system calls for a joint action to occur, it sends facilitory signals to the motor neurons that control the movers, causing them to contract, at the same time that it sends inhibitory signals to the motor neurons that control the antagonists, causing them to relax (see accompanying figure).

RI is an important reflex for the manual therapist to understand because it allows the therapist to perform a deeper stretch with the client than would have been possible otherwise. The therapist asks the client to actively contract a functional group of muscles, and the active contraction results in the inhibition/relaxation of the functional muscle group's antagonists. These relaxed antagonists are the target muscles to be stretched. Once they are relaxed, the therapist can take advantage of the RI reflex to perform an increased stretch.

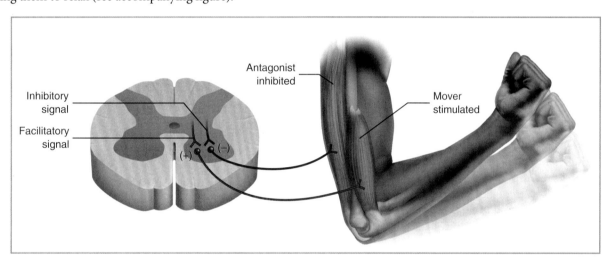

MECHANISM

AC stretching works by having the client perform active concentric contraction of agonist musculature hence the name of the stretching technique. Contracting the agonist musculature that creates a joint action triggers the neurologic reflex known as *reciprocal inhibition*, which relaxes (inhibits) the antagonists of that joint action. This allows the therapist to perform more effective stretching of the antagonist muscles. With AC stretching, the target muscles to be relaxed and stretched are the antagonists of the joint action that the client is actively creating.

When the client begins the AC stretch protocol by actively moving the body part in one direction, the stretch of the target muscles on the opposite side of the joint has already begun because the joint movement lengthens them. At the same time, the target muscles are being relaxed by the RI reflex, which allows them to then be stretched farther by the therapist. This is done by passively moving the client's body part farther in the same direction that the client has already moved it. It is customary to hold the stretch for 1 to 2 seconds and then repeat the procedure approximately

8 to 10 times. AC stretching is the basis for the stretching technique known as **active isolated stretching (AIS)**, which was developed by Aaron Mattes.

Note that, as explained in earlier chapters, the hand that performs the stretch on the client is known as the **treatment hand** or **stretching hand**, while the other hand that stabilizes the client's pelvis or trunk is the **stabilization hand**.

OVERVIEW OF TECHNIQUE

If the neurologic reflex of RI is the science of AC stretching, then the art of AC stretching lies in how the protocol is carried out. The following is an overview of the AC stretching technique protocol using the right hamstring muscle group as the target muscles being stretched. The overview describes **assisted AC stretching**, in which the client is stretched with the assistance of a therapist. However, it is often possible for a client to perform **unassisted AC stretching** without a therapist. For more on unassisted AC stretching, please see Chapter 11 (available online at thePoint.lww.com).

Communicating with the Client

As with CR stretching, AC stretching involves a number of steps and utilizes a specific breathing pattern. For these reasons, it is best to practice it before using it with clients. For clients who have never done AC stretching, it is also helpful to give a brief overview of the protocol before performing it. Explain that the client will need first to actively move the body part you are working on, and then relax as you move/stretch the body farther and then bring it back to the starting position. You should also describe the breathing protocol and let the client know approximately how many repetitions you will perform. This will allow the client to give you informed verbal consent before beginning the technique and also help the client to carry out the AC protocol more easily once you begin.

Starting Position:
- The client is supine and positioned as far to the right side of the table as possible; you are standing at the right side of the table (Fig. 8-1).
- When the client begins the AC protocol, he will flex his right thigh at the hip joint, so it is important to not lean over the table or you might be hit by the movement of the client's thigh. Having said that, it is important to be close so that you can immediately lean in to both stretch the client's thigh and stabilize the client's pelvis.

Step 1: Client Contraction and Stretch:
- Have the client perform active concentric contraction of the flexors of the right thigh at the hip joint, bringing the thigh into flexion as far as is comfortably possible; it is important that the client maintains his knee joint in full extension.

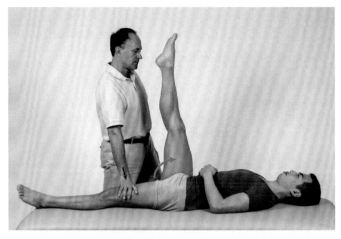

Figure 8-2 Step 1: Client contraction and stretch. Therapist steps in quickly to stabilize the pelvis and to be in position for Step 2, to further stretch the client.

- As the client begins to flex the right thigh up into the air, you need to lean in and position yourself to stabilize the client's pelvis by placing your right hand on the distal anterior surface of the client's left thigh (Fig. 8-2). It is important to make sure that the client's pelvis is stabilized before the client reaches the end of thigh flexion; otherwise, the pelvis will move into posterior tilt, and the stretch of the right hamstrings will be lessened.
- An alternate contact to stabilize the client's pelvis is to use your right knee (Fig. 8-3).
- It is also important to lean in quickly so that you can make sure that the client's right knee joint remains extended and also to be in position to further stretch the client during the next step of the routine.
- The client flexing the right thigh begins the stretch of the target muscles (the hamstrings) and also engages the RI reflex, relaxing the target muscles that are antagonistic to the joint action.
- The breathing protocol for this step is to have the client exhale while actively moving the thigh.

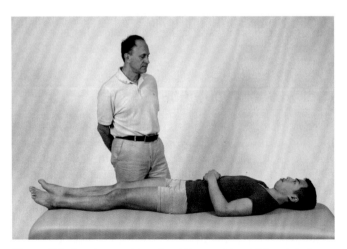

Figure 8-1 Starting position for AC stretching of the right hamstring group.

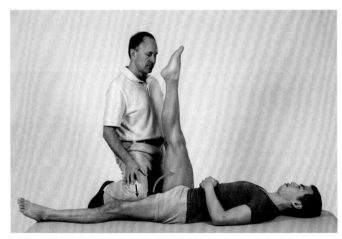

Figure 8-3 Alternate stabilization contact.

If the client contracts too forcefully or too suddenly, a pulled or torn muscle is possible.

Advise the client to initiate the muscle contraction in a smooth and gradual manner. Further, when maintaining the client's knee joint in extension, be sure to not force the client's knee joint into hyperextension.

8.2   THERAPIST TIP

Stabilizing the Client's Pelvis

As discussed in Chapter 7, when stretching musculature that crosses the client's hip joint, the thigh is moved and the pelvis must be stabilized. To stabilize the pelvis, the direction of the stabilization pressure must be opposite of how the pelvis would have moved. Stretching the right hamstrings would pull the pelvis into posterior tilt, which would cause the client's left thigh to lift from the table. Therefore, you stabilize the client's pelvis by placing your stabilization contact (right hand or right knee) on the anterior surface of his left thigh.

Step 2: Further Stretch of Client:

- From the position achieved at the end of step 1, the client relaxes while you passively move the client's thigh farther into flexion (maintaining the client's knee joint in extension), causing an even greater stretch of the right hamstring (target) muscles (Fig. 8-4).
- Hold the position of stretch for approximately 1 to 2 seconds.
- Your stabilization contact continues to hold down the client's left thigh so that his pelvis does not posteriorly tilt during the stretch.
- The breathing protocol for the client for this step is to finish exhaling.

8.3   THERAPIST TIP

Using Your Core

The advantages of working with the elbows tucked into the core have already been discussed in Chapters 4, 6, and 7. Although the position may seem uncomfortable at first, the effort is well worthwhile because it permits you to use your core strength for both your stabilization and treatment hands. For overweight therapists and large-breasted female therapists, if it is difficult to tuck the elbows in front of your body, the closer to the front of your core you can place them, the better. If you find that it is difficult to get both of your elbows in front, then focus on getting in front the one that will be exerting the most effort. With some clients and some stretches, this may be the treatment hand; with other clients, it may be the stabilization hand. Consciously laterally rotating your arms at the glenohumeral joints helps you to keep your elbows in. Once you have practiced the position for a little while, it will come naturally.

Step 3: Passively Return the Client to Starting Position:

- The client remains relaxed as you support and move the thigh passively back to the starting position (Fig. 8-5).
- The breathing protocol for this step is for the client to inhale in order to be ready to begin exhaling for the next repetition.

Further Repetitions:

- Repeat steps 1, 2, and 3 until you have performed a total of approximately 8 to 10 repetitions.
- With each successive repetition, you can add slightly more pressure to the stretch.
- At the end of the last repetition, you may choose to hold the stretch for a longer period, 5 to 20 seconds or more.

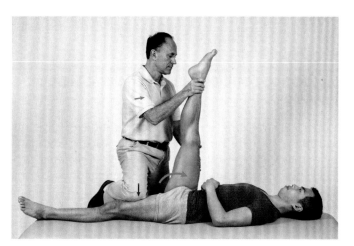

Figure 8-4 Step 2: Further stretch of client.

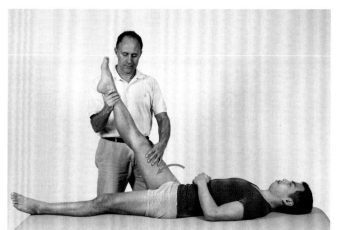

Figure 8-5 Passively return client to starting position.

8.1 **PRACTICAL APPLICATION**

Multiplane Stretching of the Hamstrings

The AC stretching protocol for the hamstring group can be transitioned to become a multiplane stretch by simply adding in a transverse plane rotation component or a frontal plane abduction/adduction component, or both. Each additional transverse or frontal plane component will focus the stretch toward specific fibers of the hamstring musculature. For more on multiplane stretching, see Chapter 6. The accompanying figure demonstrates the position of the stretch at the end of step 1 if the client flexes, abducts, and laterally rotates the thigh instead of performing pure flexion. *Note: Caution should be exercised when stretching the client's thigh into flexion and adduction and/or medial rotation, especially for clients who have had a hip replacement.*

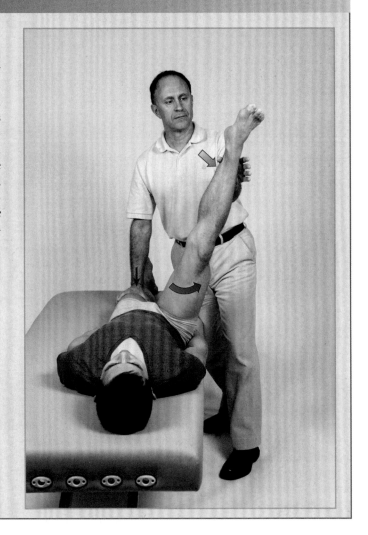

PERFORMING THE TECHNIQUE

When performing AC stretching, it is important to keep the following guidelines in mind. Each point addresses a specific aspect of the AC stretching technique. Understanding and applying these guidelines will aid in more effectively performing AC stretches.

8.1 Client Positioning

Any musculature can be stretched with the AC stretching technique. However, the client is usually positioned such that his or her contraction in step 1 is upward against gravity or at least horizontal and therefore gravity neutral. If the client's motion in step 1 of the protocol is downward, gravity will likely create the motion instead of the "agonist" musculature contracting to create it; if the agonist musculature does not contract, then the RI reflex will not be engaged, and the AC technique will not be successful. For this reason, it can be more challenging to transition a stretch to the AC tech-

nique than the CR technique. Gravity, and therefore client positioning, is irrelevant with the CR technique because the therapist provides the resistance for the client's contraction, whereas AC stretching requires the consideration of gravity, so most AC protocols position the client so that the contraction and motion are up against gravity.

8.2 Starting Position: Return to Neutral Starting Position

When AC stretching is done for the right hamstrings, the starting position of the client's thigh for each repetition is neutral anatomic position. With some AC stretching routines, it is possible to start a successive repetition from a position in which the client's body part (thigh, pelvis, or low back) is not fully back to neutral anatomic position. What is important is that there is a range of motion through which the client can move the body part. This concept is true for all AC stretches.

8.4   **THERAPIST TIP**

Starting Position

Unlike CR stretching (see Chapter 7), each successive repetition of AC stretching does not start from the position of stretch attained with the previous repetition. Instead, the client is returned back to the same or approximately the same starting position for every repetition.

8.3 Client Contraction: Concentric and Active

With AC stretching, it is crucially important that it is the client's own muscle effort that concentrically contracts and actively moves the body part through the range of motion. While your hand may be on the client's body part to further the stretch at the end of the client's active movement, you must be sure to not actually move the client passively. It can be very helpful for your hand to guide the direction of the client's motion, but if the client is moved passively and does not actually contract the agonist musculature, the RI reflex will not be engaged.

8.4 Protocol: Make It Dynamic

AC stretching tends to be performed in a very dynamic manner, with the stretch held statically for only 1 to 2 seconds during each repetition. It should take no more than 3 to 5 seconds total to complete an entire repetition of the client's actively moving, being further stretched, and then having the thigh (or pelvis/low back) moved back to the starting position. Keeping each repetition short allows for a greater number of repetitions to be performed.

8.5   **THERAPIST TIP**

Hold the Last Repetition

The principle known as **creep** accounts for the fact that stretched tissues adapt to their newly stretched length better if held for a sustained period. You can take advantage of this when stretching a client. At the end of the last repetition of the AC stretching protocol for a target muscle or muscle group, you may want to hold the position of the stretch for a longer period, perhaps 5 to 20 seconds or more.

8.5 Dynamic Stretching: Benefits

AC stretching offers advantages beyond those of regular passive stretching, thanks to the dynamic nature of the stretch. **Dynamic stretching** involves the client concentrically contract-

ing the musculature of the region and actively moving the joint through a range of motion, with less time spent in a static position. Consequently, local blood circulation to the region is increased, which offers the benefit of bringing needed nutrients to the local tissues as well as draining the waste products of metabolism away from them. Joint movement also helps to lubricate and nourish the joint by promoting greater secretion and movement of the synovial joint fluid as well as by decreasing the formation of adhesions in the fascial planes of the tissues surrounding the joint. It also reinforces neural pathways of motion. Further, the client's active concentric contraction of the agonists of the joint action strengthens these muscles.

8.6 Intensity of Stretch: Increase Gradually

It is crucially important that the intensity of the stretch increases gradually from one repetition to the next. Each repetition should add only a few ounces of pressure, with the client brought only slightly farther into a position of stretch of the target musculature than was achieved with the previous repetition. Stretching a target muscle too fast or too far can trigger the **muscle spindle reflex**, also known as the **stretch reflex**, a neurologic reflex that is protective in nature. The muscle spindle reflex prevents a muscle from being overstretched and possibly torn by ordering it to contract. This will cause a spasm of the target muscle, defeating the purpose of the stretch. Therefore, stretching should always be performed slowly and within the comfort zone of the client. It is important to emphasize that when you begin to feel the client's target tissues offering resistance to your stretch, you should add only a very small additional stretching force. Because there are so many repetitions (8 to 10), the cumulative effect of the AC stretching technique results in a great stretch of the target musculature.

8.7 Hand Placement: Treatment Hand

When performing the AC stretching technique, it is important that the placement of your treatment hand is comfortable for the client. To achieve this, offer as broad a contact with your hand as possible so that its pressure against the client is distributed as evenly as possible.

8.8 Hand Placement: Stabilization Hand

The position of your stabilization hand (or other stabilization contact) is also crucial. Without it, the client's pelvis and/or trunk would often move in such a manner as to lose the stretch of the target musculature. As with your treatment hand, placement of your stabilization hand should also be comfortable for the client and offer as broad a contact as possible. When performing AC stretching of the hamstring group, it is necessary to remove the stabilization contact with each repetition to get out of the way and make room for the client's thigh to move. However, even when it is not necessary for you to remove the stabilization hand for this reason, it is still usually necessary to remove the stabilization hand from its stabilization position to assist the treatment hand in supporting and returning the client's body part back to the starting position (step 3) for the next repetition.

The placement of the treatment and stabilization hands often requires your wrist joint to be extended. For the health of your wrists, your point of contact through which pressure is transmitted into the client should be the heel of your hand (the carpal region). If you direct the pressure through your palm or fingers, you may hyperextend and injure your wrist. Given how vulnerable the wrist joint can be, proper biomechanical positioning of the hand/wrist is crucially important.

8.9 Breathing

The usual breathing protocol for AC stretching is to have the client exhale while actively moving the body part. A mnemonic device that can help you remember the breathing protocol is "*exhale* on *exertion*" because both begin with the letter "e." Having the client exhale when actively contracting the agonist muscles to create the joint action also works very well logistically when AC stretching is combined with the CR stretching technique to perform contract relax agonist contract (CRAC) stretching (see Chapter 9).

The client usually completes the exhalation as the target musculature is relaxed and you stretch it; the client then inhales as you return the client to the starting position for the next repetition. If the client has already completed the exhalation while contracting and moving, the client can begin the inhalation when relaxing and being further stretched and then complete the inhalation while being returned to the starting position for the next repetition. What is most important is that the client has completed inhaling once you return him or her to the starting position in order to be ready to exhale again during the exertion and movement of the next repetition. If you find that the client has not exhaled completely when a repetition is finished, perhaps the client is inhaling too deeply. The inhalation at the beginning of each repetition should not be too deep.

It often takes a little while for the client to become accustomed to the AC stretching breathing protocol. However, once the client is comfortable and familiar with the breathing protocol, the repetitions proceed smoothly.

8.10 Flow of Repetitions

As mentioned previously, an entire repetition, consisting of client movement, further stretch, and return to the starting position to be ready to begin the next repetition, should take only 3 to 5 seconds. The means that a set of 10 repetitions can be accomplished in less than 1 minute. To help ensure that an AC repetition is performed within a time frame of 3 to 5 seconds, it is important to begin each successive repetition immediately at the conclusion of the previous repetition. This is a point at which time is often wasted. As soon as you return a client back to the starting position at the end of a repetition, the client should learn to begin his or her active movement immediately for the next repetition without your having to repeat the instruction every time.

| 8.6 | THERAPIST TIP |

Pace Yourself

Accomplishing an AC repetition within the recommended 3 to 5 seconds can be difficult for the therapist and/or client who are first learning and practicing the technique. As a result, therapists and clients often feel rushed when AC stretching is first introduced. Although AC stretching is usually performed at a moderate pace, it should never feel rushed to the therapist or the client. Having a sense of urgency is likely to cause anxiety and result in the client's tightening up, which is counterproductive to effective stretching. As you are first learning the technique, take a little more time if needed to perform each repetition until you have gained a sense of proficiency.

8.11 Direction of Stretch

When AC stretching is performed, the client's motion can be carried out in a cardinal plane or in an oblique plane. The three cardinal planes are the sagittal, frontal, and transverse planes. An oblique plane is any plane that is not perfectly sagittal, frontal, or transverse; in other words, it has a component of two or three cardinal planes (see Fig. 1-8 in Chapter 1 for a review of planes). This chapter presents cardinal plane AC stretches in the routines, with numerous multiplane/oblique AC stretches discussed and demonstrated in Practical Application boxes.

8.12 Electric Lift Table

As discussed in Chapters 6 and 7, when stretching the low back and pelvis/hip joint, the value of an electric lift table for optimal body mechanics cannot be overstated. Most AC routines for the low back and pelvis/hip joint require the table to be low. If the table was higher for the performance of other manual therapy techniques, having an electric lift table so that table height can be easily adjusted for AC stretching is essential for efficient clinical orthopedic work.

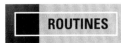

AGONIST CONTRACT ROUTINES

The routines that follow demonstrate 13 different applications of AC stretching to the low back and pelvis/hip joint. They are organized according to the functional groups of muscles being stretched. The routine for the hamstring hip joint extensors has already been shown in the "Overview of Technique" section. For all the other routines, the following steps are explained and illustrated: client contraction and stretch, further stretch of client, and passively return client to starting position. An explanation is then given on how to perform further repetitions.

8.2 PRACTICAL APPLICATION

Agonist Contract Multiplane Stretching Routines

The chapter explains how to perform the AC stretching technique and then presents the technique applied to each of the major functional groups of muscles of the LSp and pelvis/hip joint. However, the AC technique can be applied to any stretch, including the multiplane stretches presented in Chapter 6. A number of multiplane stretches for the AC routines of this chapter are presented in Practical Application boxes that follow the AC stretching routine steps. However, it should be kept in mind that just as with CR stretching, any musculature, including musculature that needs to be stretched across multiple planes (multiplane stretching), can be stretched with the AC technique. What is required to transition a stretch to the AC stretching technique is to consider the relationship with gravity so that the agonist musculature contracts when the motion in step 1 is done and then to add in the protocol steps involved with the AC technique.

SECTION 1: LUMBAR SPINE AGONIST CONTRACT ROUTINES

AC stretches of the LSp can be performed in two ways. One method is to stabilize the client's pelvis and move the upper trunk downward toward the pelvis, thereby stretching the LSp. This method begins the stretch of the LSp superiorly, and as the stretching force is increased and the LSp is increasingly moved downward, the stretch moves into the lower LSp. The second method is to stabilize the client's upper trunk and move the pelvis and lower LSp upward toward the thoracic trunk. This method begins the stretch of the LSp inferiorly, and as the stretching force is increased and the pelvis and lower spine are increasingly moved upward, the stretch moves into the upper LSp.

The following AC stretching routines for the LSp are presented in this chapter:

- Routine 8-1—LSp extensors
- Routine 8-2—LSp flexors
- Routine 8-3—LSp right lateral flexors
- Routine 8-4—LSp left lateral flexors
- Routine 8-5—LSp right rotators
- Routine 8-6—LSp left rotators

8.7 THERAPIST TIP

Stretching the Thoracic Spine

Some of the lumbar AC stretching routines presented in this chapter spread their line of tension into the thoracic spine and therefore also stretch this region. These tend to be the stretches that move the upper trunk down toward the lower trunk and pelvis. Even if a lumbar AC stretching routine does not necessarily stretch the thoracic spine, it can be transitioned to do this by altering the movement and/or stabilization so that the line of tension of the stretch enters the thoracic region. These tend to be the stretches that move the thigh, pelvis, and lower LSp up toward the upper LSp. If the upper LSp is allowed to leave the table, the stretching force will move up into the thoracic region.

ROUTINE 8-1: LUMBAR SPINE EXTENSORS

Figure 8-6 shows the functional group of muscles that extend the LSp. These muscles are located on the posterior side of the trunk in the lumbar region. The AC stretching routine presented here is essentially the double knee-to-chest stretch that is presented in Chapter 11 (Self-Care Routine 11-6; available online at thePoint.lww.com), with the AC stretching protocol added.

The Lumbar Spine Extensor Functional Group
This functional group comprises the following muscles bilaterally:
Erector spinae group
Transversospinalis group
Quadratus lumborum

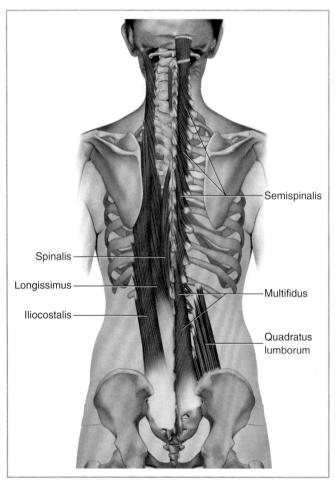

Figure 8-6

Starting Position:

- The client is supine toward the right side of the table with the hip and knee joints flexed. You are standing on the right side of the table (Fig. 8-7A).

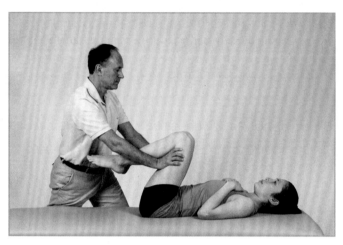

Figure 8-7A

- *Note:* The stretching routine could also be performed from the other (left) side of the table. Simply reverse the positioning of your lower extremities.
- Both of your hands are treatment hands and are placed on the distal posterior surface of the client's thighs.
- The client's upper trunk is stabilized by body weight and contact with the table. *Note:* The client's upper trunk is also stabilized by the direction that you push on her thighs when performing the stretch.
- An alternative position is for you to have your left foot on the floor, and your right lower extremity positioned on the table to be in line with the force of the stroke. The client can also place her feet on your clavicle (Fig. 8-7B).

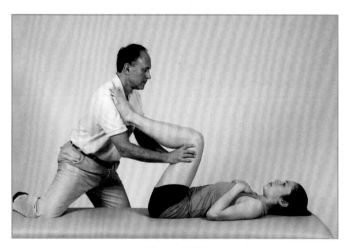

Figure 8-7B

Step 1: Client Contraction and Stretch:

- Begin by asking the client to actively bring her knees toward her chest (move the pelvis into posterior tilt and the LSp into flexion) as far as is comfortable.
- This begins the stretch of the lumbar extensor muscles (target muscle group) (Fig. 8-8A).

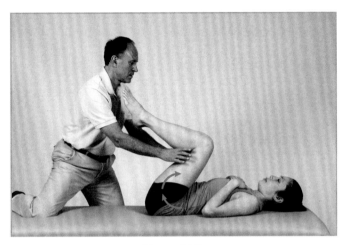

Figure 8-8A

Step 2: Further Stretch of Client:

- Once the position of stretch at the end of step 1 is reached, the client relaxes, and you further stretch the client's target extensor musculature by gently moving the client's pelvis and trunk farther into flexion until you meet tissue resistance (Fig. 8-8B).

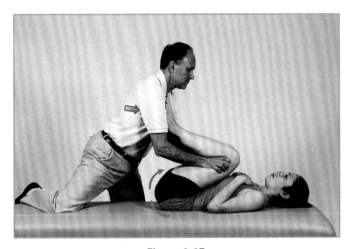

Figure 8-8B

- Hold the position of stretch for 1 to 2 seconds.
- *Note:* To maintain stabilization of the client's trunk on the table, be sure to not press the client's thighs too horizontally (parallel with table) because that would cause her trunk to excessively lift from the table, moving the stretch into the thoracic region, thereby losing the stretch in the lumbar region. It is important to press her thighs somewhat downward toward her chest.

Step 3: Passively Return Client to Starting Position:

- Once you have completed step 2, the client remains relaxed as you support and passively bring her trunk and pelvis back to the starting position.
- When you are bringing the trunk and pelvis back down to the table, it is important that you support the client comfortably but securely so that the client feels safe enough to relax her body weight into your hands, allowing you to move the client passively (Fig. 8-8C).

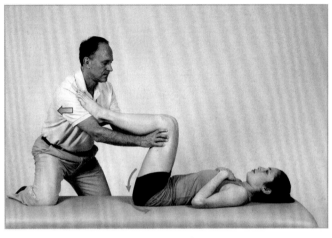

Figure 8-8C

Further Repetitions:

- Repeat this procedure for each repetition.
- With each successive repetition, you can add slightly more pressure to the stretch.
- At the end of the last repetition (usually 8 to 10 repetitions are done), you may choose to hold the position of stretch for a longer period, 5 to 20 seconds or more.
- Note that the breathing protocol is for the client to exhale when concentrically contracting.
- The client continues exhaling as the target musculature is relaxed and you stretch it, and then inhales as you return the client to the starting position for the next repetition.

| 8.3 | **PRACTICAL APPLICATION** |

Multiplane Stretching of the Lumbar Spine Extensors

The AC stretching protocol for the LSp extensors can be transitioned into a multiplane stretch. Instead of having the client bring her knees directly up toward the chest (perfectly in the sagittal plane), ask the client to bring her knees up toward the chest and deviate toward one side of the body. This will add rotation of the pelvis and lower LSp to the same side as the knees were deviated (which is rotation of the upper LSp to the opposite side of the body). This could then be performed in the other direction as well. To add lateral flexion to the stretch, simply begin the client's supine starting position with the client's LSp laterally flexed to one side (**Fig. A**). Have the client maintain that lateral flexion as the knees are brought up to the chest (**Fig. B**).

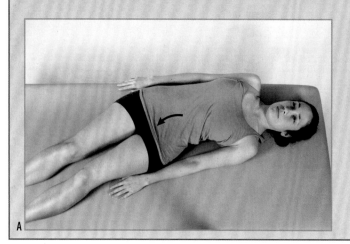

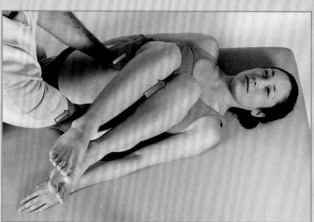

ROUTINE 8-2: LUMBAR SPINE FLEXORS

Figure 8-9 shows the functional group of muscles that flex the LSp. These muscles are often described as muscles of the anterior abdominal wall and are located on the anterior side of the trunk in the lumbar region. Although it is not often necessary to stretch the client's anterior abdominal wall, when it is indicated, it is important to know how to effectively accomplish this. The following AC stretch involves the therapist climbing onto the table. For more on stretching the LSp flexor group, including alternative positioning, see Routine 6-4. *Note*: Using the client's upper body to stretch the LSp into extension will also stretch the thoracic spine into extension as well.

The Lumbar Spine Flexor Functional Group
This functional group comprises the following muscles bilaterally:
Rectus abdominis
External abdominal oblique
Internal abdominal oblique
Psoas major
Psoas minor

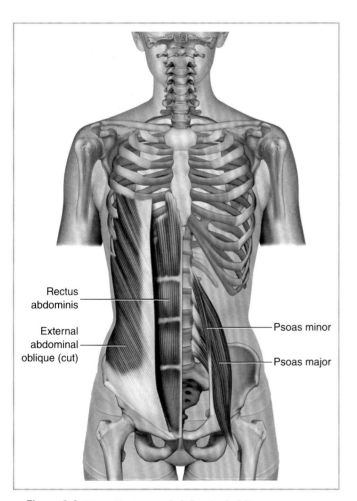

Figure 8-9 *Note*: The internal abdominal oblique is not seen.

Starting Position:

- The client is prone with her hands clasped behind her head. You are seated on the client's buttocks. Note the placement of the cushion for client and therapist modesty and comfort (Fig. 8-10).

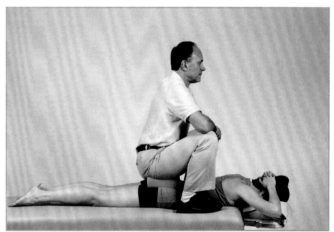

Figure 8-10

- Both of your hands are treatment hands.
- The client's pelvis is stabilized by your body weight.
- Alternative positions that do not involve sitting on the client's buttocks are shown in Chapter 6, Figures 6-18 and 6-19.

Caution must be exercised when performing these stretches for the anterior abdominal wall.

- *Bringing the client's LSp into extension approximates the facet joints and narrows the intervertebral foramina and is therefore contraindicated if the client has facet syndrome or a space-occupying lesion, such as pathologic disc or a large bone spur.*
- *The client's glenohumeral joints must be healthy enough to reach behind him or her and have a pulling force placed through them.*
- *How you position your body weight on the client's buttocks is important. If you sit too far superiorly on the pelvis, it can push it into anterior tilt, increasing the client's lumbar lordosis. If you sit too far inferiorly, the pelvis will not be securely stabilized.*

Step 1: Client Contraction and Stretch:

- Begin by asking the client to actively bring her trunk up into the air (move the trunk into extension) as far as is comfortable.
- This begins the stretch of the lumbar flexor muscles (target muscle group) (Fig. 8-11A).

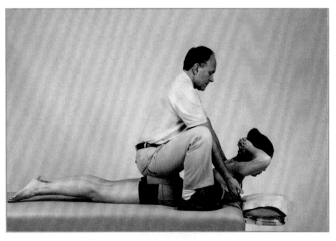

Figure 8-11A

Step 2: Further Stretch of Client:

- Once the position of stretch at the end of step 1 is reached, the client relaxes, and you further stretch the client's target flexor musculature by gently pulling up on the client's arms, bringing the trunk farther into extension until you meet tissue resistance (Fig. 8-11B).
- Hold the position of stretch for 1 to 2 seconds.

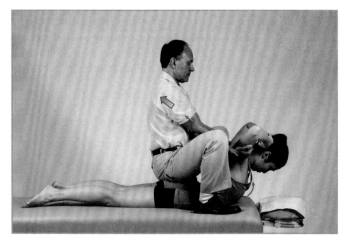

Figure 8-11B

8.8   **THERAPIST TIP**

Lean Back with Your Core

For better body mechanics, when stretching the client's trunk into extension, be sure to do this by leaning back with your core body weight instead of using your upper extremity musculature.

Step 3: Passively Return Client to Starting Position:

■ Once you have completed step 2, the client remains relaxed as you support and passively bring her trunk back down onto the table to the starting position.

■ When you are bringing the trunk back down to the table, it is important that you support the client comfortably but securely so that the client feels safe enough to relax her body weight into your hands, allowing you to move the client passively (Fig. 8-11C).

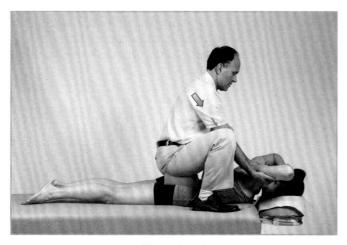

Figure 8-11C

Further Repetitions:

■ Repeat this procedure for each repetition.

■ With each successive repetition, you can add slightly more pressure to the stretch.

■ At the end of the last repetition (usually 8 to 10 repetitions are done), you may choose to hold the position of stretch for a longer period, 5 to 20 seconds or more.

■ Note that the breathing protocol is for the client to exhale when concentrically contracting.

■ The client continues exhaling as the target musculature is relaxed and you stretch it, and then inhales as you return the client to the starting position for the next repetition.

8.4   PRACTICAL APPLICATION

Multiplane Stretching of the Lumbar Spine Flexors

The AC stretching protocol for the LSp flexors can be transitioned into a multiplane stretch. Instead of having the client lift her trunk directly up in the sagittal plane, ask the client to lift up to one side. Depending on how the client is instructed to move, a frontal plane lateral flexion component to one side can be added, a transverse plane rotation component can be added, or both frontal and transverse plane components can be added (see figure). This could then be performed for movement into the other lateral flexion. **Note**: *Caution should always be exercised when rotating and/or extending the client's LSp.*

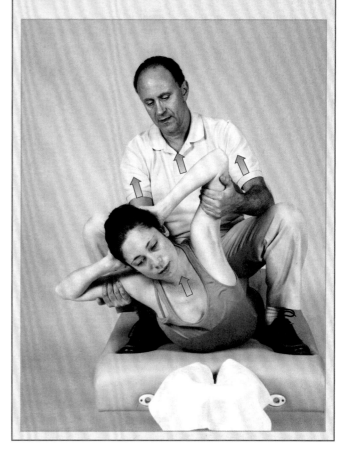

ROUTINE 8-3: LUMBAR SPINE RIGHT LATERAL FLEXORS

Figure 8-12 shows the functional group of muscles that right laterally flex the LSp. These muscles are located on the right side of the trunk in the lumbar region.

The Lumbar Spine Right Lateral Flexor Functional Group
This functional group comprises the following right-sided muscles:
Erector spinae group
Transversospinalis group
Quadratus lumborum
Rectus abdominis
External abdominal oblique
Internal abdominal oblique
Psoas major
Psoas minor

Starting Position:

- Have the client seated at the right end of the table with her arms crossed so that her hands are on the opposite shoulders.
- Stand to the right side of the client.
- Your left hand is the treatment hand and will be placed on the client's right upper trunk.
- Your right hand is the stabilization hand and functions to stabilize the client's pelvis. It is placed across the top of the client's right iliac crest or on the anterior surface of the client's proximal right thigh; if desired, a cushion can be used for comfort to broaden the pressure of the stabilization contact (Fig. 8-13).

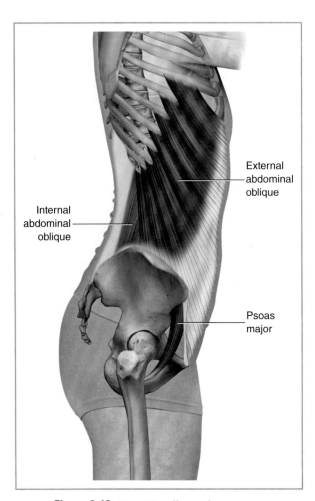

Figure 8-12 *Note*: Not all muscles are seen.

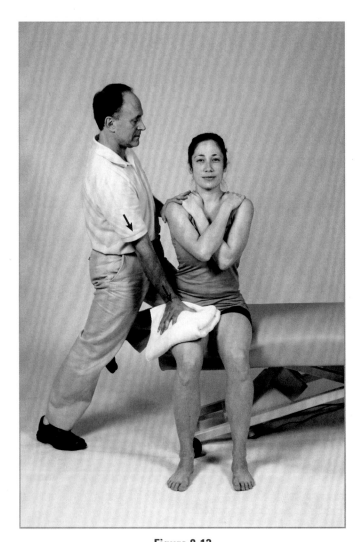

Figure 8-13

Step 1: Client Contraction and Stretch:

■ Begin by asking the client to actively side bend her trunk down to the left (move the trunk into left lateral flexion) as far as is comfortable. To focus this stretch to the LSp, the client should try to initiate the movement from the low back and not the upper back.

■ *Note*: It is important that the client actively contracts her left lateral flexors to move her trunk down to the left; she should not relax and let gravity move her.

■ This begins the stretch of the lumbar right lateral flexor muscles (target muscle group) (Fig. 8-14A).

Step 2: Further Stretch of Client:

■ Once the position of stretch at the end of step 1 is reached, the client relaxes, and you further stretch the client's target right lateral flexor musculature by gently pushing the client farther into left lateral flexion until you meet tissue resistance (Fig. 8-14B).

■ Hold the position of stretch for 1 to 2 seconds.

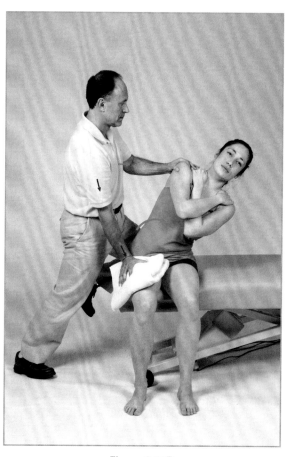

Figure 8-14B

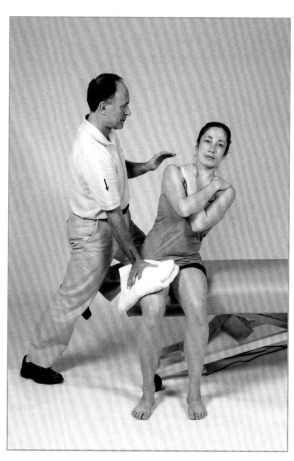

Figure 8-14A

Step 3: Passively Return Client to Starting Position:

■ Once you have completed step 2, the client remains relaxed as you support and passively bring her trunk back up to the starting position (Fig. 8-14C).

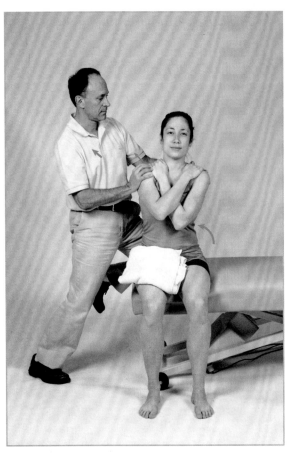

Figure 8-14C

Further Repetitions:

■ Repeat this procedure for each repetition.
■ With each successive repetition, you can add slightly more pressure to the stretch.
■ At the end of the last repetition (usually 8 to 10 repetitions are done), you may choose to hold the position of stretch for a longer period, 5 to 20 seconds or more.
■ Note that the breathing protocol is for the client to exhale when concentrically contracting.
■ The client continues exhaling as the target musculature is relaxed and you stretch it, and then inhales as you return the client to the starting position for the next repetition.

8.5   **PRACTICAL APPLICATION**

Broaden the Stretch to the Thoracic Spine

If you want to broaden the stretch to include the thoracic spine, instead of having the client cross the arms, it is beneficial to have the client place the right arm over her head. When furthering her stretch, contact her right arm instead of her upper trunk.

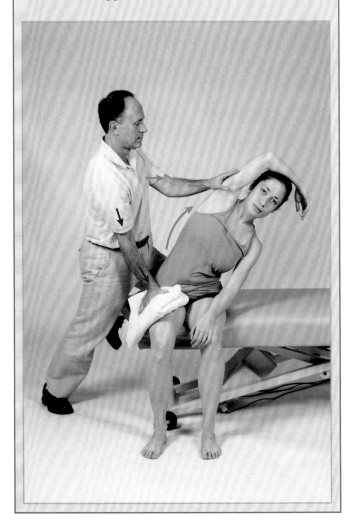

ROUTINE 8-4: LUMBAR SPINE LEFT LATERAL FLEXORS

Figure 8-15 shows the functional group of muscles that left laterally flexes the LSp. These muscles are located on the left side of the trunk in the lumbar region. To use AC stretching to stretch this functional group of muscles, follow the directions given in Figures 8-13 through 8-14 to stretch the right lateral flexor group but switch for the left side of the body.

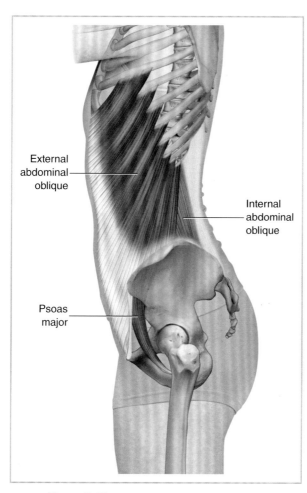

External abdominal oblique

Internal abdominal oblique

Psoas major

Figure 8-15 *Note*: Not all muscles are seen.

ROUTINE 8-5: LUMBAR SPINE RIGHT ROTATORS

Figure 8-16 shows the functional group of muscles that right rotate the LSp. These muscles are located both anteriorly and posteriorly and on both the right and left sides of the trunk in the lumbar region.

The Lumbar Spine Right Rotator Functional Group

This functional group comprises the following muscles:

Left transversospinalis group
Right erector spinae group
Left external abdominal oblique
Right internal abdominal oblique

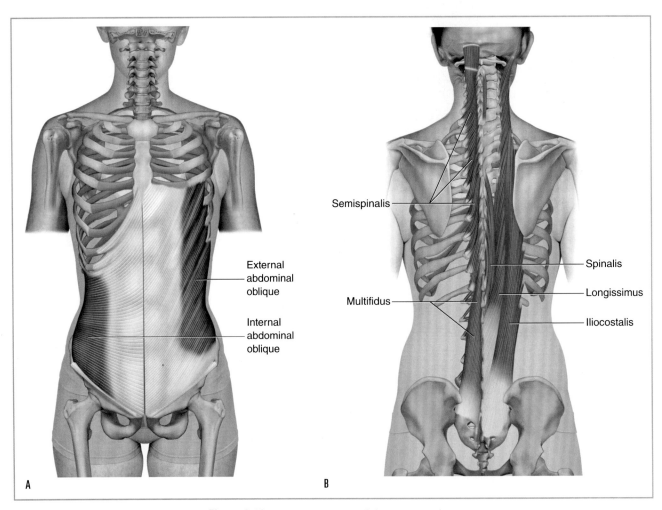

Figure 8-16 (**A**) Anterior view. (**B**) Posterior view.

Starting Position:

- Have the client seated at the right end of the table with her arms crossed so that her hands are on the opposite shoulders, but her arms should be adducted at the glenohumeral joints so that her elbows meet at the center of the body.
- Stand to the right side of the client.
- Your right hand is the treatment hand and will be placed on the client's elbows.
- Your left hand is the stabilization hand and functions to stabilize the client's pelvis. It is placed across the top of the client's right iliac crest or, as with the lateral flexion routines, it can be placed on the anterior surface of the client's proximal right thigh; if desired, a cushion can be used for comfort to broaden the pressure of the stabilization contact (Fig. 8-17).

Step 1: Client Contraction and Stretch:

- Begin by asking the client to actively rotate her trunk to the left as far as is comfortable. To focus this stretch to the LSp, the client should try to initiate the movement from the low back and not the upper back.
- This begins the stretch of the lumbar right rotator muscles (target muscle group) (Fig. 8-18A).

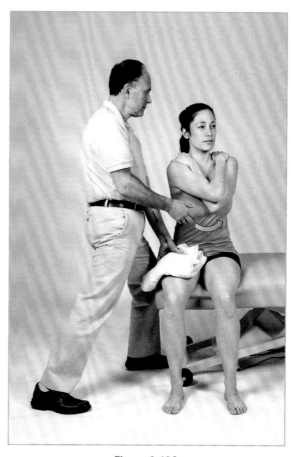

Figure 8-18A

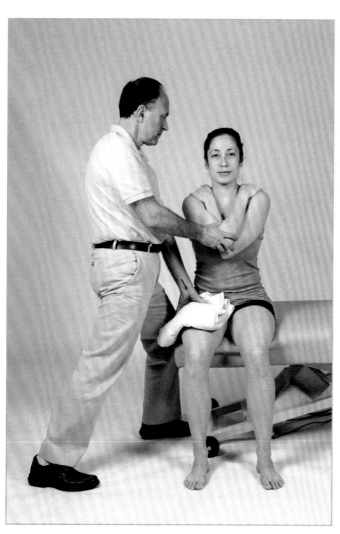

Figure 8-17

Step 2: Further Stretch of Client:

- Once the position of stretch at the end of step 1 is reached, the client relaxes, and you further stretch the client's target right rotator musculature by gently pushing the client farther into left rotation until you meet tissue resistance (Fig. 8-18B).
- Hold the position of stretch for 1 to 2 seconds.

Step 3: Passively Return Client to Starting Position:

- Once you have completed step 2, the client remains relaxed as you support and passively bring her trunk back to the starting position (Fig. 8-18C).

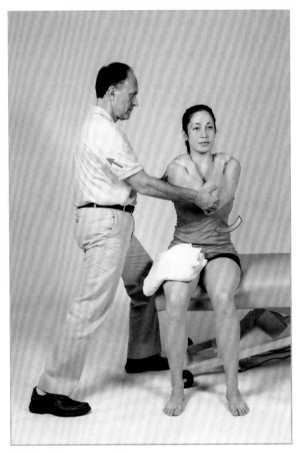

Figure 8-18C

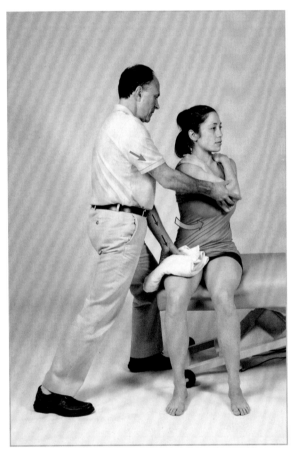

Figure 8-18B

Further Repetitions:

- Repeat this procedure for each repetition.
- With each successive repetition, you can add slightly more pressure to the stretch.
- At the end of the last repetition (usually 8 to 10 repetitions are done), you may choose to hold the position of stretch for a longer period, 5 to 20 seconds or more.
- Note that the breathing protocol is for the client to exhale when concentrically contracting.
- The client continues exhaling as the target musculature is relaxed and you stretch it, and then inhales as you return the client to the starting position for the next repetition.

ROUTINE 8-6: LUMBAR SPINE LEFT ROTATORS

Figure 8-19 shows the functional group of muscles that left rotate the LSp. These muscles are located anteriorly and posteriorly and on both the left and right sides of the trunk in the lumbar region. To use AC stretching to stretch this functional group of muscles, follow the directions given in Figures 8-17 through 8-18 to stretch the right rotator group but switch for the left side of the body.

The Lumbar Spine Left Rotator Functional Group
This functional group comprises the following muscles:
Right transversospinalis group
Left erector spinae group
Right external abdominal oblique
Left internal abdominal oblique

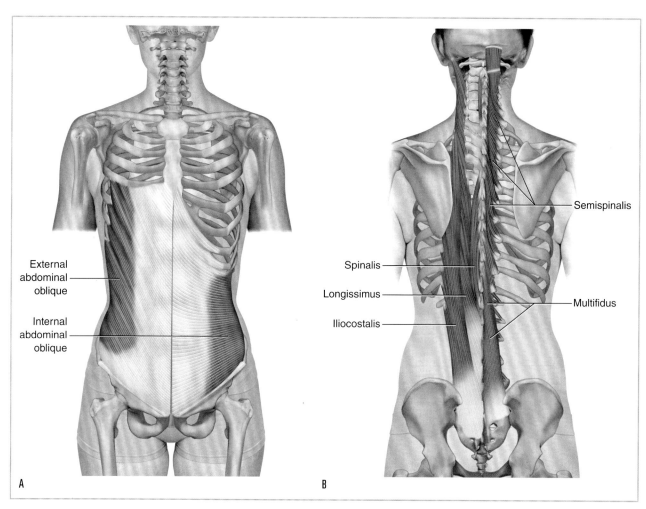

Figure 8-19 (**A**) Anterior view. (**B**) Posterior view.

8.6   PRACTICAL APPLICATION

Multiplane Stretching of the Lumbar Spine Rotators

The AC stretching protocol for the LSp rotators can be transitioned into a multiplane stretch. For a stretch of the right rotators, instead of having the client only left rotate her LSp, ask her to also flex forward in the sagittal plane as she rotates (**Fig. A**) or laterally flex to the left in the frontal plane as she rotates as seen in **Figure B** (lateral flexion to the right could be done instead of left lateral flexion).

Because these additional motions are aided by gravity, it is important to ask the client to actively engage musculature when performing these oblique plane motions. As usual for the AC protocol, once the client has relaxed, stretch the client farther into the range of motion being performed. These same multiplane stretches can be done for the left rotators of the LSp.

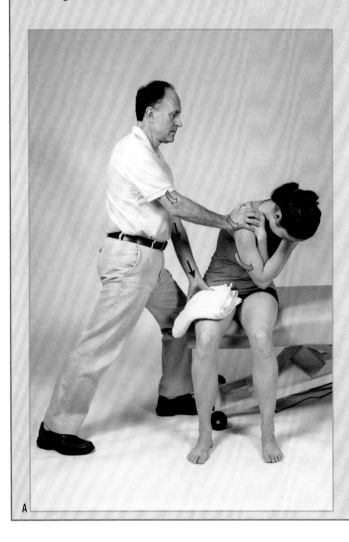

A

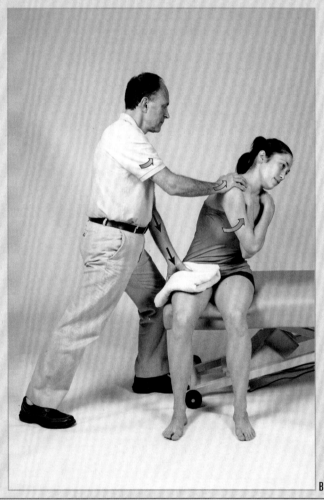

B

SECTION 2: HIP JOINT/PELVIS AGONIST CONTRACT ROUTINES

As a rule, AC stretches to the muscles of the pelvis that cross the hip joint are performed by stabilizing the client's pelvis and moving his or her thigh to create the stretch. For the stretch to be effective, it is extremely important that the pelvis is securely stabilized. Otherwise, the stretching force will enter the LSp. This will not only dissipate the stretching force at the hip joint causing it to lose its effectiveness but might also place a torque (rotary force) into the LSp that can cause pain or injury.

The following AC stretching routines for muscles of the pelvis that cross the hip joint are presented in the chapter:

- Routine 8-7—hip abductors
- Routine 8-8—hip adductors
- Routine 8-9—hip flexors
- Routine 8-10—hip extensors: hamstrings
- Routine 8-11—hip extensors: gluteals
- Routine 8-12—hip deep lateral rotators
- Routine 8-13—hip medial rotators

For most stretches of the client's hip joint musculature presented in this chapter, the leg is shown as the contact for the therapist's stretching/treatment hand. Contacting the leg increases the leverage force, making it easier for the therapist to move the client's thigh to create the stretch. However, if the client's knee joint is unhealthy, the contact should be moved from the leg to the thigh itself so that no force is placed through the knee joint. This can make the performance of the stretch more logistically challenging, especially if the therapist is small and the client is large, but is necessary to preserve the health of the client's knee.

ROUTINE 8-7: HIP ABDUCTORS

Figure 8-20 shows the functional group of muscles that abduct the right thigh at the hip joint. These muscles are located on the lateral side of the pelvis and thigh, crossing the hip joint between them. As with all stretches for hip joint musculature, it is extremely important that the pelvis is securely stabilized. Following is the AC stretching routine shown for the hip abductor functional group on the right side of the body.

The Pelvis/Hip Joint Abductor Functional Group
This functional group comprises the following muscles:
Gluteus medius
Gluteus minimus
Gluteus maximus (upper fibers)
Tensor fasciae latae (TFL)
Sartorius

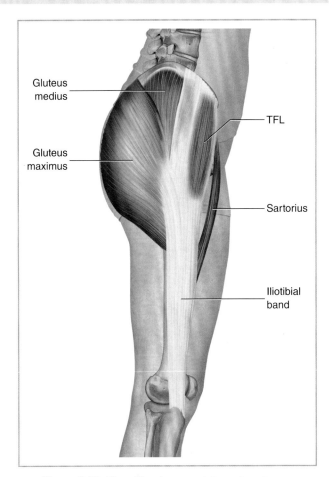

Figure 8-20 *Note*: The gluteus minimus is not seen.

Starting Position:

- Have the client supine toward the left side of the table. Her right thigh is slightly medially rotated at the hip joint, and her right leg is extended at the knee joint. Her left thigh is also slightly medially rotated at the hip joint.
- Stand to the left side of the client.
- Your left hand is the treatment hand and will be placed on the lateral side of the client's right leg.
- Your right hand is the stabilization hand and functions to stabilize the client's pelvis. It is placed on the client's left thigh; holding the client's left thigh in medial rotation improves the pelvic stabilization. A cushion can be used for client comfort (Fig. 8-21).

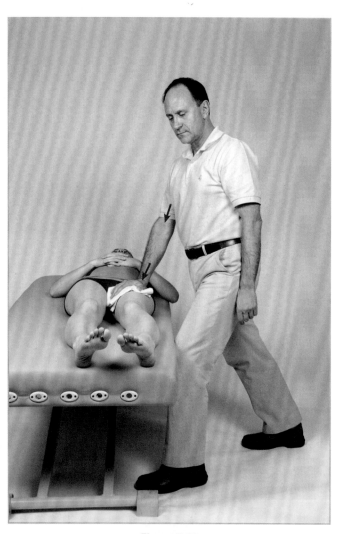

Figure 8-21

Stabilizing the Pelvis

One of the biggest challenges to performing AC stretching of the musculature of the client's hip joint is securely stabilizing the client's pelvis. One extremely efficient way to stabilize the client's pelvis is to use a strap or seat belt that is wrapped around the table and on his or her pelvis, with a cushion used to broaden the pressure for client comfort. See Practical Application Box 6.3.

Step 1: Client Contraction and Stretch:

- Begin by asking the client to actively adduct and slightly flex her right thigh across her body as far as is comfortable.
- This begins the stretch of the right abductor muscles (target muscle group) (Fig. 8-22A).

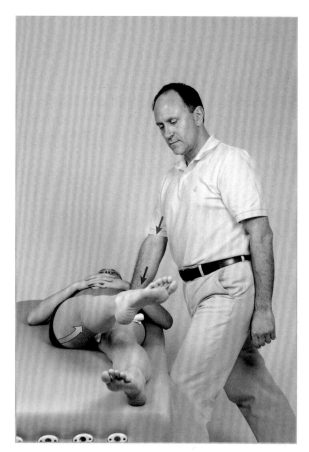

Figure 8-22A

Step 2: Further Stretch of Client:

■ Once the position of stretch at the end of step 1 is reached, the client relaxes, and you further stretch the client's target abductor musculature by gently pulling the client farther into adduction until you meet tissue resistance (Fig. 8-22B).

■ Hold the position of stretch for 1 to 2 seconds.

Step 3: Passively Return Client to Starting Position:

■ Once you have completed step 2, the client remains relaxed as you support and passively bring her thigh back to the starting position (Fig. 8-22C).

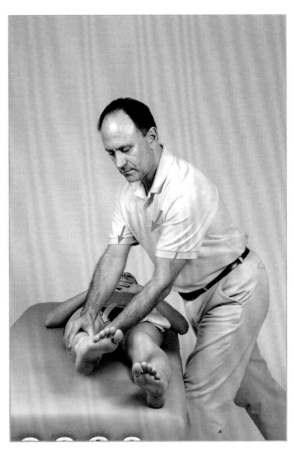

Figure 8-22C

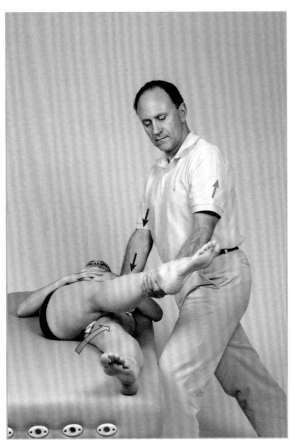

Figure 8-22B

Caution should always be employed with stretches of the hip joint with clients who have hip replacements and/or marked degenerative changes to the hip joint. Extra caution should be employed with stretches into adduction and medial rotation.

Further Repetitions:

- Repeat this procedure for each repetition.
- With each successive repetition, you can add slightly more pressure to the stretch.
- At the end of the last repetition (usually 8 to 10 repetitions are done), you may choose to hold the position of stretch for a longer period, 5 to 20 seconds or more.
- Note that the breathing protocol is for the client to exhale when concentrically contracting.
- The client continues exhaling as the target musculature is relaxed and you stretch it, and then inhales as you return the client to the starting position for the next repetition.
- *Note*: Because the stretch involves flexion of the thigh anteriorly in front of the body, it preferentially stretches the abductors that are also extensors located posteriorly, such as posterior fibers of the gluteus medius and minimus and upper fibers of the gluteus maximus. Medial rotation of the thigh was added because these abductor and extensor muscles are also lateral rotators. Given the multiple planes of movement, this stretching routine is a multi-plane stretch.

Left-Side Abductor Group:

- Repeat for the pelvis/hip joint abductor functional group on the left side of the body (Fig. 8-23).

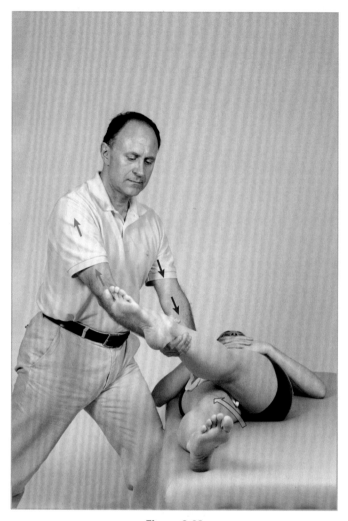

Figure 8-23

8.8	**PRACTICAL APPLICATION**

Alternate Position for Agonist Contract Stretching of the Hip Abductors

AC stretching of the functional group of hip abductors can also be performed with the client side-lying. Following are the steps to perform the AC stretch for the client's right abductor group:

- Have the client side-lying on her left side with her bottom as close to the back of the table as possible and her left shoulder as far to the opposite side of the table as possible. This positions the client diagonally on the table so that her right thigh can be dropped off the back side of the table into adduction without its path being obstructed by the table.
- Stand behind the client.
- Your right hand is the treatment hand and will be placed on the lateral surface of the client's distal right thigh.
- Your left hand is the stabilization hand and is placed on the client's pelvis just inferior to the iliac crest. It is

important to press on the iliac crest with your force directed upward toward elevation of the pelvis on that side. Otherwise, the right-side pelvic bone will depress, and the stretch at the hip joint will be lost. Note placement of a cushion to broaden the pressure of the stabilization force on the iliac crest (**Fig. A**).

- Now ask the client to actively adduct her right thigh down toward the floor. Because gravity aids the movement, it is important to emphasize to the client that adductor muscular effort must be used to move her thigh (**Fig. B**).
- At the end of the range of motion, the client relaxes, and you further stretch the abductors by pushing the client's thigh farther into adduction toward the floor (**Fig. C**).
- You then passively bring the client's thigh back to the starting position for further repetitions.

continued

8.8   PRACTICAL APPLICATION *(continued)*

- The breathing protocol follows the usual pattern for AC stretching.
- Because the stretch involves extension of the thigh posteriorly behind the body, it preferentially stretches the abductors that are also flexors located anteriorly. Given that most of these anteriorly placed abductors are also medial rotators, if the client's thigh can be held in lateral rotation during the protocol, it will increase the effectiveness of the stretch.
- *Note*: The stretch is essentially identical to the stretch shown for CR stretching of the abductor musculature in Chapter 7 (see Routine 7-7).

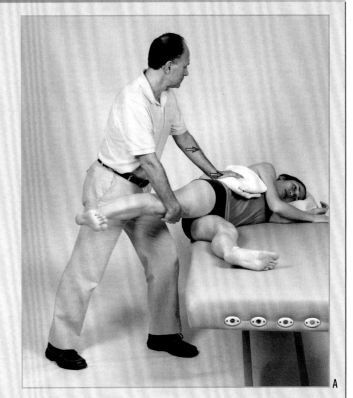

A

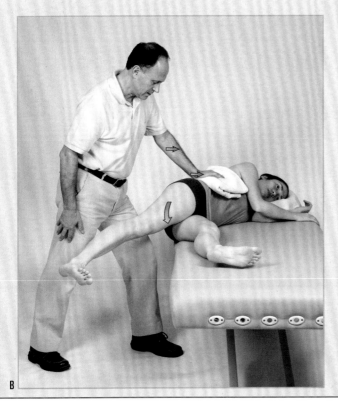

B

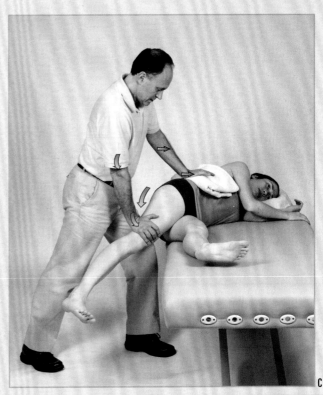

C

ROUTINE 8-8: HIP ADDUCTORS

Figure 8-24 shows the functional group of muscles that adduct the right thigh at the hip joint. These muscles are located on the medial side of the pelvis and thigh, crossing the hip joint between them. As with all stretches for hip joint musculature, it is extremely important that the pelvis is securely stabilized. Following is the AC stretching routine shown for the hip adductor functional group on the right side of the body.

The Pelvis/Hip Joint Adductor Functional Group
This functional group comprises the following muscles:
Pectineus
Adductor longus
Adductor brevis
Gracilis
Adductor magnus
Gluteus maximus (lower fibers)
Quadratus femoris

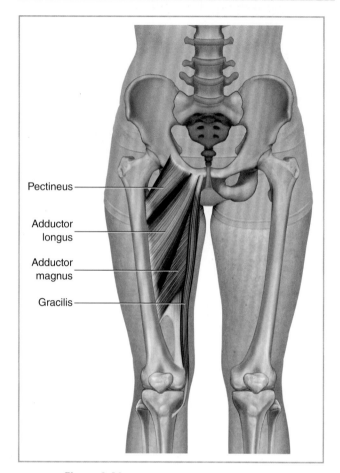

Figure 8-24   *Note*: Not all muscles are seen.

Starting Position:
- Have the client supine toward the right side of the table.
- Stand to the right side of the client (Fig. 8-25).
- Your right hand is the treatment hand and will be placed on the medial side of the client's distal right leg.
- Your left hand is the stabilization hand and functions to stabilize the client's pelvis and other (left) thigh. It will be placed on the client's anteromedial left thigh.

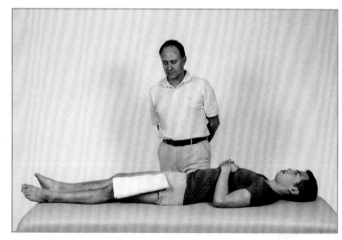

Figure 8-25

Step 1: Client Contraction and Stretch:

- Begin by asking the client to actively abduct his right thigh as far as is comfortable.
- This begins the stretch of the right adductor muscles (target muscle group) (Fig. 8-26A).

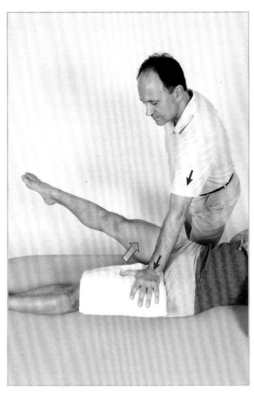

Figure 8-26A

Step 2: Further Stretch of Client:

- Once the position of stretch at the end of step 1 is reached, the client relaxes, and you further stretch the client's target adductor musculature by gently pulling the client's thigh farther into abduction until you meet tissue resistance (Fig. 8-26B).
- Hold the position of stretch for 1 to 2 seconds.

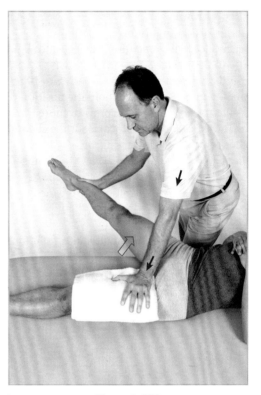

Figure 8-26B

Step 3: Passively Return Client to Starting Position:

- Once you have completed step 2, the client remains relaxed as you support and passively bring his thigh back to the starting position (Fig. 8-26C).

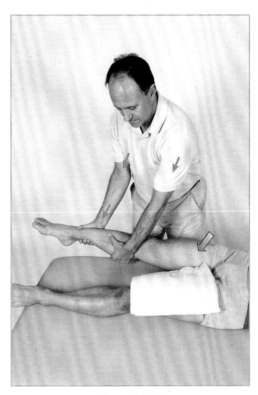

Figure 8-26C

Further Repetitions:

- Repeat this procedure for each repetition.
- With each successive repetition, you can add slightly more pressure to the stretch.
- At the end of the last repetition (usually 8 to 10 repetitions are done), you may choose to hold the position of stretch for a longer period, 5 to 20 seconds or more.
- Note that the breathing protocol is for the client to exhale when concentrically contracting.
- The client continues exhaling as the target musculature is relaxed and you stretch it, and then inhales as you return the client to the starting position for the next repetition.

Left-Side Adductor Group:

- Repeat for the pelvis/hip joint adductor functional group on the left side of the body (Fig. 8-27).

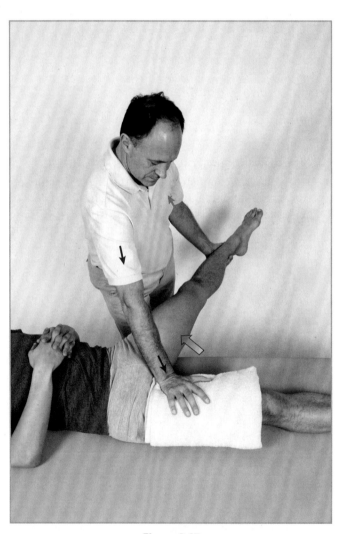

Figure 8-27

8.9 **PRACTICAL APPLICATION**

Multiplane Stretching of the Hip Joint Adductors

The AC stretching protocol for the adductors of the hip joint can be transitioned into a multiplane stretch. Following are AC multiplane stretches of the adductors on the right side: Instead of having the client only abduct his thigh, ask him to abduct and flex or to abduct and extend; because extension of the thigh is downward with gravity, be sure to instruct him to actively create this motion with muscular contraction. Adding thigh flexion would focus the stretch on the posterior adductor musculature fibers; adding thigh extension would focus the stretch on the anterior adductor musculature fibers. Lateral rotation can also be added to increase the stretch for the adductors. If the knee joint is extended, the gracilis will be maximally stretched because it is knee joint flexor; if the knee joint is bent, the gracilis will be knocked out of the stretch, perhaps allowing other adductor muscles to be maximally stretched. The accompanying figure shows flexion and lateral rotation in addition to abduction.

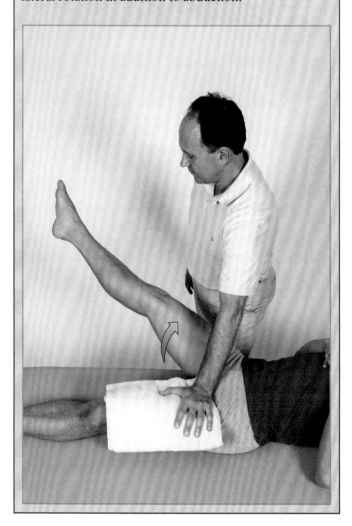

ROUTINE 8-9: HIP FLEXORS

Figure 8-28 shows the functional group of muscles that flex the right thigh at the hip joint. These muscles are located on the anterior side of the pelvis and thigh, crossing the hip joint between them. With all AC stretches to the hip joint, it is important to stabilize the pelvis. With this stretch, it is especially important because if the pelvis is not securely stabilized, it will anteriorly tilt, causing increased lordosis of the LSp. Following is the AC stretching routine shown for the hip flexor functional group on the right side of the body with the client prone. *Note*: Alternate positions to perform stretching of the hip flexor group (side-lying and prone with the therapist seated on the client) are shown in Routine 6-7 in Chapter 6. These stretches can be easily transitioned to AC stretching by adding the protocol steps for AC stretching.

The Pelvis/Hip Joint Flexor Functional Group
This functional group comprises the following muscles:
Gluteus medius (anterior fibers)
Gluteus minimus (anterior fibers)
TFL
Rectus femoris
Sartorius
Iliacus
Psoas major
Pectineus
Adductor longus
Adductor brevis
Gracilis

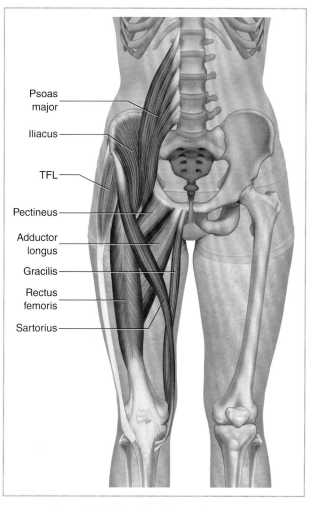

Psoas major
Iliacus
TFL
Pectineus
Adductor longus
Gracilis
Rectus femoris
Sartorius

Figure 8-28 *Note*: Not all muscles are seen.

Starting Position:
- Have the client prone toward the right side of the table.
- Stand to the right side of the client (Fig. 8-29).
- Your left hand is the treatment hand and will be placed on the anterior side of the client's right thigh.
- Your right hand is the stabilization hand and functions to stabilize the client's pelvis. It will be placed on the client's right posterior superior iliac spine (PSIS).

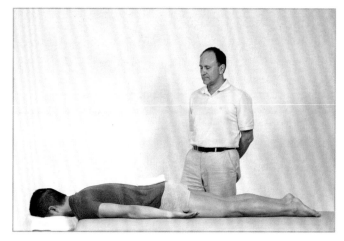

Figure 8-29

Step 1: Client Contraction and Stretch:
- Begin by asking the client to actively extend his right thigh as far as is comfortable.
- This begins the stretch of the right flexor muscles (target muscle group) (Fig. 8-30A).

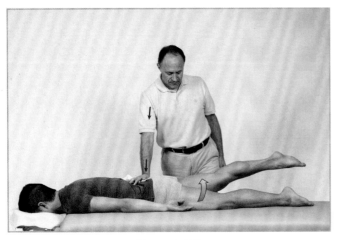

Figure 8-30A

Step 2: Further Stretch of Client:
- Once the position of stretch at the end of step 1 is reached, the client relaxes, and you further stretch the client's target flexor musculature by gently pulling the client's thigh farther into extension until you meet tissue resistance (Fig. 8-30B).
- Hold the position of stretch for 1 to 2 seconds.

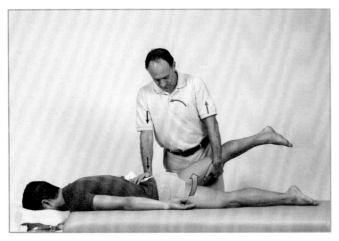

Figure 8-30B

Step 3: Passively Return Client to Starting Position:
- Once you have completed step 2, the client remains relaxed as you support and passively bring his thigh back to the starting position (Fig. 8-30C).

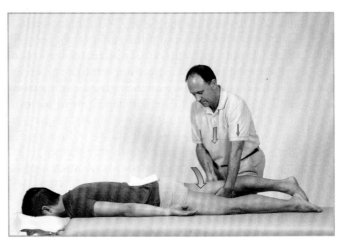

Figure 8-30C

Further Repetitions:
- Repeat this procedure for each repetition.
- With each successive repetition, you can add slightly more pressure to the stretch.
- At the end of the last repetition (usually 8 to 10 repetitions are done), you may choose to hold the position of stretch for a longer period, 5 to 20 seconds or more.
- Note that the breathing protocol is for the client to exhale when concentrically contracting.
- The client continues exhaling as the target musculature is relaxed and you stretch it, and then inhales as you return the client to the starting position for the next repetition.

Left-Side Flexor Group:
- Repeat for the pelvis/hip joint flexor functional group on the left side of the body (Fig. 8-31).

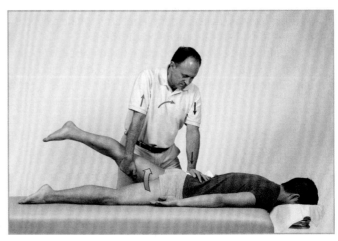

Figure 8-31

8.10   PRACTICAL APPLICATION

Multiplane Stretching of the Flexors of the Hip Joint

The AC stretching protocol for the flexors of the hip joint can be transitioned into a multiplane stretch. Following are AC multiplane stretches of the flexors on the right side: Instead of having the client to perform pure extension of his thigh in the sagittal plane, transverse plane medial rotation or lateral rotation and/or frontal plane adduction or abduction can be added. Given that the thigh will be moved in a different plane, the direction of the stabilization pressure on the client's PSIS might need to be slightly changed; it is important when extending the client's thigh to make sure that the pelvis is securely stabilized to prevent increased lumbar lordosis. Any combination of transverse plane and frontal plane components can be performed. **Figures A and B** demonstrate medial rotation and adduction being added to the sagittal plane extension motion of the thigh. In Figure A, the client actively moves the thigh to initiate the stretch and trigger the RI reflex. In Figure B, the therapist adds to the stretch once the client has relaxed. **Figure C** demonstrates adding flexion to the client's knee joint. This becomes a multijoint stretch and will maximally stretch the client's rectus femoris. If you want to knock out the rectus femoris so that the stretch can be focused on other muscles of the flexor functional group, make sure that the client's knee joint remains extended.

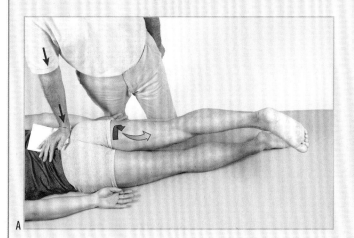

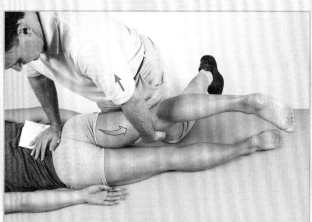

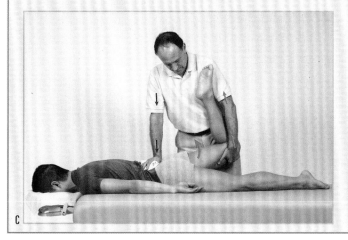

ROUTINE 8-10: HIP EXTENSORS: HAMSTRINGS

 View the video "Agonist Contract Stretching of the Hamstring Group" online on thePoint.lww.com

Figure 8-32 shows the hamstring muscles on the right side. They are located in the posterior thigh, crossing from the pelvis to the proximal leg. The hamstrings are hip extensor muscles because they cross the hip joint posteriorly with a vertical orientation to their fibers. However, unlike the gluteal muscles, which also cross the hip joint posteriorly with somewhat of a vertical orientation to their fibers, the hamstrings also cross the knee joint posteriorly; therefore, they also flex the knee joint. This is important to know when stretching them. AC stretching routine of the hamstring group was demonstrated in the "Overview of Technique" section, Figures 8-1 through 8-5.

The Hamstring Group
The group comprises the following muscles:
Biceps femoris
Semitendinosus
Semimembranosus

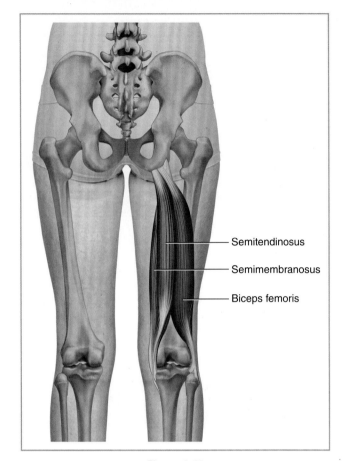

Semitendinosus

Semimembranosus

Biceps femoris

Figure 8-32

ROUTINE 8-11: HIP EXTENSORS: GLUTEALS

Figure 8-33 shows the functional group of gluteal muscles on the right side of the body. These muscles are located in the posterior pelvis in the buttock region and cross the hip joint between the pelvis and thigh. The gluteal muscles are extensors of the hip joint as are the hamstrings (see Routine 8-10). The difference is that the hamstrings cross the knee joint posteriorly, whereas the gluteals do not cross the knee joint. So to most efficiently stretch the gluteals, the knee joint is flexed to slacken and knock the hamstrings out of the stretch.

Following is the AC stretching routine shown for the gluteal group on the right side of the body. *Note*: The gluteus medius and minimus also have middle and anterior fibers that are located laterally and anteriorly in the pelvis/thigh region. These fibers are stretched with Routines 8-7 and 8-9, respectively. Routine 8-11 presented here stretches the posterior fibers of the gluteal group.

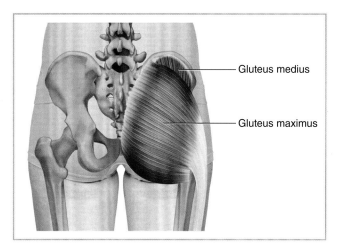

Figure 8-33 *Note*: The gluteus minimus is not seen.

The Gluteal Group
This functional group comprises the following muscles:
Gluteus maximus
Gluteus medius
Gluteus minimus

- Have the client flex his right thigh at the hip joint and flex his right leg at the knee joint; his right foot will be flat on the table.
- Your left hand is the treatment hand and will be placed on the posterior side of the client's right thigh.
- Your right hand is the stabilization hand and functions to stabilize the client's pelvis. It will be placed on the anterior surface of the client's left thigh.
- An alternate stabilization contact is to use your right knee on the anterior surface of the client's left thigh (see Fig. 8-3).

Step 1: Client Contraction and Stretch:
- Begin by asking the client to actively bring his right knee to his chest (flex his right thigh at the hip joint and leg at the knee joint) as far as is comfortable.
- This begins the stretch of the right gluteal muscles (target muscle group) (Fig. 8-35A).

Starting Position:
- Have the client supine toward the right side of the table.
- Stand to the right side of the client (Fig. 8-34).

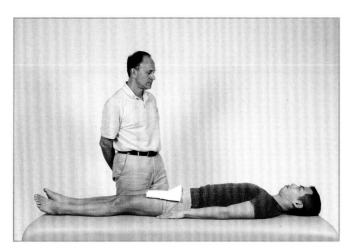

Figure 8-34

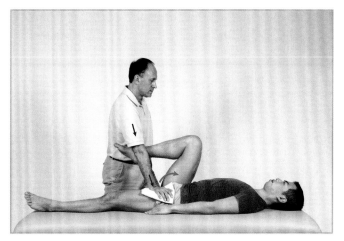

Figure 8-35A

Step 2: Further Stretch of Client:

- Once the position of stretch at the end of step 1 is reached, the client relaxes, and you further stretch the client's target gluteal musculature by gently pushing the client's thigh farther into flexion until you meet tissue resistance (Fig. 8-35B).
- Hold the position of stretch for 1 to 2 seconds.

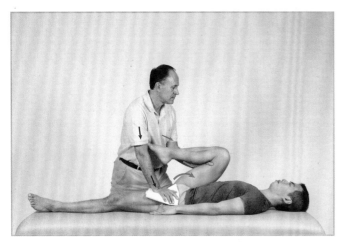

Figure 8-35B

Step 3: Passively Return Client to Starting Position:

- Once you have completed step 2, the client remains relaxed as you support and passively bring his thigh back to the starting position (Fig. 8-35C).

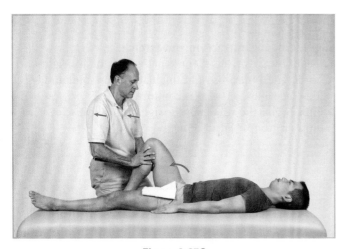

Figure 8-35C

- Instead of returning the client all the way to the initial starting position, the client can be returned part of the way (Fig. 8-35D). The advantage to this is that you do not have to step away completely and remove your treatment and stabilization hands before beginning the next repetition. What is important is that the client still has enough room to concentrically contract and bring the knee to the chest so that the RI reflex will be triggered to inhibit the gluteal musculature.

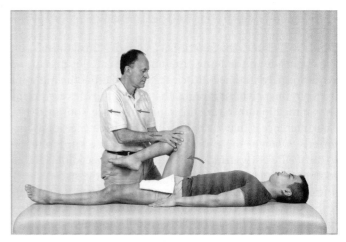

Figure 8-35D

Further Repetitions:

- Repeat this procedure for each repetition.
- With each successive repetition, you can add slightly more pressure to the stretch.
- At the end of the last repetition (usually 8 to 10 repetitions are done), you may choose to hold the position of stretch for a longer period, 5 to 20 seconds or more.
- Note that the breathing protocol is for the client to exhale when concentrically contracting.
- The client continues exhaling as the target musculature is relaxed and you stretch it, and then inhales as you return the client to the starting position for the next repetition.
- *Note*: As discussed in Chapter 6, if the client is asked to bring the knee up to the chest and over to the opposite of the body, making this a multiplane stretch, it begins to resemble the stretch for the deep lateral rotators. Routine 8-12 demonstrates the AC stretching technique for the deep lateral rotator group.

Left-Side Gluteal Group:

- Repeat for the pelvis/hip joint gluteal group on the left side of the body (Fig. 8-36).

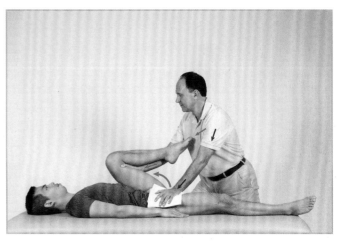

Figure 8-36

ROUTINE 8-12: HIP DEEP LATERAL ROTATORS

Figure 8-37 shows the functional group of deep lateral rotator muscles on the right side of the body. These muscles are located in the posterior pelvis in the buttock region, deep to the gluteus maximus, and cross the hip joint between the pelvis and thigh. *Note*: The posterior capsular ligament of the hip joint (ischiofemoral ligament) is stretched with medial rotation, as are the deep lateral rotator muscles. Therefore, the stretching protocol presented here for the deep lateral rotators is also very effective at stretching and loosening a taut posterior hip joint capsule. Following is the AC stretching routine shown for the deep lateral rotator group on the right side of the body.

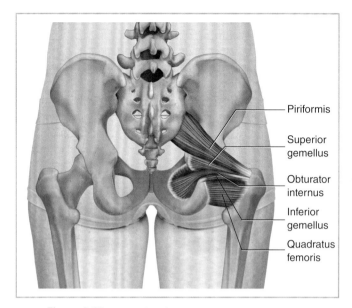

Figure 8-37 *Note*: The obturator externus is not seen.

The Deep Lateral Rotator Group
This functional group comprises the following muscles:
Piriformis
Superior gemellus
Obturator internus
Inferior gemellus
Obturator externus
Quadratus femoris

Starting Position:

- Have the client prone with her right leg flexed at the knee joint.
- Stand to the right side of the table (Fig. 8-38).
- Your left hand is the treatment hand and will grasp around the medial side of the client's distal right leg.
- Your right hand is the stabilization hand and functions to stabilize the client's pelvis. It is placed on the client's left PSIS.

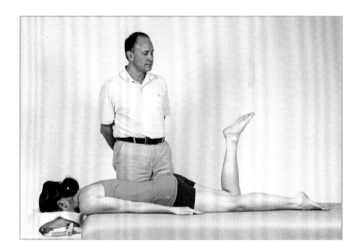

Figure 8-38

Step 1: Client Contraction and Stretch:

- Begin by asking the client to actively bring her right foot outward by medially rotating her right thigh at the hip joint as far as is comfortable.
- This begins the stretch of the right deep lateral rotator muscles (target muscle group) (Fig. 8-39A).

Step 2: Further Stretch of Client:

- Once the position of stretch at the end of step 1 is reached, the client relaxes, and you further stretch the client's target deep lateral rotator musculature by gently pushing the distal end of the client's leg farther laterally, increasing the medial rotation of her thigh at the hip joint, until you meet tissue resistance (Fig. 8-39B).
- Hold the position of stretch for 1 to 2 seconds.

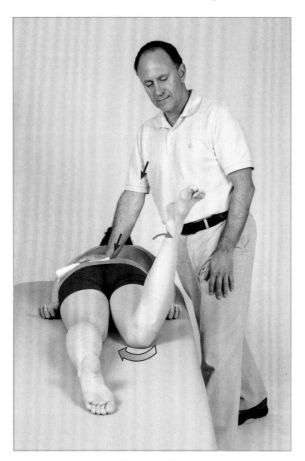

Figure 8-39A

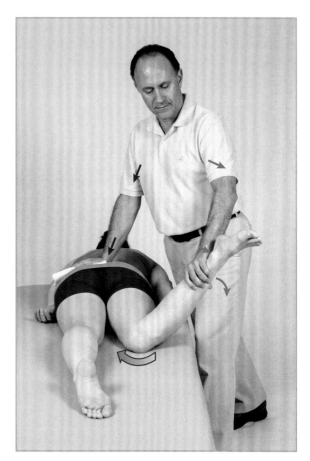

Figure 8-39B

By using the client's leg as a lever to medially rotate the thigh at the hip joint, a torque (rotary force) is placed through the client's knee. If the client has an unhealthy knee, this stretch is contraindicated, and the supine AC deep lateral rotator stretch in Practical Application Box 8.11 should be performed instead.

Step 3: Passively Return Client to Starting Position:

■ Once you have completed step 2, the client remains relaxed as you support and passively bring her lower extremity back to the starting position (Fig. 8-39C).

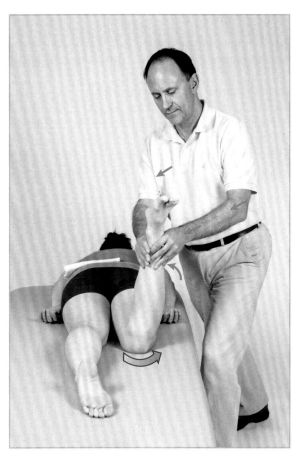

Figure 8-39C

Further Repetitions:

■ Repeat this procedure for each repetition.
■ With each successive repetition, you can add slightly more pressure to the stretch.
■ At the end of the last repetition (usually 8 to 10 repetitions are done), you may choose to hold the position of stretch for a longer period, 5 to 20 seconds or more.
■ Note that the breathing protocol is for the client to exhale when concentrically contracting.
■ The client continues exhaling as the target musculature is relaxed and you stretch it, and then inhales as you return the client to the starting position for the next repetition.

Left-Side Deep Lateral Rotator Group:

■ Repeat for the pelvis/hip joint deep lateral rotator group on the left side of the body (Fig. 8-40).

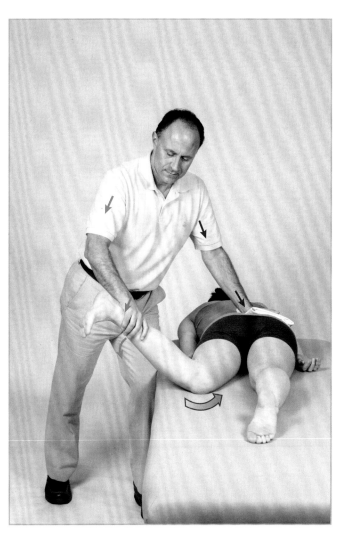

Figure 8-40

8.11 PRACTICAL APPLICATION

Alternate Agonist Contract Stretch for the Deep Lateral Rotator Group

The deep lateral rotator group can also be stretched with the client lying supine with the hip and knee joints flexed.

If the client has an unhealthy knee joint, then her leg should not be used as a lever to create the medial rotation force to stretch the deep lateral rotators. Following is an alternative AC stretch for the deep lateral rotators that does not involve the client's knee joint. This stretch is demonstrated and explained for the client's right side.

■ Have the client supine with her right hip and knee joints flexed and her foot flat on the table. You stand to her right side.

■ Begin by asking the client to actively bring her right knee up and across her body toward the opposite shoulder by further flexing and horizontally adducting her thigh at the hip joint (**Fig. A**). This begins the stretch of the deep lateral rotators and triggers the RI reflex to inhibit and relax them.

■ Now ask the client to relax and you increase the stretch of the client's deep lateral rotators by gently pushing her knee further toward her opposite shoulder (**Fig. B**).

■ After holding the position for 1 to 2 seconds, passively bring the client's thigh back to the starting position (**Fig. C**).

■ Repeat for a total of 8 to 10 repetitions.

■ *Note*: It is helpful to purposely change the angle that you ask the client to bring the thigh up and across her body. After bringing the knee toward the opposite shoulder, instruct the client to change the angle to be more across the body, in other words, less flexion and more horizontal adduction. Each different angle within the quadrant between straight up toward the chest and directly horizontally across her body will preferentially stretch different fibers of the deep lateral rotator group.

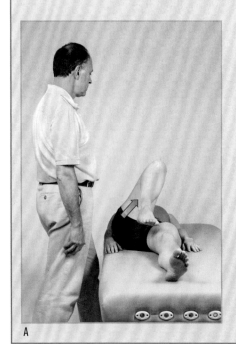

A

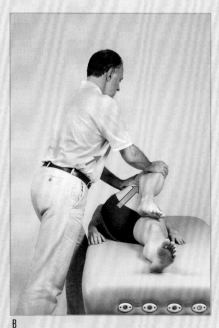

B

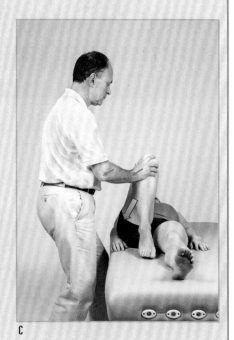

C

ROUTINE 8-13: HIP MEDIAL ROTATORS

Figure 8-41 shows the functional group of medial rotator muscles on the right side of the body. These muscles are located in the anterior pelvis and cross the hip joint between the pelvis and thigh. Following is the AC stretching routine shown for the medial rotator group on the right side of the body.

The Medial Rotator Group
This functional group comprises the following muscles: TFL
Gluteus medius (anterior fibers)
Gluteus minimus (anterior fibers)
Pectineus
Adductor longus
Adductor brevis
Gracilis
Adductor magnus

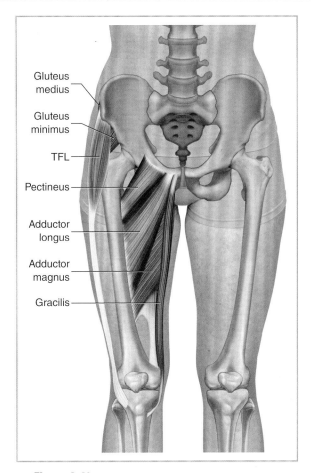

Gluteus medius

Gluteus minimus

TFL

Pectineus

Adductor longus

Adductor magnus

Gracilis

Figure 8-41 *Note*: The adductor brevis is not seen.

Starting Position:

- Have the client prone with her right leg flexed at the knee joint.
- Stand on the (opposite) left side of the table (Fig. 8-42).
- Your left hand is the treatment hand and will grasp around the posterior side of the client's distal right leg.
- Your right hand is the stabilization hand and functions to stabilize the client's pelvis. It will be placed on the client's right PSIS.

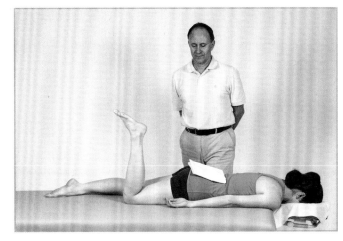

Figure 8-42

Step 1: Client Contraction and Stretch:

- Begin by asking the client to actively bring her right foot inward by laterally rotating her right thigh at the hip joint as far as is comfortable.
- This begins the stretch of the right medial rotator muscles (target muscle group) (Fig. 8-43A).

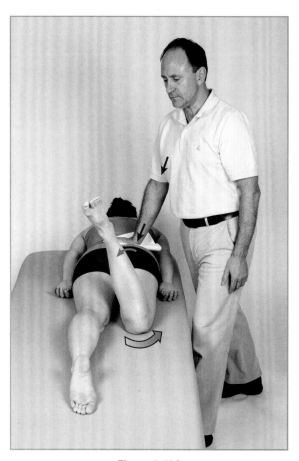

Figure 8-43A

Step 2: Further Stretch of Client:

- Once the position of stretch at the end of step 1 is reached, the client relaxes, and you further stretch the client's target medial rotator musculature by gently pushing the distal end of the client's leg farther medially, increasing the lateral rotation of her thigh at the hip joint, until you meet tissue resistance (Fig. 8-43B).
- Hold the position of stretch for 1 to 2 seconds.

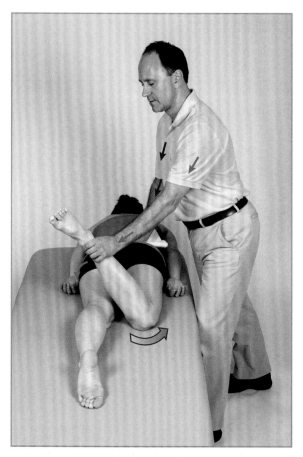

Figure 8-43B

By using the client's leg as a lever to medially rotate the thigh at the hip joint, a torque (rotary force) is placed through the client's knee. If the client has an unhealthy knee, the stretch is contraindicated and the AC medial rotator stretch in Practical Application Box 8.12 should be performed instead.

Step 3: Passively Return Client to Starting Position:

■ Once you have completed step 2, the client remains relaxed as you support and passively bring her lower extremity back to the starting position (Fig. 8-43C).

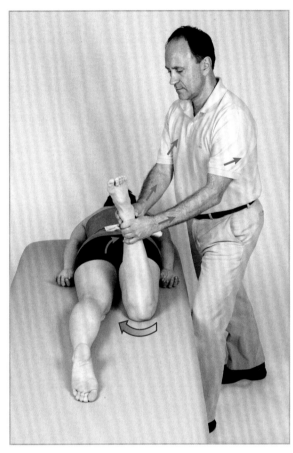

Figure 8-43C

Further Repetitions:

■ Repeat this procedure for each repetition.
■ With each successive repetition, you can add slightly more pressure to the stretch.
■ At the end of the last repetition (usually 8 to 10 repetitions are done), you may choose to hold the position of stretch for a longer period, 5 to 20 seconds or more.
■ Note that the breathing protocol is for the client to exhale when concentrically contracting.
■ The client continues exhaling as the target musculature is relaxed and you stretch it, and then inhales as you return the client to the starting position for the next repetition.

Left-Side Medial Rotator Group:

■ Repeat for the pelvis/hip joint medial rotator group on the left side of the body (Fig. 8-44).

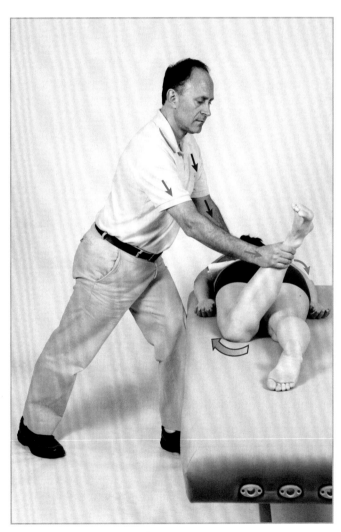

Figure 8-44

8.12 PRACTICAL APPLICATION

Alternate Agonist Contract Stretch for the Medial Rotator Group

Having the client supine is an excellent alternative position to stretch her medial rotator functional group. The advantage of this position is that it allows the therapist to primarily use the client's thigh instead of her leg to further the stretch. This minimizes the involvement of the client's knee joint, which is important if the client's knee is unhealthy. The supine stretch is demonstrated and explained for the client's right side.

- Have the client supine toward the right side of the table with her thigh flexed at the hip joint and her knee flexed at the knee joint. Stand to the right of the client.

- Have the client initiate the AC stretching protocol by laterally rotating the thigh at the hip joint (**Fig. A**).

- Then ask the client to relax and you quickly step in, grasping the client's right thigh with your left forearm and placing your right hand on the distal lateral surface of her right leg. Now increase the stretch of the medial rotator musculature by stretching the client's thigh farther into lateral rotation (**Fig. B**). It is important that the majority of your stretching force is applied to the client's thigh with your forearm and not to her leg with your hand.

- Then passively return the client to the starting position for the next repetition.

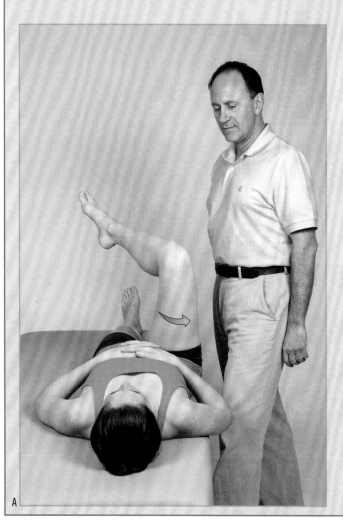

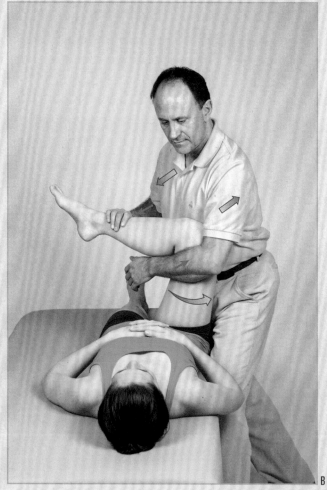

Agonist Contract Stretching of Both Functional Groups within a Plane in One Routine

It is not always necessary to perform AC stretching for only one functional group at a time. In fact, it can be more efficient and beneficial to perform AC stretching for both functional muscle groups within a plane—thereby stretching two target groups of muscles during the same procedure. To do this, it is necessary that both functional group actions can be performed with the same client position and that you can position yourself to be able to efficiently participate in both stretching protocols with regard to your body mechanics. An example of this is stretching the client's right hip joint musculature into medial rotation and lateral rotation during the same procedure.

When stretching the client's right hip joint into medial rotation, the lateral rotation group (the first target muscle group) is stretched; when stretching the client's right hip joint into lateral rotation, the medial rotation group (the second target muscle group) is stretched. This procedure begins similarly no matter the side to which the rotation stretch begins. The following example is shown on the client's right side and is based on starting the stretch for the lateral rotators.

Starting Position:

- Have the client supine toward the right side of the table with her thigh flexed at the hip joint and her leg flexed at the knee joint. Stand to the right of the client.

First Repetition: Client Contraction and Stretch of Target Muscle Group #1:

- Begin by asking the client to actively move the thigh into medial rotation at the hip joint as far as is comfortable (**Fig. A**).
- This begins the stretch of the target lateral rotator muscles (target muscle group #1).

Further Stretch of Client:

- When the position of stretch is reached at the end of the first repetition, the client relaxes, and you further stretch the client's target lateral rotator musculature by gently moving the client's thigh farther into medial rotation until you meet tissue resistance (**Fig. B**).
- Hold the position of stretch for 1 to 2 seconds.

continued

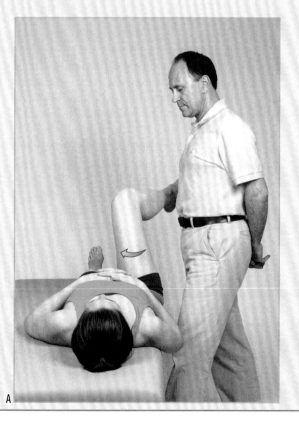

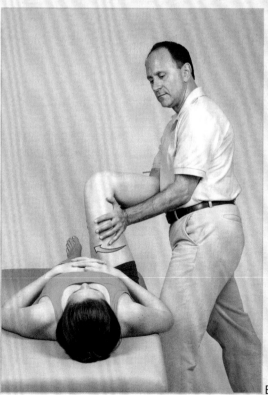

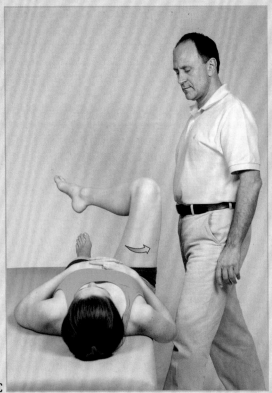
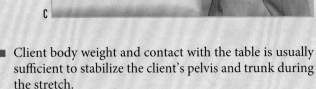
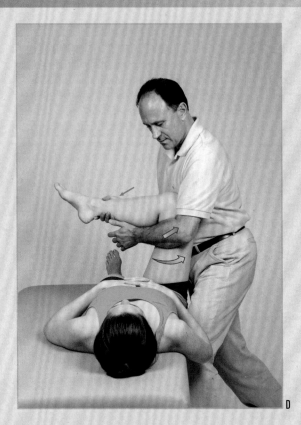

- Client body weight and contact with the table is usually sufficient to stabilize the client's pelvis and trunk during the stretch.

Client Contraction and Stretch of Target Muscle Group #2:

- At this point, instead of bringing the client back to the starting position for the next repetition, ask the client to actively move the thigh all the way into lateral rotation as far as is comfortable, beginning the stretch of the target medial rotator muscles (target muscle group #2) **(Fig. C)**.

Further Stretch of Client:

- Once this position of stretch is reached, the client relaxes, and you further stretch the client's target medial rotator musculature by gently moving the client's thigh farther into lateral rotation until you meet tissue resistance **(Fig. D)**.
- Hold the position of stretch for 1 to 2 seconds.
- This completes one repetition in which both groups of hip joint rotation musculature (both target muscle groups) have been stretched.

Further Repetitions:

- All further repetitions are carried out in the same manner as the first repetition, except that the starting position is different. The starting position for the first repetition was neutral anatomic position. However, the starting position for the second and all successive repetitions is with the client stretched into lateral rotation. Therefore, the client begins the second and all successive repetitions by moving the thigh from the position of lateral rotation all the way to medial rotation.
- Note that the breathing protocol is for the client to exhale when concentrically contracting.
- The client completes the exhalation and inhales as the target musculature is relaxed and you stretch it. Because there is no step in which you return the client to the initial starting position, the client must also inhale while being stretched. For this reason, when performing AC stretching technique for both functional groups within a plane in one routine, the client's inhalation should not be too deep.

8.9 THERAPIST TIP

When Should You Use Agonist Contract Stretching?

The AC stretching technique is an advanced technique that can and should be employed whenever a client does not respond well to standard stretching techniques. Although it is not necessary to wait until a client stops responding to regular stretching to use AC stretching, there are several factors to take into consideration when deciding whether it is appropriate to use this technique.

First, because AC stretching does tend to require more time to carry out, it makes sense to choose carefully when and for which areas of the client's body it is used. Another consideration is that AC stretching requires the client's active participation. If a client expects to come to a session and remain passive while you work his or her muscles, AC stretching may not be appropriate. Alternatively, you may need to educate the client about his or her possible role during a treatment session.

A question that is often asked is, "Which advanced neural inhibition technique is the better stretching technique, CR or AC?" Although each technique has its proponents, each technique works well for a particular subset of the client population, and neither is inherently better than the other for stretching any particular muscle or muscle group. Which method you choose should be based on how well it works for each particular client, how well the client enjoys the particular technique, and/or which technique you find biomechanically easier to employ for that particular muscle/muscle group.

Because the AC technique does require more active motion on the part of the client, it is likely the better technique with regard to warming up the client's body because local fluid circulation (blood, lymph, and synovial joint fluid) would be increased. AC technique's movements would also better enforce neural patterns of movement. On the other hand, because AC technique requires more active client participation and effort than CR, CR technique might be preferred over AC for the client looking for a more passive treatment session. Also, it is generally easier to transition a stretch to CR technique than AC technique because regardless of the client position, the therapist can add the resistance needed for the CR technique, whereas AC technique usually requires the client to contract and move the body part either up against gravity or at least parallel with gravity. Therefore, the client position in relation to gravity matters with AC stretching but does not for CR stretching.

A case probably could be made that CRAC stretching (see Chapter 9) is more effective at stretching target musculature than either CR or AC stretching alone because it combines the effectiveness of both techniques. However, it does take twice as long to perform, and spending more time stretching one muscle means that there is less time left to work on other areas of the client's body. Ultimately, which technique is chosen is a clinical decision that will depend on the unique circumstances of each scenario.

CHAPTER SUMMARY

AC stretching is an advanced stretching technique that can often provide the key to helping clients with tight muscles. Although the exact manner in which the technique is performed can vary, it is most commonly carried out as described in the following summary:

- The client first actively moves into a position that stretches the target muscle group, which both begins the stretch of the target musculature and initiates the RI reflex that inhibits/relaxes the target musculature.
- The client then relaxes, and the therapist takes advantage of the RI reflex to stretch the client's target musculature farther than would have been possible otherwise.
- The therapist completes the technique by passively bringing the client back to the starting position for the beginning of the next repetition.
- The most important aspect of the breathing protocol is for the client to exhale when actively contracting.
- An entire repetition usually takes approximately 3 to 5 seconds; 8 to 10 repetitions are typically done.

Essentially, any stretch can be carried out using the AC technique. As with all stretching, AC stretching is most effective when performed after the client's tissues are first warmed up.

CASE STUDY

HYESUN

■ History and Physical Assessment

A new client, Hyesun Alexander, age 42 years, comes to your office complaining of low back pain and stiffness. She tells you that the symptoms began 1 week ago after she spent a long time standing and bending over, working on a project for work. She says that other than an occasional mild tightness in her low back, she has never experienced any low back problems before now. She tried stretching on her own, but it only seemed to make the pain worse. After 3 days, she saw her medical doctor, who sent her for radiography. The radiographs were negative for fracture and dislocation, and she was released with a recommendation to use over-the-counter analgesics as needed. She then went to a massage therapist that a friend recommended, but she felt that the massage was very light and not effective at relieving her pain.

In addition to strong dull pain with prolonged sitting (more than 20 minutes) and prolonged standing (more than 30 minutes), she is having difficulty sleeping because she cannot find a comfortable position. Her pain level (on a scale of 0 to 10, in which 0 is no pain and 10 is the worst pain that she can imagine) is 4 when lying down, 5 to 6 with prolonged standing, and 7 to 8 with prolonged sitting, including driving. Bending forward or to either side causes immediate sharp pain at a level of 9. She normally works out five times a week, employing a combination of aerobic training and weights, but has not been able to work out since the pain began. She points to her lumbar region on both sides of the spine as the source of her pain. She reports no pain down either lower extremity. She has come to you because she has heard that you do effective clinical orthopedic manual therapy.

Your assessment shows that low back flexion is decreased to 5 degrees and that both right and left lateral flexions are decreased to 10 degrees. All other ranges of motion are within normal limits. The results of your assessments are also negative for cough test and Valsalva maneuver (for a review of assessment procedures, see Chapter 3). Active straight leg raise causes immediate pain bilaterally in her lumbar region. Passive straight leg raise causes no pain but is tight and pulls bilaterally in her lumbar region. Nachlas' and Yeoman's tests are negative. Palpation of Hyesun's lumbar region reveals extremely tight paraspinal musculature (erector spinae and transversospinalis) bilaterally as well as a tight and tender quadratus lumborum bilaterally. Gluteal musculature is mildly to moderately tight, but when palpating this region, Hyesun reports no pain or discomfort.

■ Think-It-Through Questions:

1. Should an advanced stretching technique such as AC stretching be included in your treatment plan for Hyesun? If so, why? If not, why not?

2. If AC stretching would be of value, is it safe to use with her? If yes, how do you know? If not, why not?

3. If AC stretching is done, which specific stretching routines should be done? Why did you choose the ones you did?

Answers to these Think-It-Through Questions and the Treatment Strategy employed for the client are available online at thePoint.lww.com/MuscolinoLowBack

CHAPTER 9 Contract Relax Agonist Contract Stretching

OBJECTIVES

After completing this chapter, the student should be able to:

1. Describe the mechanism of contract relax agonist contract (CRAC) stretching.
2. Describe in steps an overview of the usual protocol for carrying out the CRAC stretching technique.
3. Describe the roles of the treatment hand and the stabilization hand.
4. Describe the usual breathing protocol for the client during the CRAC stretching technique.
5. Explain why stretching should never be performed too fast or too far.
6. Define each key term in this chapter and explain its relationship to the CRAC stretching technique.
7. Perform the CRAC stretching technique for each of the functional groups of muscles of the lumbar spine and pelvis/hip joint.

KEY TERMS

agonist contract (AC) stretching
contract relax agonist contract (CRAC) stretching

contract relax (CR) stretching
creep
Golgi tendon organ reflex

muscle spindle reflex
reciprocal inhibition
resistance hand

stabilization hand
stretching hand
treatment hand

INTRODUCTION

Contract relax agonist contract (CRAC) stretching is an advanced stretching technique that is performed by combining **contract relax (CR) stretching** (see Chapter 7) with **agonist contract (AC) stretching** (see Chapter 8). CRAC stretching is not difficult for the therapist to perform once the CR and AC stretching techniques have each been mastered. It requires only a small additional step to synthesize these two techniques into the CRAC stretching technique. As the acronym itself indicates, the therapist simply performs the techniques sequentially, beginning with CR stretching and immediately following with AC stretching. As with any hands-on method, practice is the key to a comfortable, smooth, and efficient application. Even though performing CRAC stretching requires more time than does either of the two techniques alone, it might prove to be the only technique that is effective for some difficult cases in which the client's target musculature is resistant to relaxing and stretching. In these cases, the extra time spent will be well worth it.

Note: In the Technique and Self-Care chapters of this book (Chapters 4 to 12), green arrows indicate movement, red arrows indicate stabilization, and black arrows indicate a position that is statically held.

BOX 9.1

Contract Relax Agonist Contract Routines

The following CRAC stretching routines are presented in the chapter:
- Section 1: lumbar spine (LSp):
  - Routine 9-1—LSp extensors
  - Routine 9-2—LSp right rotators
- Section 2: hip joint/pelvis:
  - Routine 9-3—hip flexors
  - Routine 9-4—hip extensors: hamstrings (in the "Overview of Technique" section)
  - Routine 9-5—hip deep lateral rotators

MECHANISM

The proposed mechanism of CRAC stretching is a combination of the mechanism for CR stretching, which is classically stated as the **Golgi tendon organ reflex**, and the mechanism for AC stretching, which is **reciprocal inhibition** (RI). Chapter 7's Box 7.2 presents the Golgi tendon organ reflex in more detail, and Chapter 8's Box 8.2 focuses on RI.

The Golgi tendon organ reflex of CR stretching and the RI reflex of AC stretching each work to inhibit musculature from contracting (in other words, to relax it). Both of these reflexes can be utilized in CRAC stretching to relax and stretch the target muscle. It stands to reason that if both of these stretching techniques are employed together when stretching a client's target muscle, that muscle's relaxation will be increased, allowing for an even greater stretch than would have been possible with either technique alone.

It is important to note that, as with CR and AC stretching, the therapist's hand that resists the client's contraction and performs the stretch is known as the **treatment hand** or the **stretching hand**; it is also known as the **resistance hand**. The therapist's other hand is known as the **stabilization hand** and is used to stabilize the client's pelvis or trunk.

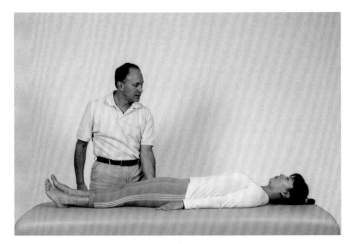

Figure 9-1 Starting position for CRAC stretching of the right hamstring group.

| 9.1 | THERAPIST TIP |

Learn the Contract Relax Agonist Contract Stretching Technique before Using It with Clients

CRAC stretching is not difficult to perform, but it does involve a number of steps and can be confusing at first to learn and use with clients. For this reason, it is helpful first to learn and master working with the CR and AC stretching techniques independently as well as the combined CRAC technique before attempting to learn and apply the CRAC stretching technique with clients.

OVERVIEW OF TECHNIQUE

View the video "Contract Relax Agonist Contract Stretching of the Hamstring Group" online on thePoint.lww.com

The artful performance of CRAC stretching involves a seamless integration of the CR and AC stretching techniques. For this reason, it is strongly recommended that Chapters 7 and 8, which discuss CR and AC stretching individually, be read and practiced before attempting CRAC stretching.

The following is an overview of the CRAC stretching technique using the right hamstring muscle group as the target muscle group being stretched.

Starting Position:
- The client is supine and positioned as far to the right side of the table as possible; you are standing at the right side of the table (Fig. 9-1).

Step 1: Client Isometric Contraction:
- Begin by asking the client to gently contract the target right hamstring musculature in an attempt to extend the thigh at the hip joint and the leg at the knee joint down against the table. If you would like, you can place your left hand under the client's thigh or leg to monitor that she is pressing in the correct manner and direction (Fig. 9-2).
- The client's body weight and contact with the table provides stabilization of the pelvis for this step of the protocol.
- Have the client hold this isometric contraction for approximately 5 to 8 seconds and then ask the client to relax.
- This aspect of the CRAC stretch is the CR protocol, engaging the Golgi tendon organ reflex to inhibit and relax the target right hamstring musculature.
- *Note*: It is identical to the CR protocol explained in Chapter 7, except that CR stretching usually begins from a position in which the target musculature is first stretched (i.e., the thigh is already flexed).

| 9.2 | THERAPIST TIP |

Communicate with the Client

For clients who have never experienced the CRAC stretching technique, it can be helpful first to give them a brief overview of how you will perform the technique. Let the client know that he or she will need to press against your resistance in one direction, then move his or her body (thigh, pelvis, and/or low back) in the opposite direction, and then relax as you perform the stretch. In addition, inform the client about how long to press against your resistance, how many repetitions there will be, and what the breathing protocol is to be. This will allow the client to give you informed verbal consent before beginning the technique and also will help the client carry out the CRAC protocol more easily once you begin.

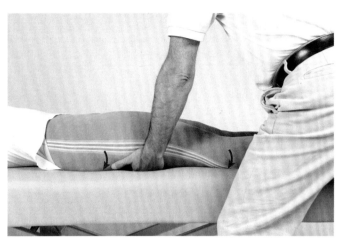

Figure 9-2 Step 1: Isometric contraction of the client's right hamstring musculature against the resistance of the table.

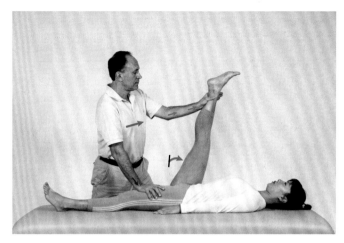

Figure 9-4 Step 3: The client relaxes and is stretched further by the therapist.

Step 2: Client Concentric Contraction and Stretch:

- As soon as the client relaxes, have the client perform active concentric contraction of the flexors of the right thigh at the hip joint, bringing the thigh into flexion as far as is comfortably possible; it is important that the client maintains her knee joint in full extension.
- As the client begins to flex her right thigh up into the air, you need to lean in and position yourself to stabilize the client's pelvis with your right hand by pressing on the client's anterior left thigh (Fig. 9-3A). It is important to make sure that the client's pelvis is stabilized before the client reaches the end of her flexion motion; otherwise, her pelvis will move into posterior tilt and the stretch of the right hamstrings will not be optimal. An alternate position to stabilize the client's pelvis is to use your right knee (Fig. 9-3B).
- It is also important to lean in quickly so that you can make sure that the client's knee joint remains extended and also

to be in position to further stretch the client during the next step of the routine.

- This step adds in the AC protocol, beginning the stretch of the target right hamstring musculature and engaging the RI reflex to further inhibit and relax the target musculature.
- *Note*: This step differs from the usual CR stretching protocol, in which the client relaxes and the therapist stretches the client's target musculature by passively moving the client's thigh into flexion.

Step 3: Client Relaxation and Further Stretch:

- Continuing with the AC protocol, once the client has actively moved the thigh into flexion, the client relaxes, and you now increase the stretch of the client's target right hamstring musculature by gently and passively moving the client's thigh farther into flexion until you meet tissue resistance (Fig. 9-4).
- Hold this position of stretch for 1 to 2 seconds.

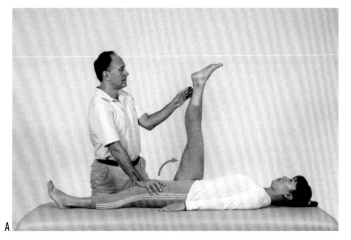
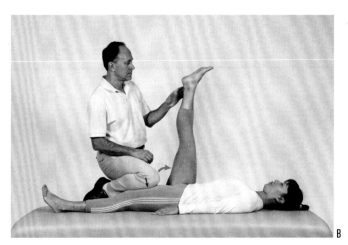

Figure 9-3 Step 2: Client actively moves into flexion of the right thigh at the hip joint. **(A)** Stabilization of the client's pelvis with the right hand. **(B)** Alternate stabilization contact: the right knee.

9.1 **PRACTICAL APPLICATION**

Return Only Part Way in Step 4

It is typical for stretching routines that include the AC stretching protocol to return the client all the way back to anatomic position for the beginning of the next repetition. When stretching the hamstrings, this requires the therapist to continually step away so that the thigh can be lowered back to the table, only to have to step back in to further stretch the client's thigh and stabilize her pelvis in the next repetition. However, it is not necessary to return the client all the way to the table; the client can be returned only part way. What is important is that the client is returned far enough so that there is a range of motion of flexion through which she can actively move her thigh so that the RI reflex is initiated. When performing CRAC stretching for the hamstring group, it is much more practical during step 4 to return the client only part way so that you can remain in one position during the entire stretching protocol. **Figures A and B** demonstrate the end and beginning positions of the stretching routine when the client is returned only part way.

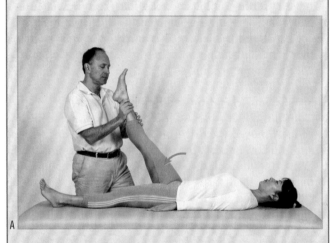

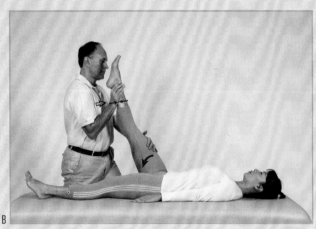

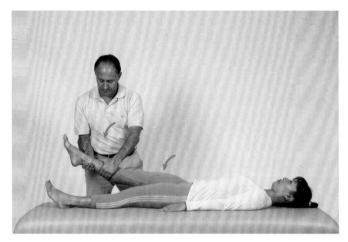

Figure 9-5 Step 4: The client's thigh is passively returned to the starting position.

Step 4: Passively Return Client to Starting Position:
- After holding the client's right thigh in this stretch position as indicated, support and passively bring the thigh back to the starting position for the next repetition (Fig. 9-5).

Further Repetitions:
- Repeat this CRAC protocol for additional repetitions as needed.
- The number of repetitions typically performed varies from 3 to 10.

PERFORMING THE TECHNIQUE

When performing CRAC stretching, it is important to keep the following guidelines in mind. Each point addresses a specific aspect of the CRAC stretching technique. Understanding and applying them consistently will enhance the effectiveness of this technique.

9.1 Position: Select an Appropriate Starting Position

There is no single correct starting position for the client. It is typical to ask the client to begin in neutral anatomic position. However, the client's body part can be returned only part way toward that position—in other words, for this example with the hamstrings, to a position of partial flexion of the thigh. What is most important is that (1) the client is in a position in step 1 that is comfortable when contracting his or her musculature isometrically during the CR phase of the protocol and that (2) the client has a range of motion in step 2 to move (the thigh into flexion in this example) during the AC phase of the protocol. The client's range of motion in step 2 is important because the RI reflex is engaged only if the client concentrically contracts and moves his or her body.

Start from the Correct Position

CRAC stretching is similar to AC stretching in that all repetitions begin from approximately the same starting position. CRAC stretching differs from CR stretching, which usually begins each successive repetition from the position of stretch attained during the previous repetition.

9.2 Resistance: Your Role

When you offer resistance as the client isometrically contracts in step 1 during the CR phase of the protocol, keep in mind that it is not a contest between you and the client. It is your role to meet the client's resistance, not to exceed it. Thus, to ensure that the client's contraction of the target muscle is isometric, you must equal whatever force the client generates. Also, as soon as you ask the client to relax, it is important that you immediately ease off your pressure so that the client's body is not suddenly pushed into the stretch.

9.3 Client Concentric Contraction: Instruct the Client to Move Actively

When performing CRAC stretching, it is crucial during the AC phase of the protocol in step 2 that the client concentrically contracts and actively moves through the range of motion without your assistance. Although your hand may be on the client's body part to increase the stretch at the end of the client's active movement, you must be sure to not actually move the client passively. It can be helpful for your hand to guide the direction of the client's motion, but if the client is passively moved and does not actually contract the agonist musculature, the RI reflex will not be engaged.

9.4 Repetition Time: Keep It Dynamic

Like AC stretching, CRAC stretching tends to be performed in a dynamic manner, with the stretch held statically in step 3 for only 1 to 2 seconds. However, because of the isometric contraction required in step 1, a repetition of CRAC stretching will last longer than an AC repetition. Typically, a CRAC repetition lasts approximately 8 to15 seconds.

9.5 Stretch: Slow and Easy

When stretching the client's target musculature, it is extremely important that the stretch is performed slowly and is never forced. If a target muscle is stretched too fast or too far, the **muscle spindle reflex** may be triggered. The muscle spindle reflex is a protective reflex that tightens a muscle to prevent overstretching and possible muscle tearing. This will cause a spasm of the target muscle, defeating the purpose

Use Your Core

When performing CRAC stretching, there may be times when a client contracts so forcefully that you feel overpowered. Using the larger muscles of your core can help to remedy this. To align your body weight behind your forearms and hands, bring your elbows in front of your core by laterally rotating the arms at the glenohumeral joints and placing your elbows inside (or close to) your anterior superior iliac spines. If you cannot bring your elbows in front of your body, bring them in as far as possible. If this is still insufficient, try either placing a foot behind you on the floor or place your knee on the table so you can engage your lower extremity muscles to brace your core (see accompanying figure).

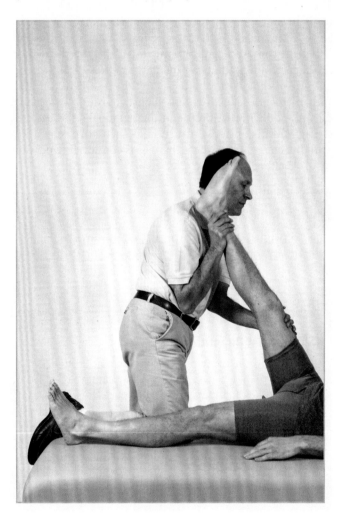

of the stretch. Stretching should always be done slowly and within the comfort zone of the client. When you first meet tissue resistance, add only a small additional stretch to the client's tissues. Because a number of repetitions are performed, gaining a small incrementally increased stretch at each repetition will allow for an excellent degree of stretch at the end of the CRAC stretching technique protocol.

9.6 Number of Repetitions

The number of repetitions performed for CRAC stretching varies. Because CR stretching usually involves 3 to 4 repetitions and AC stretching usually involves 8 to 10 repetitions, some therapists treat CRAC stretching like an add-on to CR stretching and perform 3 to 4 CRAC repetitions. Other therapists treat it more like an add-on to AC stretching and perform 8 to 10 CRAC repetitions. As with all clinical work, the response of the client's tissues is the best guideline for applying the CRAC technique.

9.7 Contraction: Increase Gradually

The goal for each successive CRAC stretch repetition is to build on the previous one so that the degree of stretch achieved gradually increases. For the CR portion, in which the client contracts against your resistance, the strength of the client's contraction can increase gradually from the beginning of the set of repetitions to the end. To accomplish this, instruct the client to press against your resistance gently during the first repetitions and then gradually increase the strength of his or her contraction in successive repetitions until the client is pressing as hard as is comfortably possible by the last repetitions.

*If the client contracts too forcefully or too suddenly, a pulled or torn muscle is possible. It may be helpful during the final or last few repetitions to tell the client, "Contract as hard as you **comfortably** can without hurting yourself."*

| 9.5 | THERAPIST TIP |

Hold the Last Repetition

According to the principle known as **creep**, stretched tissues adapt to their newly stretched length more effectively if the stretch is held for a sustained period. For this reason, when you reach the end of the last repetition of the CRAC stretching protocol for a target muscle or muscle group, you may decide to hold the position of the stretch for a longer than usual period, perhaps 10 to 20 seconds or more.

9.8 Hand Placement: Treatment Hand

When performing the CRAC stretching technique, it is important that you place your treatment hand in a comfortable manner for the client. To do this, try to offer a broad contact so that the pressure against the client is distributed as evenly as possible.

9.9 Hand Placement: Stabilization Hand

The position of your stabilization hand (or other stabilization contact) is also crucial. Without it, the client's pelvis and/or trunk would often move in such a manner as to lose the stretch of the target musculature. As with your treatment hand, placement of your stabilization hand should also be comfortable for the client and offer as broad a contact as possible. When performing CRAC stretching of the hamstring group, it is usually necessary to remove the stabilization contact with each repetition to get out of the way and make room for the client's thigh to move. However, even when it is not necessary for you to remove the stabilization contact for this reason, it is still usually necessary to remove the stabilization contact from its stabilization position to assist the treatment hand in supporting and returning the client's body part back to the starting position (step 4) for the next repetition.

The placement of the treatment and stabilization hands often requires your wrist joint to be extended. For the health of your wrists, your point of contact through which pressure is transmitted into the client should be the heel of your hand (the carpal region). If you direct the pressure through your palm or fingers, you may hyperextend and injure your wrist. Given how vulnerable the wrist joint can be, proper biomechanical positioning of the hand/wrist is crucially important.

9.10 Breathing

The usual breathing protocol for CRAC stretching is to have the client hold the breath in step 1 when performing isometric contraction during the CR phase of the protocol. In step 2, the client exhales when actively moving into the stretch

---

| 9.6 | THERAPIST TIP |

Explain the Breathing Protocol to the Client

Chapter 7's discussion of the CR stretching technique stated that when the client isometrically contracts against your resistance, the client can either hold the breath or exhale. However, when performing CR as part of CRAC stretching, the client must hold the breath during this step because the client needs to exhale during the AC portion of the stretch.

Because this breathing protocol is a bit complicated, it often takes a while for the client to become accustomed to it. To help facilitate a smooth performance of the CRAC technique, start by talking the client through when to inhale, when to hold the breath, and when to exhale. Have the client practice this breathing protocol for as many repetitions as is necessary. Once the client is comfortable with and has mastered the breathing protocol, CRAC repetitions proceed smoothly and efficiently.

at the beginning of the AC phase of the protocol. During step 3, the client usually continues exhaling as he or she is relaxed and you further the stretch. In step 4, the client must inhale as you passively return the client's body part back to the starting position so that the client is ready to hold his or her breath for step 1 of the next repetition.

9.11 Direction of Stretch

As with CR or AC stretching, when CRAC stretching is performed, the client can carry out the motion in a cardinal plane or in an oblique plane that combines any two or all three cardinal planes. The precise directions that you choose

for the stretches should be determined by the restrictions that you feel when you assess the client's ranges of motion.

9.12 Electric Lift Table

As discussed in Chapters 6, 7, and 8, when stretching the low back and pelvis/hip joint, the value of an electric lift table for optimal body mechanics cannot be overstated. Most CRAC routines for the LSp and pelvis/hip joint require the table to be low. If the table was higher for the performance of other manual therapy techniques, having an electric lift table so that table height can be easily adjusted for CRAC stretching is essential for efficient clinical orthopedic work.

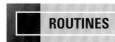

ROUTINES

CONTRACT RELAX AGONIST CONTRACT ROUTINES

Chapters 7 and 8 provided a thorough application of the individual CR and AC stretches of the neck. This chapter covers five examples to clarify the flow of combining CR and AC stretching into the CRAC stretching technique. CRAC stretching for the hamstring group was shown in "Overview of Technique" section. Four additional examples follow here in the "Contract Relax Agonist Contract Routines" section. You can then apply this flow to perform CRAC stretching for the other functional muscle groups of the LSp and pelvis/hip joint.

Contract Relax Agonist Contract Multiplane Stretching Routines

This chapter explains how to perform the CRAC stretching technique and then presents the technique applied to a few of the major functional groups of muscles of the LSp and pelvis/hip joint. However, the CRAC technique can be applied to any stretch, including the multiplane stretches presented in Chapter 6. A couple of multiplane stretches for the CRAC routines of this chapter are presented in Practical Application boxes that follow the CRAC stretching routine steps. However, it should be kept in mind that just as with CR and AC stretching, any musculature, including musculature that needs to be stretched across multiple planes (multiplane stretching), can be stretched with the CRAC technique. What is required to transition a stretch to the CRAC stretching technique is to consider the relationship with gravity so that the agonist musculature concentrically contracts when the motion in step 2 is done and then to add in the protocol steps involved with the CRAC technique.

SECTION 1: LUMBAR SPINE CONTRACT RELAX AGONIST CONTRACT ROUTINES

As with CR and AC stretching, CRAC stretches of the LSp can be performed in two ways. One method is to stabilize the client's pelvis and move his or her upper trunk downward toward the pelvis, thereby stretching the LSp. This method begins the stretch of the LSp superiorly, and as the stretching force is increased and the LSp is increasingly moved downward, the stretch moves into the lower LSp. The second method is to stabilize the client's upper trunk and move his or her pelvis and lower LSp upward toward the thoracic trunk. This method begins the stretch of the LSp inferiorly, and as the stretching force is increased and the pelvis and lower spine are increasingly moved upward, the stretch moves into the upper LSp.

The following CRAC stretching routines for the LSp are presented in this chapter:

- Routine 9-1—LSp extensors
- Routine 9-2—LSp right rotators

Stretching the Thoracic Spine

CRAC stretches that move the upper trunk down toward the lower trunk and pelvis tend to stretch the thoracic spine as well as the LSp. However, any LSp stretch can be transitioned to also stretch the thoracic spine by altering either the movement and/or stabilization of the client's body so that the line of tension of the stretch enters the thoracic region.

ROUTINE 9-1: LUMBAR SPINE EXTENSORS

Figure 9-6 shows the functional group of muscles that extend the LSp. These muscles are located on the posterior side of the trunk in the lumbar region. The CRAC stretching routine presented here is essentially the double knee-to-chest stretch that is presented in Chapter 11 (Self-Care Routine 11-6; available online at thePoint.lww.com), with the CRAC stretching protocol added.

The Lumbar Spine Extensor Functional Group

This functional group comprises the following muscles bilaterally:

Erector spinae group
Transversospinalis group
Quadratus lumborum

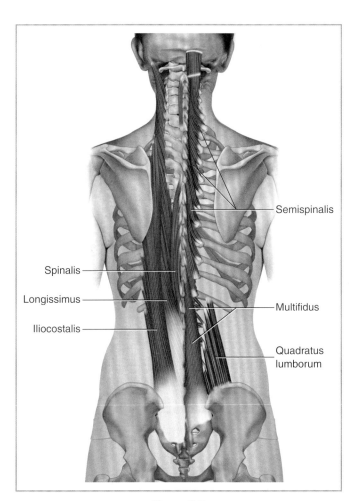

Figure 9-6

Starting Position:

■ The client is supine toward one side of the table with his hip and knee joints flexed. You are standing on the right side of the table. Your left foot is on the floor; your right lower extremity is positioned on the table so that your core is in line with the force of the stroke.

■ *Note*: The stretching routine could also be performed from the other (left) side of the table. Simply reverse the positioning of your lower extremities.

■ Both of your hands are treatment hands and are placed on the distal posterior surface of the client's thighs.

■ The client can place his feet on your clavicle as seen in Figure 9-7.

■ The client's upper trunk is stabilized by body weight and contact with the table as well as the direction that you push on his thighs when performing the stretch in step 3).

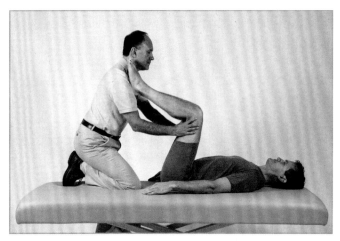

Figure 9-7

Step 1: Client Isometric Contraction:

■ Ask the client to perform a gentle isometric contraction of the target muscles for approximately 5 to 8 seconds (in an attempt to extend the lower trunk back down toward the table) against your resistance (Fig. 9-8A).

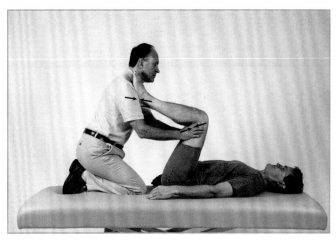

Figure 9-8A

■ Ask the client to relax.

■ This phase of the CRAC stretch is the CR protocol.

■ Please note that the breathing protocol for every repetition is to have the client hold the breath when contracting against your resistance.

Step 2: Client Concentric Contraction and Stretch:

■ As soon as the client relaxes, ask him to concentrically contract the LSp flexor musculature to actively bring his knees toward his chest (move the pelvis into posterior tilt and the LSp into flexion) as far as is comfortable (Fig. 9-8B).

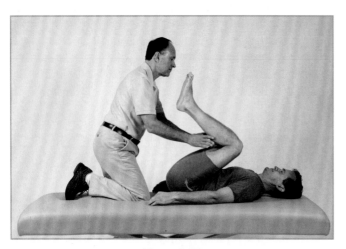

Figure 9-8B

■ This differs from CR stretching technique, in which the client would relax, and you would stretch the client's target musculature by passively moving the client's trunk into flexion.

■ This stage of CRAC stretching begins the AC protocol.

Step 3: Client Relaxation and Further Stretch:

■ Once the client has finished actively moving into flexion, the client relaxes.

■ As soon as the client relaxes, you now increase the stretch of the client's target LSp extensor musculature by gently and passively moving the client's LSp farther into flexion until you meet tissue resistance (Fig. 9-8C).

■ Hold the client in this position of stretch for 1 to 2 seconds.

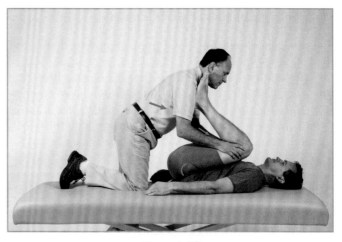

Figure 9-8C

Step 4: Passively Return Client to Starting Position:

■ Support the client's trunk as you passively bring the client back to the starting position for the next repetition.

■ Use both of your hands to support and move the client's body back to starting position (Fig. 9-8D).

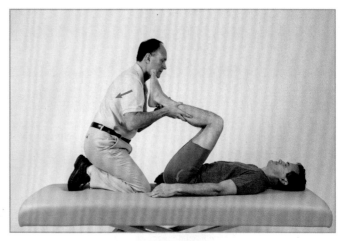

Figure 9-8D

Further Repetitions:

■ This CRAC protocol can be repeated for a total of 3 to 10 repetitions.

■ Once the final position of stretch is reached at the end of the last CRAC repetition, many therapists like to hold this position of stretch for a longer period, often 10 to 20 seconds or more.

9.3   PRACTICAL APPLICATION

Multiplane Stretching of the Lumbar Spine Extensors

The CRAC stretching protocol for the LSp extensors can be transitioned into a multiplane stretch. For example, during step 1 of the protocol, instead of having the client contract the target muscles against your resistance directly down toward the table (perfectly in the sagittal plane), ask the client to press down toward extension and also to one side (Fig. A). Then during step 2, instead of directing him to actively bring his knees directly up toward the chest (again, perfectly in the sagittal plane), ask him to bring his knees up toward the chest and deviate toward the other side of the body (Fig. B). This protocol can then be repeated for the other side of the body.

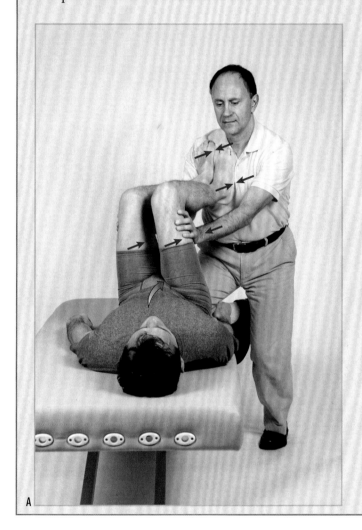

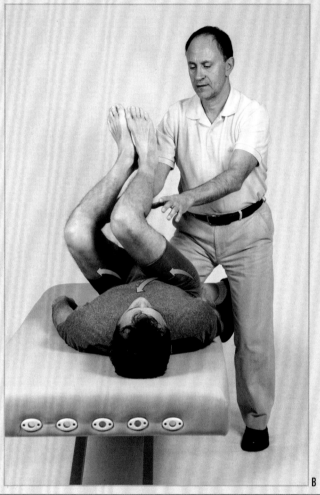

A   B

ROUTINE 9-2: LUMBAR SPINE RIGHT ROTATORS

Figure 9-9 shows the functional group of muscles that right rotate the LSp. These muscles are located both anteriorly and posteriorly and on both the right and left sides of the trunk in the lumbar region.

The Lumbar Spine Right Rotator Functional Group

This functional group comprises the following muscles:

Left transversospinalis group
Right erector spinae group
Left external abdominal oblique
Right internal abdominal oblique

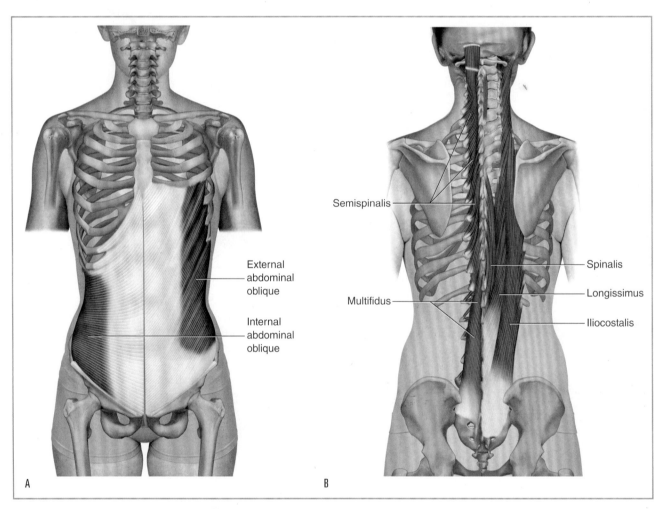

External abdominal oblique

Internal abdominal oblique

Semispinalis

Multifidus

Spinalis

Longissimus

Iliocostalis

A

B

Figure 9-9 (**A**) Anterior view. (**B**) Posterior view.

Starting Position:

- Have the client seated at the right end of the table with her arms crossed so that her hands are on the opposite shoulders, but her arms should be adducted at the glenohumeral joints so that her elbows meet at the center of the body.
- Stand to the right side of the client.
- Your right hand is the treatment hand and is placed on the client's elbows.

- Your left hand is the stabilization hand and functions to stabilize the client's pelvis. It is placed across the top of the client's right iliac crest; if it is not possible to grasp the client's iliac crest, the stabilization hand can be placed on the proximal anterior surface of the client's right thigh; if desired, a cushion can be used for comfort to broaden the stabilization contact (Fig. 9-10).

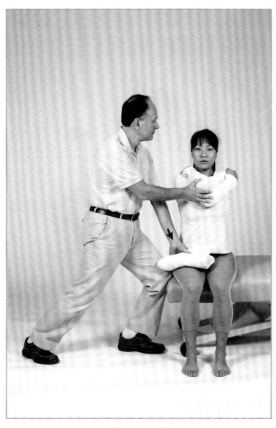

Figure 9-10

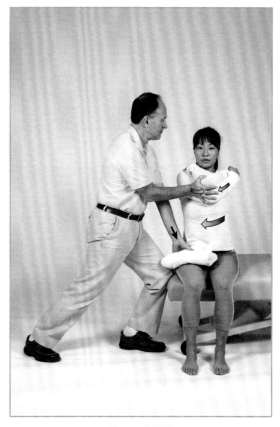

Figure 9-11A

Step 1: Client Isometric Contraction:

■ Ask the client to perform a gentle isometric contraction of the target muscles for approximately 5 to 8 seconds (in an attempt to rotate the LSp to the right) against your resistance (Fig. 9-11A).

■ Ask the client to relax.

■ This phase of the CRAC stretch is the CR protocol.

■ Please note that the breathing protocol for every repetition is to have the client hold the breath when contracting against your resistance.

Step 2: Client Concentric Contraction and Stretch:

■ As soon as the client relaxes, ask her to concentrically contract the lumbar left rotator musculature to actively rotate her LSp to the left as far as is comfortable (Fig. 9-11B).

■ This differs from CR stretching technique, in which the client would relax, and you would stretch the client's target musculature by passively moving the client's trunk into left rotation.

■ This stage of CRAC stretching begins the AC protocol.

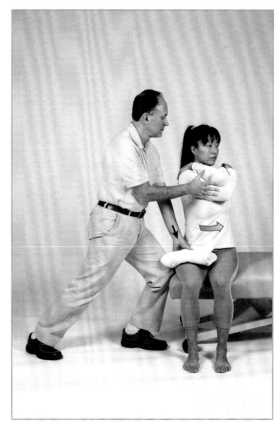

Figure 9-11B

Step 3: Client Relaxation and Further Stretch:

- Once the client has finished actively moving into left rotation, the client relaxes.
- As soon as the client relaxes, you now increase the stretch of the client's target LSp right rotator musculature by gently and passively moving the client's LSp farther into left rotation until you meet tissue resistance (Fig. 9-11C).
- Hold the client in this position of stretch for 1 to 2 seconds.

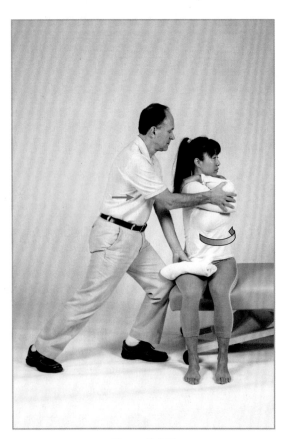

Figure 9-11C

Step 4: Passively Return Client to Starting Position:

- Support the client's trunk as you passively bring the client back to the starting position for the next repetition.
- Use both of your hands to support and move the client's body back to starting position (Fig. 9-11D).

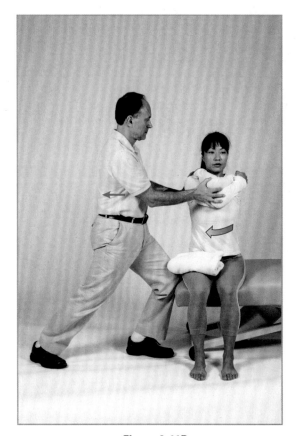

Figure 9-11D

Further Repetitions:

- This CRAC protocol can be repeated for a total of 3 to 10 repetitions.
- Once the final position of stretch is reached at the end of the last CRAC repetition, many therapists like to hold this position of stretch for a longer period, often 10 to 20 seconds or more.

Lumbar Spine Left Rotators:

- *Note*: To use CRAC stretching to stretch the LSp left rotator functional group of muscles, follow the directions given in Figures 9-10 through 9-11 to stretch the right rotator group but switch for the left side of the body.

SECTION 2: HIP JOINT/PELVIS CONTRACT RELAX AGONIST CONTRACT ROUTINES

As a rule, CRAC stretches to the muscles of the pelvis that cross the hip joint are performed by stabilizing the client's pelvis and moving his or her thigh to create the stretch. For the stretch to be effective, it is extremely important that the pelvis is securely stabilized. Otherwise, the stretching force will enter the LSp. This will not only dissipate the stretching force at the hip joint causing it to lose its effectiveness but might also place a torque (rotary force) into the LSp that can cause pain or injury.

The following CRAC stretching routines for muscles of the pelvis that cross the hip joint are presented in the chapter:

- Routine 9-3—hip flexors
- Routine 9-4—hip extensors: hamstrings (in the "Overview of Technique" section)
- Routine 9-5—hip deep lateral rotators

For many stretches of the client's hip joint musculature presented in this book, the leg is shown as the contact for the therapist's stretching/treatment hand. Contacting the leg increases the leverage force, making it easier for the therapist to move the client's thigh to create the stretch. However, if the client's knee joint is unhealthy, the contact should be moved from the leg to the thigh itself so that no force is placed through the knee joint. This can make the performance of the stretch more logistically challenging, especially if the therapist is small and the client is large but is necessary to protect the client's knee from injury.

ROUTINE 9-3: HIP FLEXORS

Figure 9-12 shows the functional group of muscles that flex the right thigh at the hip joint. These muscles are located on the anterior side of the pelvis and thigh, crossing the hip joint between them. With all CRAC stretches to the hip joint, it is important to stabilize the pelvis. With this stretch, it is especially important because if the pelvis is not securely stabilized, it will anteriorly tilt, causing increased lordosis of the LSp. Following is the CRAC stretching routine shown for the hip flexor functional group on the right side of the body with the client prone. *Note*: Alternate positions to perform stretching of the hip flexor group (prone with the therapist seated on the client and side-lying) are shown in Routine 6-7 in Chapter 6. These stretches can be easily transitioned to CRAC stretching by adding the protocol steps for CRAC stretching.

The Pelvis/Hip Joint Flexor Functional Group
This functional group comprises the following muscles:
Gluteus medius (anterior fibers)
Gluteus minimus (anterior fibers)
Tensor fasciae latae
Rectus femoris
Sartorius
Iliacus
Psoas major
Pectineus
Adductor longus
Adductor brevis
Gracilis

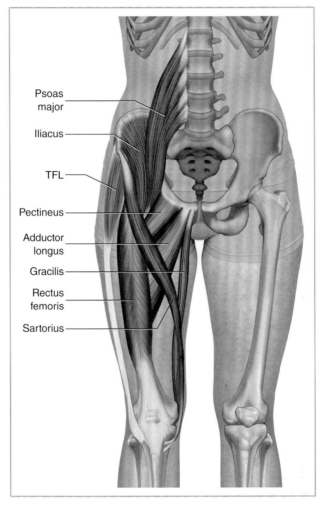

Figure 9-12 *Note*: Not all muscles are seen.

Starting Position:

- Have the client prone toward the right side of the table.
- Stand to the right side of the client.
- Your left hand is the treatment hand and is placed under (on the anterior surface of) the client's right thigh.
- Your right hand is the stabilization hand and functions to stabilize the client's pelvis. It is placed on the client's right posterior superior iliac spine (PSIS) (Fig. 9-13).

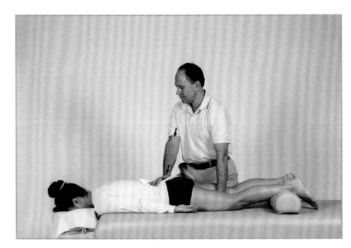

Figure 9-13

Step 1: Client Isometric Contraction:

- Ask the client to perform a gentle isometric contraction of the target muscles for approximately 5 to 8 seconds in an attempt to flex the thigh at the hip joint down against the resistance of the table. Your left hand under the client's thigh monitors that she is pressing in the correct manner and direction (Fig. 9-14A).

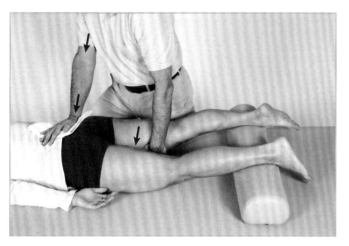

Figure 9-14A

- Ask the client to relax.
- This phase of the CRAC stretch is the CR protocol.
- Please note that the breathing protocol for every repetition is to have the client hold the breath when contracting against your resistance.

Step 2: Client Concentric Contraction and Stretch:

- As soon as the client relaxes, ask her to concentrically contract the extensors of the right thigh at the hip joint to actively extend the right thigh as far as is comfortable (Fig. 9-14B).

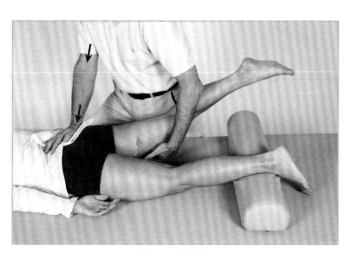

Figure 9-14B

- This differs from CR stretching technique, in which the client would relax, and you would stretch the client's target musculature by passively moving the client's thigh into extension.
- This stage of CRAC stretching begins the AC protocol.

Step 3: Client Relaxation and Further Stretch:

- Once the client has finished actively moving into extension, the client relaxes.
- As soon as the client relaxes, you now increase the stretch of the client's target right hip flexor musculature by gently and passively moving the client's right thigh farther into extension until you meet tissue resistance (Fig. 9-14C).
- Hold the client in this position of stretch for 1 to 2 seconds.

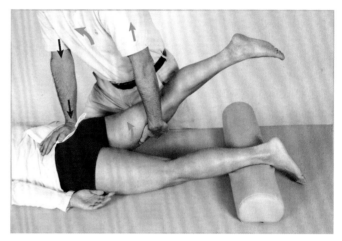

Figure 9-14C

Step 4: Passively Return Client to Starting Position:

- Support the client's trunk as you passively bring the client back to the starting position for the next repetition.
- Use one or both of your hands to support and move the client's thigh back to starting position (Fig. 9-14D).

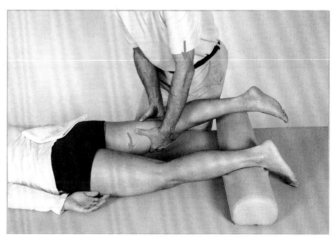

Figure 9-14D

Further Repetitions:

■ This CRAC protocol can be repeated for a total of 3 to 10 repetitions.

■ Once the final position of stretch is reached at the end of the last CRAC repetition, many therapists like to hold this position of stretch for a longer period, often 10 to 20 seconds or more.

Left-Side Flexor Group:

■ Repeat for the pelvis/hip joint flexor functional group on the left side of the body (Fig. 9-15).

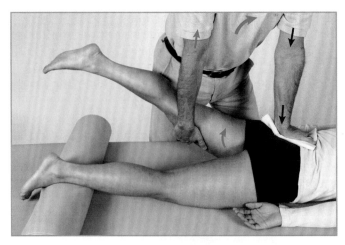

Figure 9-15

9.4	**PRACTICAL APPLICATION**

Multiplane Stretching of the Hip Joint Flexors

The CRAC stretching protocol for the flexors of the hip joint can be transitioned into a multiplane stretch. For example, during step 1 of the protocol, instead of having the client contract the target (hip flexor) muscles and press her thigh against your resistance directly down toward the table (perfectly in the sagittal plane), ask the client to press down toward flexion and toward abduction **(Fig. A)**. Then during step 2, instead of directing her to actively bring her thigh directly up in the air (again, perfectly in the sagittal plane), ask her to bring her thigh up and deviate medially toward adduction **(Fig. B)**. This will focus the stretch toward the flexors that are also abductors located anterolaterally in the thigh (e.g., TFL). This could be done instead for flexors that are also adductors by deviating up toward abduction. To add in transverse plane rotation, have the client preset the thigh in rotation before beginning the routine and then maintain the rotation during the routine. Figure B demonstrates medial rotation in addition to extension and adduction. Figure C demonstrates the addition of lateral rotation.

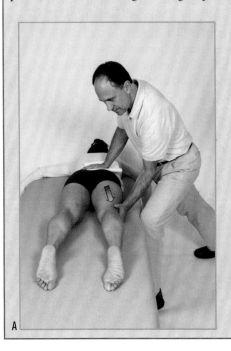
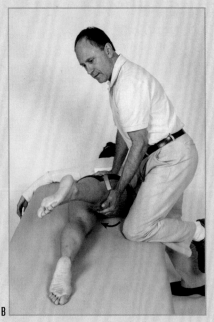
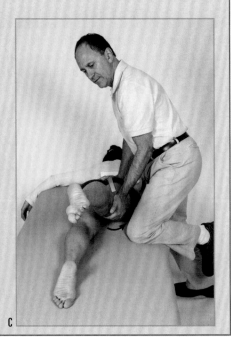

ROUTINE 9-4: HIP EXTENSORS: HAMSTRINGS

 View the video "Contract Relax Agonist Contract Stretching of the Hamstring Group" online on thePoint.lww.com

Figure 9-16 shows the hamstring muscles on the right side. They are located in the posterior thigh, crossing from the pelvis to the proximal leg. The hamstrings are hip extensor muscles because they cross the hip joint posteriorly with a vertical orientation to their fibers. However, unlike the gluteal muscles, which also cross the hip joint posteriorly with somewhat of a vertical orientation to their fibers, the hamstrings also cross the knee joint posteriorly; therefore, they also flex the knee joint. This is important to know when stretching them. CRAC stretching routine of the hamstring group was demonstrated in the "Overview of Technique" section, Figures 9-1 through 9-5.

The Hamstring Group
This group comprises the following muscles:
Biceps femoris
Semitendinosus
Semimembranosus

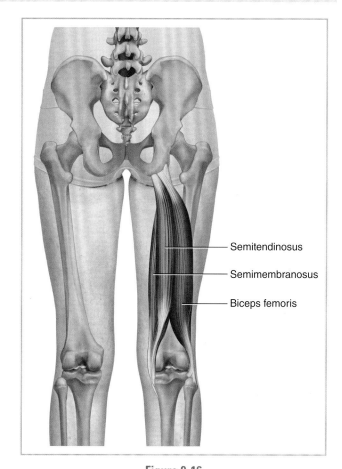

Semitendinosus

Semimembranosus

Biceps femoris

Figure 9-16

ROUTINE 9-5: HIP DEEP LATERAL ROTATORS

Figure 9-17 shows the functional group of deep lateral rotator muscles of the hip joint on the right side of the body. These muscles are located in the posterior pelvis in the buttock region, deep to the gluteus maximus, and cross the hip joint between the pelvis and thigh. *Note*: The posterior capsular ligament of the hip joint (ischiofemoral ligament) is stretched with medial rotation, as are the deep lateral rotator muscles. Therefore, the stretching protocol presented here for the deep lateral rotators is also very effective at stretching and loosening a taut posterior hip joint capsule. Following is the CRAC stretching routine shown for the deep lateral rotator group on the right side of the body.

Starting Position:

- Have the client supine toward the right side of the table.
- Position yourself at the right side of the table.
- Flex the client's right hip and knee joints and place his right foot flat on the table.
- Both of your hands will be treatment hands and can be placed against the lateral surface of the client's distal right thigh (Fig. 9-18).
- No stabilization hand is necessary; the client's body weight and contact with the table, as well as the direction that you move his thigh, stabilize his pelvis.

The Deep Lateral Rotator Group
This functional group comprises the following muscles:
Piriformis
Superior gemellus
Obturator internus
Inferior gemellus
Obturator externus
Quadratus femoris

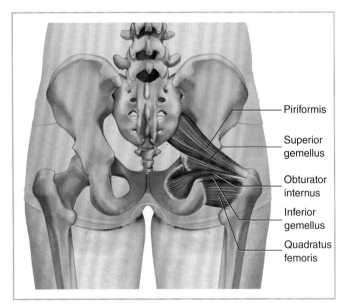

Figure 9-17 *Note*: The obturator externus is not seen.

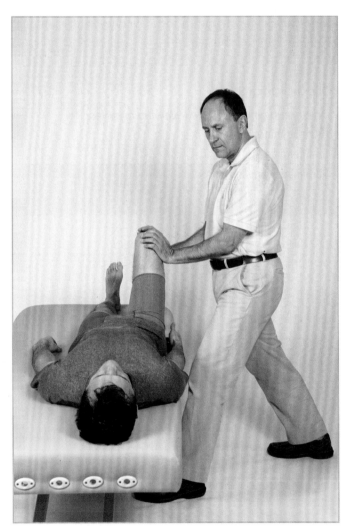

Figure 9-18

Step 1: Client Isometric Contraction:

- Ask the client to perform a gentle isometric contraction of the target muscles for approximately 5 to 8 seconds in an attempt to horizontally abduct the thigh at the hip joint against your resistance (Fig. 9-19A).

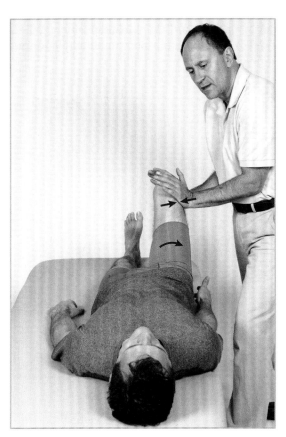

Figure 9-19A

- Ask the client to relax.
- This phase of the CRAC stretch is the CR protocol.
- Please note that the breathing protocol for every repetition is to have the client hold the breath when contracting against your resistance.

Step 2: Client Concentric Contraction and Stretch:

- As soon as the client relaxes, ask him to concentrically contract the horizontal adductors of the right thigh at the hip joint to actively bring his right thigh up and across his body (horizontally adduct) as far as is comfortable (Fig. 9-19B).

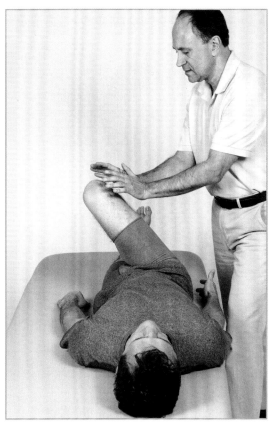

Figure 9-19B

- This differs from CR stretching technique, in which the client would relax, and you would stretch the client's target musculature by passively moving the client's thigh into horizontal adduction.
- This stage of CRAC stretching begins the AC protocol.

Step 3: Client Relaxation and Further Stretch:

- Once the client has finished actively moving into horizontal adduction, the client relaxes.
- As soon as the client relaxes, you now increase the stretch of the client's target right hip deep lateral rotator musculature by gently and passively moving the client's right thigh farther into horizontal adduction until you meet tissue resistance (Fig. 9-19C).
- Hold the client in this position of stretch for 1 to 2 seconds.

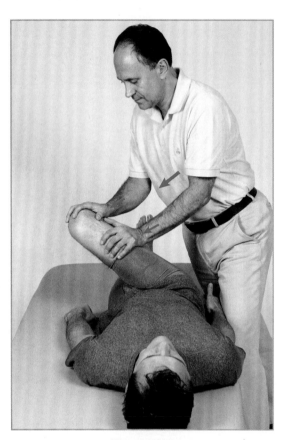

Figure 9-19C

Step 4: Passively Return Client to Starting Position:

- Support the client's thigh as you passively bring the client back to the starting position for the next repetition.
- Use both of your hands to support and move the client's thigh back to starting position (Fig. 9-19D). Alternately, the client's thigh does not have to be brought all the way back to starting position, but instead, it can be brought part way back toward the starting position. What is important is that there is a horizontal adduction range of motion possible for the client.

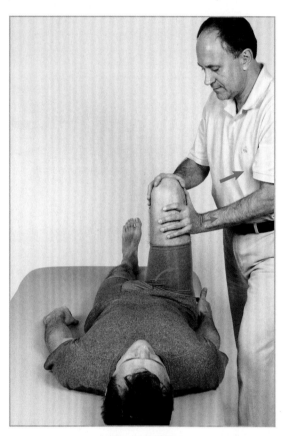

Figure 9-19D

Further Repetitions:
- This CRAC protocol can be repeated for a total of 3 to 10 repetitions.
- Once the final position of stretch is reached at the end of the last CRAC repetition, many therapists like to hold this position of stretch for a longer period, often 10 to 20 seconds or more.

Left-Side Deep Lateral Rotator Group:
- Repeat for the pelvis/hip joint deep lateral rotator functional group on the left side of the body (Fig. 9-20). As seen in the figure, you can place your knee on the table for added stabilization.

9.8	THERAPIST TIP

Use Discernment When Deciding Whether to Use Contract Relax Agonist Contract Stretching

Advanced stretches are often the best treatment option when a client presents with a tighter-than-usual low back/hip joint or has a history of not responding to standard stretching techniques. Both CR and AC stretching employ a neurologic reflex that facilitates the stretch by inhibiting and relaxing the client's tight musculature. Because CRAC stretching combines the neurologic reflexes of CR and AC stretching, it is likely the most powerful stretching option and therefore would be the stretching technique of choice for clients with the most chronic and stubborn conditions, especially those clients who have not responded to CR or AC stretching performed separately.

However, CRAC stretching is more time consuming to perform than either CR or AC stretching done alone, and spending more time stretching one muscle group means less time to work on other muscle groups in other areas of the client's body. Ultimately, the choice of stretching technique in each scenario is a clinical decision that rests on the unique circumstances with which the client presents.

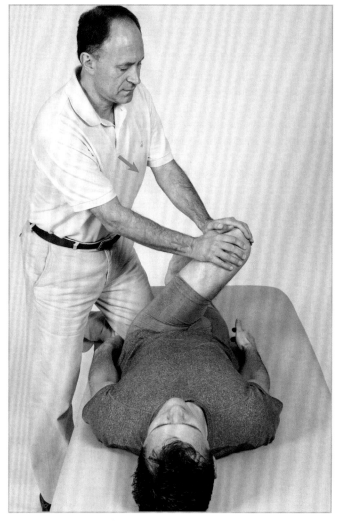

Figure 9-20

CHAPTER SUMMARY

CRAC stretching is an advanced neural inhibition stretching technique that combines the CR stretching technique with the AC stretching technique. Because it does combine these two techniques, its protocol can take some practice to master. It is strongly recommended to first learn and master the CR and AC techniques independently and then apply that knowledge (with minor modifications) to perform the CRAC technique. Because CRAC combines the effect of the CR and AC techniques, it can often help clients with tight muscles when other stretching techniques have not succeeded. As with all stretching, CRAC stretching is most effective when the client's tissues have been warmed up first.

Determine the Proper Frequency of Care

Determining the proper frequency of care is extremely important. Many manual therapists feel uncomfortable asking a client to come in more than once a week. However, examples from physical therapy, chiropractic, and athletic training all demonstrate that rehabilitation work is most efficient when treatments are performed two to three times per week. Clinical massage and other manual therapies are no different. When you are performing true clinical rehabilitation work, once-weekly visits are often not only insufficient to help the clients but are also, in fact, a disservice to them.

Each bodywork treatment continues the healing process that was gained in the previous treatment session. However, with each day that passes after a treatment, the client's body reverts more to its initial pattern of tightness,
and the healing gained in the previous treatment is increasingly lost. A good analogy is that each treatment brings the client one step forward, but if a full week passes before the next treatment, the client falls back three-quarters of a step, if not the entire step, causing the same ground to be covered repeatedly in future sessions. The result is a waste of the client's time and money.

The maximum benefit is gained when treatments are spaced no more than 2 to 4 days apart. In this manner, each treatment moves the client a step forward, and only a half-step or less is lost if the next treatment occurs within a couple of days. This timing allows for a speedier healing process for the client and actually saves time and money in the long run.

CASE STUDY

LESLIE

■ **History and Physical Assessment**

A new client, Leslie Weber, age 55 years, comes to your office complaining of a stiff low back. She tells you that over the years, she has noticed a gradual stiffening of her low back, although she has experienced no accompanying pain. She says she thinks that the increasing stiffness is probably the result of a combination of factors, including poor posture when doing desk work and working at her computer, sleeping on her stomach, and a long history of strenuous working out (Zumba and working out with weights) without commensurate stretching. She states that she has had no previous major physical traumas, operations, or major pathologic conditions of her low back. Other than an occasional "tight low back," she has never noticed any problems.

Leslie further reports that she has already tried deep tissue massage therapy once a week for the past 6 weeks and that she has also been working with a fitness trainer specifically for stretching once a week for over a month now. She says that although she has experienced some improvement with the massage and stretching at the gym, she does not feel that they have helped her sufficiently to regain her lost motion. She says she also saw her medical physician, who ordered radiography of her LSp. The physician told her that the radiographs were negative for fracture and dislocation and that they showed only mild lumbar degenerative joint disease (osteoarthritis).

Your assessment exam finds that on active and passive range of motion examination, each lateral flexion motion is decreased by 20 degrees, flexion is decreased by 25 degrees, and extension is decreased by 10 degrees. Assessment also shows negative cough test and Valsalva maneuver as well as negative active and passive straight leg raise tests for lower extremity referral. (For a review of assessment procedures, see Chapter 3.) Palpation exam reveals uniform tightness of her lumbar and lower thoracic paraspinal musculature bilaterally as well as bilateral tightness of her quadratus lumborum and psoas major. Her deep lateral rotator musculature of the hip joint is also tight bilaterally.

■ **Think-It-Through Questions:**

1. Should an advanced stretching technique such as CRAC stretching be included in your treatment plan for Leslie? If so, why? If not, why not?
2. If CRAC stretching would be of value, is it safe to use with her? If yes, how do you know? If not, why not?
3. If CRAC stretching is done, which specific stretching routines should be done and why did you choose the ones you did?

Answers to these Think-It-Through Questions and the Treatment Strategy employed for this client are available online at thePoint.lww.com/MuscolinoLowBack

OBJECTIVES

After completing this chapter, the student should be able to:

1. Describe the similarity between joint mobilization and stretching.
2. Describe the relationship between joint mobilization and pin and stretch.
3. Explain how joint mobilization differs from other forms of stretching.
4. Describe the relationship between joint hypomobilities and hypermobilities.
5. Describe the roles of the treatment hand, stabilization hand, and support hand.
6. Describe in steps an overview of the usual protocol for carrying out a joint mobilization of the sacroiliac and lumbar spinal (LSp) joints.
7. Describe the relationship between joint mobilization and passive range of motion and joint play.
8. Explain why thrusting should never be done when performing joint mobilization.
9. State conditions that contraindicate joint mobilization of the sacroiliac and LSp joints.
10. Define each key term in this chapter and explain its relationship to joint mobilization technique.
11. Perform joint mobilization technique for each of the routines presented in this chapter.
12. Describe and perform two methods of joint play distraction (traction).

KEY TERMS

active range of motion	joint mobilization
adjustment	joint play
axial distraction	joint release
distraction	manual traction
hypermobile	mobilization grading
hypomobile	motion palpation

passive range of motion	towel traction
pin and stretch	traction
"pocket to pocket"	treatment hand
segmental joint level	
stabilization hand	
support hand	

INTRODUCTION

Among the advanced techniques that are available to manual therapists, none is more underutilized than joint mobilization. In treatment sessions, most massage therapists employ massage strokes, many use hydrotherapy (e.g., hot/cold), and many stretch their clients, but very few use joint mobilization. This is unfortunate because, of all the advanced treatment techniques, none is more powerful and has more potential therapeutic benefit than joint mobilization. However, any therapy that has the power to heal also has the power to cause harm if not employed judiciously and with skill. Joint mobilization is such a skill. Ideally, this chapter should be consulted along with attendance at a hands-on joint mobilization workshop. But even without attendance at a hands-on workshop, this chapter, along with careful study and practice, provides a solid beginning foundation on how to perform this technique.

Note: In the Technique and Self-Care chapters of this book (Chapters 4 to 12), green arrows indicate movement, red arrows indicate stabilization, and black arrows indicate a position that is statically held.

MECHANISM

The mechanism of **joint mobilization** of the SIJ and LSp joints is simple. One bone is stabilized while the adjacent bone is mobilized by moving it in relation to the stabilized bone. This mobilization causes a stretch of the soft tissues located between these two bones. In essence, joint mobilization is a very precise form of stretching. It is stretching that is aimed at loosening taut intrinsic soft tissues at a **segmental joint level**. These tissues include joint capsules, ligaments, and short deep intrinsic muscles. A segmental joint level is a specific joint level; for example, the L4-L5 segmental joint level refers to the spinal disc and facet joints between L4 and L5, and the SIJ refers to the joint between the sacrum and ilium (for a review of the anatomy of the LSp and SIJ, please see Chapter 1). More specifically, a joint mobilization is aimed at a **hypomobile** segmental joint level, in other words, a joint level whose range of motion is decreased.

Joint mobilization is performed within a range of motion called **joint play**—that is, the small range of motion that is possible beyond the end of passive range of motion (Fig. 10-1). **Active range of motion** is defined as the range of motion of a joint that can be performed by the contraction of the muscles of that joint. **Passive range of motion** is defined as the range of motion of the joint that can be produced by a force other than the contraction of the muscles of that joint (passive range of motion is often performed by a therapist). In a healthy joint, passive range of motion is slightly greater than active range of motion. Joint mobilization technique is performed within the range of joint play.

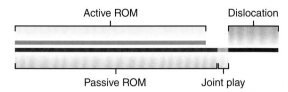

Figure 10-1 Illustration of the relationship of a joint's active range of motion, passive range of motion, and joint play. *ROM*, range of motion.

The range of motion within joint play is extremely small so the amount of stretch that you apply during a joint mobilization to a client's SIJ and LSp joints needs to be extremely small. This motion is barely measurable, literally a fraction of an inch (a quarter inch or less), and is only enough to slightly stretch the client's tissues that are located deeply around the joint. As with any stretching technique, joint mobilization should never be forced and should not be painful for the client. Because joint mobilization technique is performed within the range of motion called joint play, the technique is often called *joint play*.

Comparison of Joint Mobilization and Stretching

Joint mobilization is similar to stretching techniques; when a joint is moved in one direction, the soft tissues on the other side of the joint are stretched. These tissues are the antagonist musculature, ligaments and joint capsule fibers, and other fascial tissues. However, unlike all other stretching techniques, instead of stretching the entire low back and pelvis, and thus the larger, longer soft tissues that span the entire lumbosacral spine and posterior pelvis, joint mobilization focuses the stretch on the smaller intrinsic muscles of the spine (e.g., rotatores, intertransversarii) and the smaller ligaments and joint capsules of the segmental joint level being stretched.

All stretching techniques discussed thus far in this book involve stretching the entire LSp and pelvis. In other words, the line of tension of the stretch is spread across all the LSp joints from T12 to the sacrum and the pelvis from the lumbosacral spine to the lower extremity. The problem with this is that a client's low back may have full range of motion even if one or more segmental levels are hypomobile. For example, the L3-L4 segmental joint level can have decreased motion into right lateral flexion, yet the LSp as a whole may still exhibit full right lateral flexion. Another example might be that the left SIJ has decreased range of motion, but the joints of the pelvis as a whole exhibit may still exhibit full range of motion. This is because other lumbar and pelvic joints compensate by becoming **hypermobile** and therefore move more than normal. In the case of the lumbar example, if the low back joints above L3 and below L4 increase their flexibility in right lateral flexion, they can fully compensate for the right lateral flexion motion that is lost between L3 and L4. In the pelvic example, if the right SIJ increases its motion, it can fully compensate for the motion that is lost at the left SIJ. When the client's lumbar or pelvic range of motion is assessed, it will exhibit full motion, even though

| 10.1 | THERAPIST TIP |

Importance of Segmental Joint Hypomobilities

The following question might be asked: If the LSp and pelvis have full range of motion, why do you care if there are hypermobilities compensating for hypomobilities? After all, if the low back can move as far as is needed in each direction, is it not fully functional?

The answer is yes, but this full range of motion comes at a price. In time, the excessive motion of the compensating hypermobile joints can lead to their overuse and irritation. This can cause pain, which then triggers the pain-spasm-pain cycle to cause protective spasming of the musculature of those joints. This spasming then causes further pain, resulting in a vicious cycle. The muscular spasming that occurs also causes restriction of motion at those segmental joint levels, changing the hypermobilities into hypomobilities. Overuse of a hypermobile segment can also cause irritation and swelling, which can result in the influx of fibroblasts, which lay down scar tissue adhesions, further transitioning the hypermobility to a hypomobility. As a result, there will be even more hypomobile segmental joint levels in the low back, requiring even greater hypermobility compensation of the remaining joints. In time, these remaining hypermobilities will likely also become

hypomobilities. This is a classic domino effect pattern that occurs in the spine as compensatory hypermobilities become hypomobilities and the region of hypomobility spreads. This explains how large spinal regions can become locked up and hypomobile.

When a client has just one or two low back joint hypomobilities and the adjacent hypermobile joints "successfully" compensate, the client often is unaware of the problem and does not seek care. Regions of hypomobility usually become apparent only when they become so large that the adjacent joints are no longer capable of compensating sufficiently. As a result, the gross range of motion of the low back finally diminishes. This is usually the point at which the client realizes that there is a problem, whereas in reality, the condition likely has been progressing for months, if not years. Treatment success is more linked with the length of time (chronicity) that the client has had a condition than any other one factor. Therefore, it is important to locate these segmental hypomobilities as soon as possible before they are long-standing and before they spread. Joint mobilization assessment and treatment is the ideal technique to accomplish this.

---

one or more of its segmental joint levels are restricted and in need of stretching/mobilizing.

In this manner, hypomobilities create corresponding hypermobilities. Once formed, hypermobilities enable the persistence of hypomobilities. However, if enough hypomobile levels are present, their decreased motion might contribute to an overall decrease in gross range of the motion of the LSp or pelvis. But even this condition can be difficult to resolve with standard or advanced stretching, because if you stretch the client's low back in an attempt to lengthen and loosen these hypomobilities, the hypermobilities may "absorb" the stretch by becoming even more hypermobile. Thus, this stretch may result in a restoration of gross range of the motion, even though the underlying hypomobilities are still present. In cases such as these, which are quite common, all standard and advanced stretching techniques are usually ineffective at increasing the flexibility of these hypomobile joints. In fact, these techniques may actually be detrimental because they cause or perpetuate the hypermobile joint compensations.

Joint mobilization is the only treatment technique available to manual therapists that can address and resolve a segmental joint hypomobility. If, for example, the L3-L4 joint is decreased in right lateral flexion, joint mobilization can apply the localized force needed to address this very specific loss of motion at this specific joint level. As with regular stretching, the force used in joint mobilization is a tension force, but instead of producing a line of tension across a large swath of tissue (such as the entire LSp), this force is localized

and applied to only one segmental joint level of the low back or pelvis. In this sense, joint mobilization can be considered a very specific and focused stretching technique.

OVERVIEW OF TECHNIQUE

The following is an overview of joint mobilization technique using seated joint mobilization technique for the L2-L3 segmental level as the hypomobile joint that needs to be mobilized into left lateral flexion. In this example, because the client has a restriction in left lateral flexion at the L2-L3 joint level, you can assume that the L2 vertebra is not left laterally flexing freely on the L3 vertebra. To resolve this problem, it will be necessary to apply a force that moves L2 into left lateral flexion on L3 while L3 remains stable, thereby stretching whatever taut tissues between them are restricting this frontal plane motion. This is accomplished by using one hand to stabilize L3 while the other hand moves L2 on L3.

As with regular stretching, the **treatment hand** applies the stretching or mobilization force, and the **stabilization hand** prevents the adjacent body part from moving. Placing the hands in this manner focuses the stretch on the appropriate joint level and keeps it from being lost on other levels of the low back. In this case, the therapist's right (lower) hand is the stabilization hand that is stabilizing the client's L3 vertebra. The therapist's left (upper) hand is the treatment hand that moves the entire upper body and L2 into left lateral flexion on top of the stabilized L3.

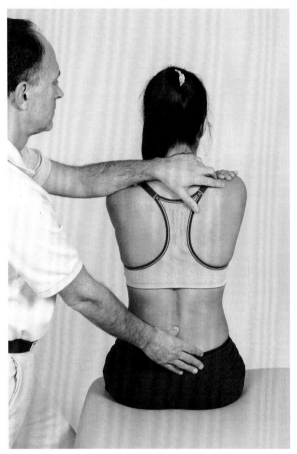

Figure 10-2 Starting position for L2-L3 left lateral flexion joint mobilization.

Starting Position:
- The client is seated, with her hands comfortably crossed to her opposite shoulders and her arms resting on her chest. You are standing (or seated) behind the client, slightly to the left side.
- Your right hand will be the lower stabilization hand, and your left hand will be the upper treatment hand.
- Note that your elbows are tucked in front of your body as much as possible so that you can use your core body weight behind your forearms and hands when pressing on the client with your treatment and stabilization hands.
- Use your left hand to hold across the top of the client's shoulders/trunk (Fig. 10-2).

Step 1: Stabilize Lower Bone:
- Stabilize/pin L3 by placing the thumb pad of your right hand against the left side of the spinous process (SP) of L3 (Fig. 10-3A).

Step 2: Bring Joint to Tension:
- After securely stabilizing L3 with your right hand, use your left hand to gently but firmly move the client's trunk into left lateral flexion on the L3 vertebra until you reach tissue tension at the end of passive range of motion (Fig. 10-3B).
- *Note*: It is extremely important that your right hand keep L3 stabilized so that it does not move at all.

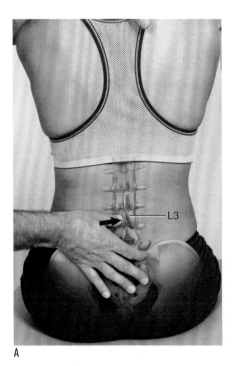
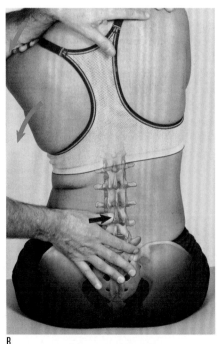
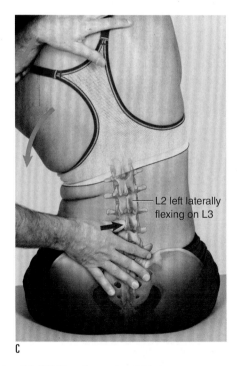

Figure 10-3 L2-L3 left lateral flexion joint mobilization steps. **(A)** Step 1, stabilizing L3. **(B)** Step 2, moving L2 into left lateral flexion until tissue tension is felt. **(C)** Step 3, joint mobilization is performed by gently increasing L2's left lateral flexion on L3.

Step 3: Perform Joint Mobilization:

- As soon as you reach the end of passive range of motion, perform the actual left lateral flexion joint mobilization of L2 on L3 by gently applying slightly more force to the client's trunk with your left hand (Fig. 10-3C). *Note*: When you move the client's trunk with your left hand, you are moving L2 and the entire trunk that is above it.
- Hold for only a fraction of a second and then release.

Further Repetitions:

- Once the joint mobilization has been performed at one level, apply it at all the other levels of the LSp so that all LSp joints are mobilized into left lateral flexion.
- This joint mobilization of the entire LSp may then be repeated for a total of two or three times, with concentration at the segmental joint levels that are least mobile.

10.1 | **PRACTICAL APPLICATION**

Transitioning Seated Lumbar Spine Lateral Flexion Mobilization to Rotation and Extension Mobilizations

The seated LSp lateral flexion mobilization technique can be modified to mobilize the LSp into rotation or extension.

If rotation mobilization is performed, the client's arms should be crossed so that her hands are on the opposite shoulders, but her arms should be adducted at the glenohumeral joints so that her elbows meet at the center of the body. For left rotation, stand behind and to the client's left side and grasp her elbows with your left hand and place the thumb of your right hand on the left side of the SP at the desired level of the LSp. Rotate the client's upper body into left rotation until the end of passive range of motion is reached. To perform the mobilization, both hands act as treatment hands: The left hand gently brings the client's spine farther into left rotation as the thumb of the right hand pushes the SP farther to the right (when the SP moves to the right, the anterior surface of the vertebral body orients to the left; therefore, this motion is defined as left rotation) **(Figs. A and B)**. The vertebrae that are below the contacted verte-

bra are stabilized by body weight. Repeat on the other side of the client for right rotation mobilization, switching the placement of your hands.

To perform extension mobilization, the client holds her arms flexed to 90 degrees at the glenohumeral joint and each hand holds the opposite-side elbow. Stand behind and to the left side of the client and grasp her forearms with your left hand and place your contact over the midline (center) of the SP at the desired level of the LSp **(Fig. C)**. Using both hands, bring the client into extension until the end of passive range of motion is reached. To perform the mobilization, both hands act as treatment hands: The left hand gently brings the client's spine farther into extension as your right hand contact pushes the vertebra farther into extension (Fig. C). The vertebrae below the contacted vertebra are stabilized by body weight.

Your contact on the client's SP can be the middle phalanx of your index finger supported by your thumb

continued

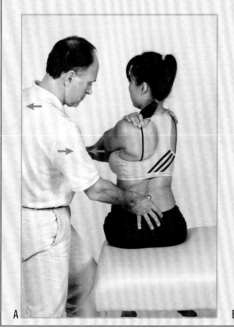
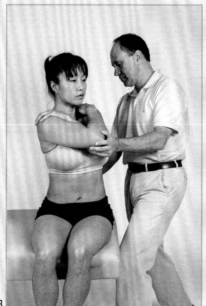
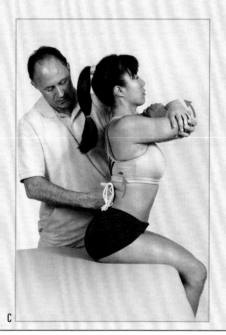

A   B   C

(Fig. D). Alternately, you can use your fist **(Fig. E)**. This is a stronger contact for the therapist. It is also less pokey because it broadens out the mobilization force across several vertebrae; however, for this reason, it is also less precise. With either contact, for client and therapist comfort, a small cushion can be placed between the therapist's contact and the client's spine. A folded towel also works well (see Fig. C). *Note*: This mobilization could have been performed with the therapist standing on the other side of the client using the right hand to support the client's forearms in front and the left hand as the vertebral contact hand.

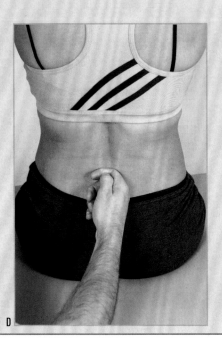

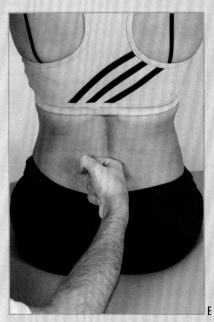

10.2   **THERAPIST TIP**

Apply the Technique Even If the Spinal Level Cannot Be Discerned

Sometimes, it is difficult to distinguish exactly which vertebral level of the LSp you are on. The most important thing is that you apply the joint mobilization technique to each hypomobile segmental level of the LSp, even if you cannot name with certainty exactly which segmental joint you are on at any given time. With continued experience, learning to distinguish and name each segmental level of the LSp will become easier.

BOX   **10.2**

Joint Mobilization and the Pin-and-Stretch Technique

Joint mobilization is not only a type of stretching but also a form of the **pin-and-stretch** technique. A pin and stretch is done by pinning, or stabilizing, one point and then stretching the soft tissues relative to that pinned point. In the example given in the "Overview of Technique" section, when the stabilization hand stabilizes the third lumbar vertebra, it is pinning L3. Then, when the trunk above L3 is moved relative to L3, the tension of the stretch is directed to the L2-L3 joint level. In effect, the *pin-point accuracy* of LSp joint mobilization occurs because one vertebral level is pinned, directing the stretch specifically to the joint adjacent to that vertebra. Generally, the lower vertebra is pinned, and the stretch is applied to the joint above.

PERFORMING THE TECHNIQUE

10.1 Stabilization Hand: Your Contact

Because joint mobilization technique is so specific, your choice of contact points on the client is crucial. This is especially true of your lower stabilization hand. Figure 10-4 shows three choices for the stabilization hand's contact on the client. One contact is the thumb pad, another is the pads of the index and middle fingers, and the third is the pisiform of the hypothenar eminence of the hand.

Each choice confers specific advantages:

- Use of the thumb pad is generally the most efficient because it is larger and stronger than the pad of the index and middle fingers but smaller than the hypothenar eminence to better fit against the vertebral SP (Fig. 10-4A). The disadvantage of the thumb pad contact is that some therapists have an interphalangeal joint of the thumb that tends to collapse into hyperextension when pressure is applied against it; excessive use of the thumb can aggravate this condition.
- Use of the finger pads tends to be the most specific and easiest to fit against the vertebral SP; however, the fingers have less strength than the thumb pad or hypothenar eminence and may also feel pokey to the client (Fig. 10-4B).
- Use of pisiform of the hypothenar eminence is the largest and strongest contact; however, because it is the largest contact, it is often hard to fit it against the SP (Fig. 10-4C).

As long as the goal of stabilization is achieved, you can use any contact that works and is comfortable for you and the client.

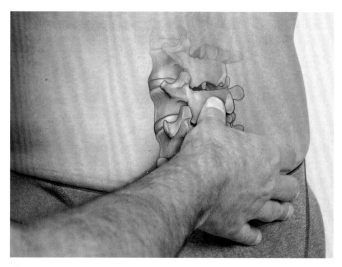

Figure 10-5 The SP is the client contact for the stabilization hand.

10.2 Stabilization Hand: Client Contact

Also important is the precise contact location on the client's LSp for your stabilization hand. Contact must be made against the SP because this is the only lumbar vertebral landmark that is easily accessible and pressure can be applied against (Fig. 10-5). If it is possible to reach deeper into the client's tissues and spread this contact over the lamina, this should be done. The more of the SP and perhaps lamina that can be contacted, the more powerful the stabilization is and the more comfortable it is for the client.

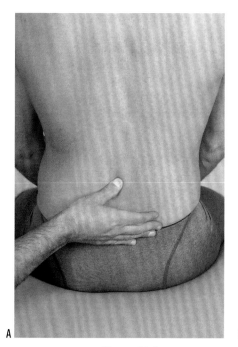 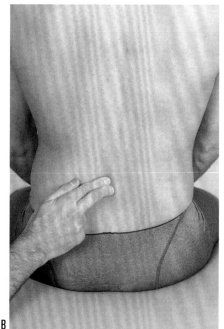 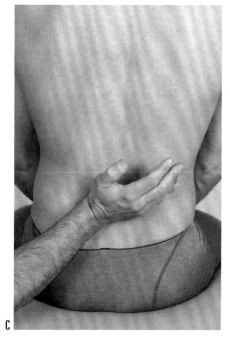

Figure 10-4 Stabilization hand contacts. **(A)** Thumb pad. **(B)** Finger pads. **(C)** Hypothenar eminence.

Locating the Spinous Process Contact

The SPs are located midline. Begin by locating the SPs in the posterior midline of the LSp with your thumb pad. Because of the lordotic curve of the LSp, this can be challenging for some of the vertebral levels; find whatever vertebral SP is easiest to find. Now drop laterally off the tip of the SP toward the side of the body to which you are standing/seated and press in against the side of the SP. Reach in as far deep against the SP toward the lamina as you can so that your contact is as firm as possible (see Fig. 10-5). Be sure to not move too far laterally off the SP and onto the laminar groove musculature. For a review of the anatomy of the LSp, see Chapter 1.

10.3 Treatment Hand: Your Contact

The placement of your upper treatment hand that moves the client's trunk does not need to be placed as specifically as the lower stabilization hand. However, the upper hand is the hand that has to support and move the client's trunk, so having a gentle but firm and secure contact on the client is important (Fig. 10-6). A client who does not feel comfortable and does not sense that you are holding the trunk securely will not relax and let you perform the joint mobilization.

10.4 Treatment Hand: Client Contact

The upper treatment hand needs to hold onto the client's trunk above the stabilization hand. The role of the treatment hand is to move L2 on L3. Because it is not possible to precisely contact L2 to move it on L3, the entire trunk is held at the shoulders/upper thoracic region. When the treatment hand moves the client's trunk into left lateral flexion, the en-

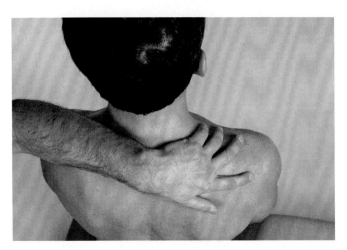

Figure 10-6 Positioning the treatment hand. The position of the treatment hand is placed on the top of the client's shoulders/upper thoracic region.

Holding the Client's Trunk

Your hold of the client's trunk must be gentle but firm and secure so that the client relaxes and allows you to support and move the trunk. To ensure the client's comfort, make sure that your contact is broad, holding the client's trunk with as much of the forearm and palmar (anterior) surface of your fingers and palm as possible (see Fig. 10-6). It is important to minimize curling your fingers to contact the client's trunk with your fingertips because this can feel pokey and uncomfortable to the client.

tire thoracic spine and any and all lumbar vertebrae that are above the stabilization pin (L3 as shown in this section) are moved relative to L3. This focuses the stretch/mobilization to the L2-L3 segmental joint level.

10.5 Using Both Hands in Concert

When first practicing joint mobilization, the easiest way is to keep the lower stabilization hand fixed and only use the upper treatment hand to move the client's trunk as previously described. However, the roles can be reversed; after tension in the joint is attained, the upper hand can be used as a stabilization hand to keep the trunk/upper vertebrae fixed as the lower hand moves the vertebra that is contacted below. Figure 10-7A shows the position attained in step 2 of the joint mobilization protocol in which the client's trunk has been brought to tension. Figure 10-7B shows the upper hand creating the joint mobilization force as usually done and described thus far in this chapter. Figure 10-7C shows the lower hand being used to create the joint mobilization force instead of the upper hand. Stabilizing the upper vertebra and moving the lower one offers another method of performing joint mobilization of the LSp. Whether the upper vertebra is moved relative to the lower one, or the lower vertebra is moved relative to the upper one, mobilization of the joint between them is accomplished.

In fact, as you become more comfortable and experienced performing joint mobilization, you can increase your proficiency by learning to move both hands in concert to apply the stretch of the mobilization. As the upper hand applies a gentle force to stretch the upper vertebra on the lower one, the lower hand applies a gentle force in the opposite direction to move the lower vertebra relative to the upper one (Fig. 10-7D). In this manner, both hands act as treatment hands, and the degree of mobilization of the segmental level between the two vertebrae is increased. Using the hands in concert as treatment hands greatly adds to the smoothness and proficiency of the joint mobilization technique. Becoming skilled at using both hands in concert, like any other technique skill, involves careful practice.

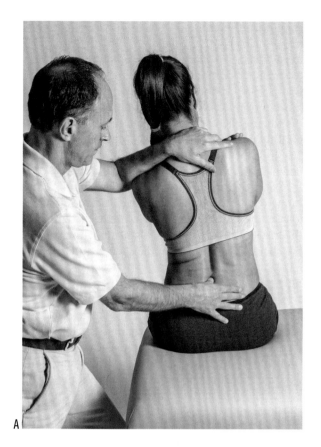
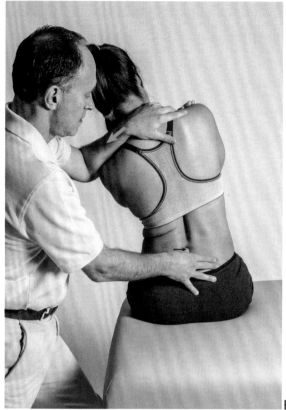
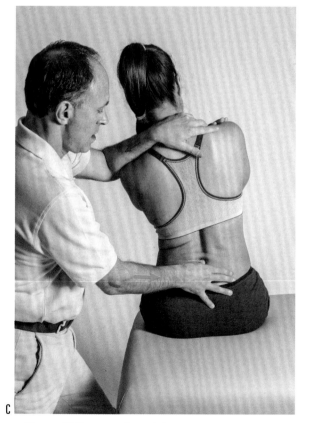
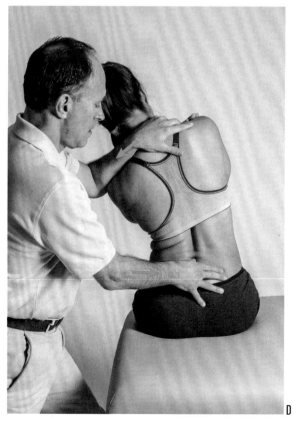

Figure 10-7 Using the stabilization hand to treat. **(A)** The client's trunk (and specifically the joint to be mobilized) has been brought to tension. **(B)** The lower vertebra is stabilized while the upper vertebra is mobilized (moved to the left) above it. **(C)** The upper vertebra is stabilized while the lower vertebra is mobilized (moved to the right) under it. **(D)** Both hands can administer the joint mobilization force simultaneously. The upper hand moves the upper vertebra to the left while the lower hand moves the lower vertebra to the right.

It is critical that you study the joint mobilization technique carefully and understand it before attempting to use it on your clients. Any technique that has the power to help also has the power to do harm, and joint mobilization is an extremely powerful technique. Joint mobilization, when applied inappropriately, can cause serious harm to the client. Inappropriate application of joint mobilization technique includes applying joint mobilization to a condition for which its use is indicated but executing the technique incorrectly—for example, performing it too forcefully. It also includes applying joint mobilization to a condition for which it is contraindicated, usually a space-occupying lesion such as a pathologic disc or advanced degenerative joint disease (see Chapter 3 for assessment of pathologic conditions). If you have any doubt about whether it is appropriate to use joint mobilization for a particular client, be sure first to obtain written permission from the client's chiropractic or medical physician.

10.6 Bring the Joint to Tension First

Before you perform the actual stretch of the joint mobilization, you must first bring the joint that is to be mobilized to tissue tension at the end of its passive range of motion. This is done by first stabilizing the lower vertebra with your stabilization hand and then using your treatment hand to move the trunk on the fixed vertebra until you reach the end of passive range of motion. The amount of motion necessary to reach this point varies depending on the region of the LSp that is being mobilized. Mobilizing the lower LSp requires more motion on the part of the treatment hand than does mobilizing the upper LSp. Note the difference in the upper treatment hand's motion by comparing Figures 10-8A and 10-8B. Joint mobilization can be performed only when the end of passive range of motion is first reached.

As the treatment hand moves the client through a greater range of motion, it becomes even more important for the lower stabilization hand to stabilize the vertebra securely. For this reason, it can be more challenging for you to mobilize the client's lower LSp than the client's upper LSp.

10.7 Degree of Stretch/Mobilization

The degree of stretch of an LSp joint mobilization is critically important. Joint mobilization is performed within the range of motion called joint play. Because the range of motion within joint play is so small, the amount of stretch that you apply during a joint mobilization to the client's LSp or SIJs needs to be extremely small. This motion is barely mea-

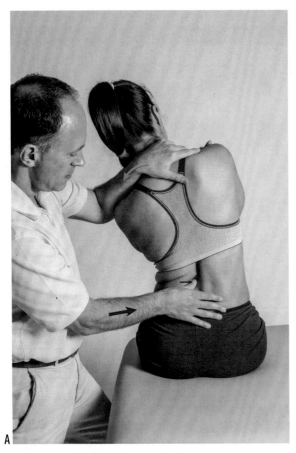
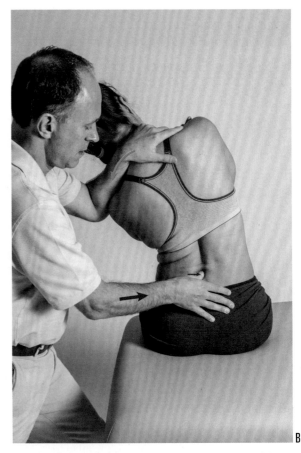

A   B

Figure 10-8 Bringing the joint to tension. Bringing the joint to tension requires less or more movement of the client's trunk depending on the level of joint mobilization. **(A)** Mobilization of the upper LSp requires less movement of the client's trunk. **(B)** Mobilization of the lower LSp requires more movement of the client's trunk.

THERAPIST TIP

Learning Joint Mobilization of the Low Back and Pelvis

When first learning joint mobilization of the LSp, learning to mobilize the lower LSp is the most challenging because the SP of L5 can be difficult to locate and contact, and the treatment hand has a larger range of motion excursion, requiring more skill to control. Learning to mobilize the middle of the LSp might also be challenging because the lordotic curve causes the SPs to be farther from reach. Therefore, mobilization of the upper LSp is usually the easiest region to learn and master. The routines for joint mobilization of the LSp in this chapter are presented by starting at the upper LSp and then working inferiorly to the lower LSp. However, when first learning and practicing this technique, it is best to begin wherever you can most easily perform this technique. If it is at the upper LSp, then begin there and work your way downward. If it is at the lower LSp, then begin there and work upward. If it is at the middle of the LSp, then begin there and work upward and downward as you please. Once you have become proficient with this technique, it is more efficient to begin at one end of the LSp and work your way methodically toward the other end.

surable, literally a fraction of an inch (a quarter inch or less), and is only enough to slightly stretch the client's tissues that are located deeply around the joint. As with any stretching technique, joint mobilization should never be forced and should not be painful for the client.

Keep in mind that the goal of joint mobilization is to mobilize hypomobile joints. There is no reason to apply joint mobilization to hypermobile joints. In fact, as a rule, it is contraindicated to mobilize hypermobile joints because it will likely increase the degree of hypermobility.

10.8 Length of Time of Stretch/Mobilization

It is also important that you hold the mobilization stretch of the client's LSp or SIJ in joint play for only a very short time, as holding for a sustained period can be very uncomfortable for the client. Proper joint mobilization technique involves bringing the client's joint into the range of joint play for a second or less and then releasing the joint; this can then be repeated approximately three to five times. As with any stretching technique, joint mobilization should not be forced and should be experienced by the client as a comfortable stretch; it should never cause the client pain.

10.9 Applying the Force

Joint mobilization technique is performed by bringing the client's joint to the end of passive range of motion and then gently applying an even and steady force that further stretches

the joint in the desired direction of motion. It cannot be emphasized too strongly that the force applied to perform a joint mobilization is gentle yet firm, even, and steady. It can be helpful to think of application of force as being gentle oscillations. Joint mobilization does not involve any type of fast or sudden thrust. A fast thrust within the realm of joint play is defined as a *chiropractic* or *osteopathic adjustment* and cannot be performed legally by most manual therapists.

THERAPIST TIP

Never Thrust

Two types of manipulations are possible within the range of motion that is termed joint play. If the force that stretches the soft tissues of the joint is applied in a slow, steady manner, it is defined as joint mobilization. A joint mobilization is often described as being a low-velocity manipulation. If, however, the force that stretches the tissue is applied in a fast thrusting manner, it is defined as a chiropractic/osteopathic **adjustment**. An adjustment is often described as being a high-velocity manipulation. Adjustments cannot be performed legally by massage therapists and most other manual therapists. For this reason, it is extremely important when doing a joint mobilization that no thrust is applied to the client's tissues.

As with any joint stretch, a **joint release** (a popping sound) occasionally may occur. This is not defined as an adjustment any more than it would be if it had occurred during a regular stretch of that joint. However, when performing joint mobilization, it should not be your intent to apply a fast thrust within the realm of joint play for the purpose of creating a joint release.

10.10 Breathing

There is no specific breathing protocol that must be used for joint mobilization. Most typically, the client is asked to breathe out and relax as the mobilization stretch is applied. However, what is most important is that the client should continue to breathe in a comfortable and relaxed manner.

10.11 Repetitions

When performing joint mobilization to the LSp, it is possible to choose to mobilize just one segmental level and then repeat the mobilization at that level a number of times. This is often done in sets of three to five oscillations. However, it is more common to mobilize the entire LSp, one segmental joint level at a time, before repeating the joint mobilization at any one joint level.

Most often, the therapist begins at either the top of the LSp at the T12-L1 joint and works down to the bottom of the LSp or begins at the bottom of the LSp at the L5-S1 joint and works up to the top of the LSp. Regardless of the direc-

Joint Mobilization/Manipulation Grades

Some sources define the term joint mobilization more generically to describe all motions of a joint. One classification of joint **mobilization grading** divides joint motion/mobilization into five grades.

- Grade I: slow, small-amplitude movement performed at the beginning of a joint's range of active/passive motion
- Grade II: slow, large-amplitude movement performed through the joint's active range of motion
- Grade III: slow, large-amplitude movement performed to the limit of the joint's passive range of motion
- Grade IV: slow, small-amplitude movement performed at the limit of a joint's passive range of motion and into resistance (joint play)
- Grade V: fast, small-amplitude movement performed at the limit of a joint's passive range of motion and into resistance (joint play)

In this grading system, Grade II is the active range of motion that a client can create at a joint. Grade III is a typical passive stretch that is performed by a therapist on a client or a passive self-stretch performed by a client (see Chapters 6 to 9 and Chapter 11, available online at thePoint.lww.com). Grade IV is joint mobilization as the term is used in this text. Grade V is a chiropractic/osteopathic high-velocity (fast thrust) manipulation that is not within the scope of practice for most manual therapists.

tion, once the entire LSp has been mobilized (i.e., all of the hypomobile joints of the LSp have been mobilized), this process can now be repeated a second and third time. In other words, instead of performing three to five repetitions at one joint level before moving on, it is more common to perform one joint mobilization repetition for the entire LSp. Then, if desired, a second repetition for the entire LSp and/or even a third repetition for the entire LSp can be done. Most often, two or three repetitions of joint mobilization of the entire LSp are done. After the LSp has been mobilized in this manner, further joint mobilizations can be repeated at the most restricted levels as needed. As with all treatment techniques, the needs of the client and the response of the tissue are the

best factors to use when determining how to apply joint mobilization technique.

10.12 Determining the Need for Joint Mobilization

Determining the need for the stretching techniques presented in Chapters 6 to 9 is accomplished by assessing the low back's gross passive range of motion in each direction. Determining the need for joint mobilization technique is accomplished by assessing the specific joint play range of motion at each segmental joint level. This is done via the assessment technique known as **motion palpation**. Motion palpation assessment is performed in the same manner as joint mobilization treatment is. One bone of the client's joint is stabilized/pinned, and the other bone is moved until tension is reached. The motion palpation assessment is then done by gently introducing a slightly increased motion at that joint level, feeling for the end-feel of motion in joint play.

A healthy joint's end-feel has a springy bounce to it. An unhealthy hypomobile joint has an end-feel that is restricted and feels like you are pushing against a hard block. An unhealthy hypermobile joint is excessive in motion and has a soft doughy/mushy feel to it. If an unhealthy restricted end-feel is found, that joint is in need of mobilization. If a healthy end-feel is present, joint mobilization may be performed at that level to proactively maintain the functional health of the joint. However, if a hypermobile joint is assessed, joint mobilization is contraindicated at that level.

It should be noted that joint mobilization treatment technique is simply an extension of motion palpation assessment technique. They are performed in an identical manner except that motion palpation is done to assess the motion that is present, and joint mobilization is done to maintain or increase that motion. When assessing and treating the client's low back, it is common to do motion palpation at a joint level and, if it is restricted, to simply add a little more force to perform the mobilization. Hence, motion palpation flows into joint mobilization.

10.13 Scope of Practice

Before adding joint mobilization to your practice, it is important to be sure that it is within the scope of practice of your profession. If there is any doubt about the ethical or legal application of joint mobilization within your profession, please check with your local, state, or provincial licensing body; your certifying body; and/or your professional organization.

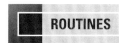

JOINT MOBILIZATION ROUTINES

As with regular and advanced stretching techniques, joint mobilizations can be done in axial cardinal plane ranges of motion. It is also possible to do multiplane joint mobilizations by combining two or more of these cardinal plane motions into an oblique plane motion. Anterior- to posterior-directed joint mobilization of the LSp into flexion usually is not done because it would require contacting and pressing on the client's anterior abdomen, which would be uncomfortable for the client.

Additionally, joint mobilizations can be done for nonaxial ranges of motion, including axial distraction, also known as distraction or traction. Nonaxial compression joint mobilization usually is not performed because it does not stretch any soft tissue and therefore does not increase mobility, which is the reason for performing joint mobilization.

Motion within the spine, both axial and nonaxial, at any particular segmental joint level is determined by the plane of the facets at that level. This must be taken into account when performing joint mobilization. Generally, the planes of the lumbar facets are sagittally oriented; therefore, lumbar motion is most free in the sagittal plane, in other words, flexion and extension. However, the facet plane of the L5-S1 joint is more frontal plane in orientation; therefore, its lateral flexion motions would theoretically be freer. When performing joint mobilization technique, it is important to palpate and feel the facet plane motion at that segmental joint level and work by mobilizing this plane of motion (see Chapter 1 for more information about the facet joint planes and range of motion of the lumbar and thoracic spine).

SECTION 1: SACROILIAC JOINT MOBILIZATION ROUTINES

View the video "Introduction to Joint Mobilization of the Sacroiliac Joint" online on thePoint.lww.com

SIJ mobilization introduces motion into the SIJ. The motion that is introduced can vary depending on which bone is mobilized and in what direction. The treatment hand contact can mobilize the ilium with the sacrum stabilized, or the sacrum can be mobilized with the ilium stabilized. Further, the contact location on the sacrum or ilium can vary, as can the direction of the mobilization force. Because very little musculature crosses directly from one bone of the SIJ to the other, musculature is not the primary target of SIJ mobilization. In all cases, the primary soft tissue target of SIJ mobilization is the ligament complex that connects the two bones.

Following are seven SIJ mobilization routines:

- Routine 10-1—SIJ prone: PSIS compression
- Routine 10-2—SIJ prone: sacrum compression
- Routine 10-3—SIJ side-lying: compression
- Routine 10-4—SIJ supine: compression
- Routine 10-5—SIJ supine: single knee to chest
- Routine 10-6—SIJ supine: horizontal adduction
- Routine 10-7—SIJ side-lying: horizontal adduction

ROUTINE 10-1: SACROILIAC JOINT PRONE: POSTERIOR SUPERIOR ILIAC SPINE COMPRESSION

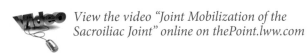 *View the video "Joint Mobilization of the Sacroiliac Joint" online on thePoint.lww.com*

As the name of the routine implies, SIJ prone PSIS compression mobilization is performed with the client lying face down and the contact mobilization force applied to the PSIS of the ilium. The direction of the mobilization force can vary from anteriorly (down toward the table/floor) and superiorly, to anteriorly and laterally, to anteriorly and inferiorly.

The following are the steps to perform prone PSIS compression mobilization of the left SIJ:

- The client is prone, and you are standing at the left side of the table.
- Place your right hand on the client's left PSIS, with the PSIS positioned in the groove between the thenar and hypothenar eminences (the intereminential groove).
- Support your right hand with the thumb web of your left hand.

- The sacrum is stabilized by body weight, so no stabilization contact is needed.
- Gently lean in with body weight, adding compression force to the PSIS anteriorly and superiorly until you reach tissue tension at the end of passive range of motion.
- Now gently stretch the SIJ into its joint play by leaning in further with body weight, adding a small increased compression force on the PSIS. This will involve a very small excursion of anterior tilt of the ilium on that side (Fig. 10-9A).
- Hold for only a fraction of a second and then release.
- This joint mobilization of the SIJ may then be repeated for a total of three to five times.
- Now repeat the mobilization routine, this time leaning in on the PSIS anteriorly and laterally, mobilizing the ilium by gapping it laterally away from the sacrum (Fig. 10-9B). Repeat for a total of three to five times. *Note:* This mobilization motion causes internal (medial) rotation of the ilium on that side and results in gapping of the posterior aspect of the SIJ.

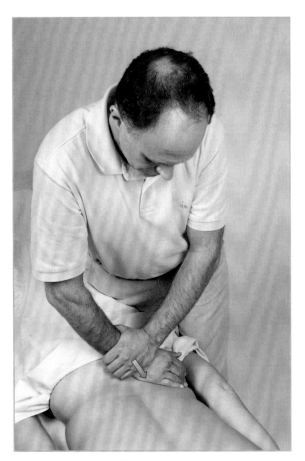

Figure 10-9A

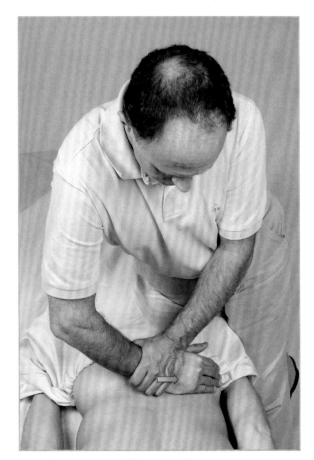

Figure 10-9B

■ If desired, the routine can be repeated again, this time pressing anteriorly and inferiorly, mobilizing the ilium toward posterior tilt. If this orientation of pressure is used, it is helpful to first place a pillow under the client's abdomen. It is also easier for the therapist to stand adjacent to the client's upper back facing toward the client's feet, and to use the left hand as the contact hand (Fig. 10-9C).

■ Repeat for the other side SIJ, switching contact and support hands and which side of the table you are standing on.

■ Repeat these routines as needed with concentration at the SIJ motions that are restricted.

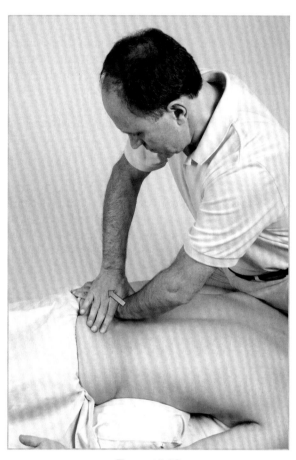

Figure 10-9C

| 10.7 | **THERAPIST TIP** |

Support Hand

Most joint mobilizations in the body involve the use of a treatment hand and a stabilization hand. However, joint mobilizations of the LSp and pelvis often do not require a stabilization hand because the client's body weight does a good job of stabilizing the other bone of the joint. When this is the case, this frees up the therapist's other hand to act as a **support hand** to brace/support the treatment hand. Given how much force is sometimes needed to mobilize a lumbar or SIJ, having the help of a support hand is good body mechanics.

| 10.2 | **PRACTICAL APPLICATION** |

Prone Posterior Superior Iliac Spine Compression with Thigh Extension

Prone PSIS compression of the SIJ into anterior tilt can be augmented with passive thigh extension. Place one hand on the PSIS (positioned in the intereminential groove between your thenar and hypothenar eminences) and your other hand on the client's anterior distal thigh. Now, as you lean in with your body weight, mobilizing the PSIS anteriorly and superiorly toward anterior tilt, augment this motion of the ilium by simultaneously extending the client's thigh. Once tissue tension has been reached, lean in further with body weight, mobilizing the ilium into anterior tilt. Via femoropelvic rhythm, thigh extension couples with anterior tilt of the ilium, adding to the mobilization force. This technique is powerful and should be performed with caution.

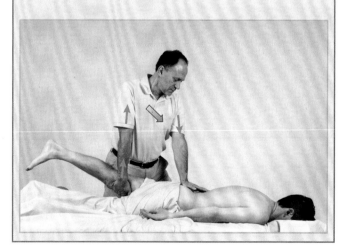

ROUTINE 10-2: SACROILIAC JOINT PRONE: SACRUM COMPRESSION

 View the video "Joint Mobilization of the Sacroiliac Joint" online on thePoint.lww.com

This routine is carried out similarly to the SIJ prone PSIS compression, except that the sacrum is contacted and mobilized instead of the PSIS of the ilium. The contact on the sacrum can be superior at its base or inferior at its apex. As with the PSIS compression, the direction of mobilization force can vary. If the base of the sacrum is contacted, it can be contacted at its midline and mobilized anteriorly and superiorly, or it can be contacted toward one side and mobilized anteriorly, superiorly, and laterally to that side. If the apex of the sacrum is contacted, it is mobilized anteriorly and inferiorly.

The following are the steps to perform prone sacrum compression mobilization of the SIJ:

- The client is prone, and you are standing at the left side of the table.
- Place the ulnar side of your left hand on the midline of the client's sacral base.
- Your right hand is placed under, on the anterior surface of the client's left thigh (as described in Practical Application 10.2).
- Gently lean in with body weight as you pull up on the client's thigh, adding compression force to the sacral base anteriorly and superiorly until you reach tissue tension at the end of passive range of motion.
- Now gently stretch the SIJ into its joint play by leaning in further with body weight, adding a small increased compression force on the sacrum. This will involve a very small excursion of anterior tilt (nutation) of the sacrum on that side (Fig. 10-10A).

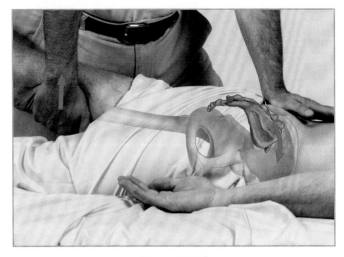

Figure 10-10A

- Hold for only a fraction of a second and then release.
- This joint mobilization of the SIJ may then be repeated for a total of two to three times.

- Alternately, one side of the sacral base can be contacted instead. If this is done, place the ulnar side of your right hand on the left side of the client's sacral base (immediately medial to the left PSIS).
- Support your right hand with the thumb web of your left hand.
- The ilium is stabilized by body weight, so no stabilization hand is needed.
- Gently lean in with body weight, adding compression force to the left side of the sacral base anteriorly, superiorly, and laterally until you reach tissue tension at the end of passive range of motion.
- Now gently stretch the SIJ into its joint play by leaning in further with body weight, adding a small increased compression force on the sacrum. This will involve a very small excursion of anterior tilt (nutation) of the sacrum on that side.
- This would then be repeated for the other (right) side of the sacral base.
- Now repeat the mobilization routine, this time, pressing anteriorly and inferiorly on the middle of the sacral apex, mobilizing the sacrum toward posterior tilt (counternutation). If this orientation of pressure is used, it is helpful to first place a pillow under the client's abdomen. It is also easier for the therapist to change orientation to face the client's feet and use the left hand as the contact hand (Fig. 10-10B).

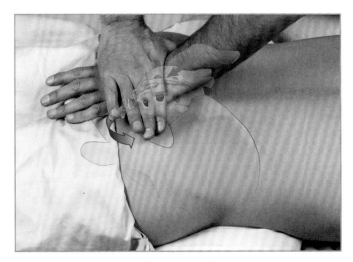

Figure 10-10B

- Repeat for the other side SIJ, switching contact and support hands and which side of the table you are standing on.
- Repeat these routines as needed with concentration at the SIJ motions that are restricted.

 When contacting the sacral apex, be sure not to contact the client too inferiorly. If pressure is placed on the coccyx instead of the sacrum, a sprain of the sacrococcygeal ligament or fracture of the coccyx could occur.

ROUTINE 10-3: SACROILIAC JOINT SIDE-LYING: COMPRESSION

Similar to prone compression, the SIJ can be mobilized with the client side-lying with pressure placed on the client's iliac crest. Although this pressure will transmit through to both SIJs, the upper SIJ (the one away from the table) is primarily mobilized. For this reason, the routine is usually repeated with the client lying on the other side.

The following are the steps to perform side-lying compression mobilization of the SIJ:

- The client is side-lying on the right side, and you are standing at the side of the table, behind the client.
- Place your left hand on the client's iliac crest.
- Support your left hand with the thumb web of your right hand.
- The sacrum is stabilized by body weight, so no stabilization hand is needed.
- Gently lean in with body weight, adding compression force to the iliac crest directly medially (down toward the table/floor) until you reach tissue tension at the end of passive range of motion.
- Now gently stretch the SIJ into its joint play by leaning in further with body weight, adding a small increased compression force on the iliac crest (Fig. 10-11A). *Note*: This mobilization motion causes internal rotation of the ilium on that side and results in gapping of the posterior aspect of the SIJ.

- Hold for only a fraction of a second and then release.
- This joint mobilization of the SIJ may then be repeated for a total of three to five times.
- Now repeat the mobilization routine, this time with the client lying on the other (left) side (Fig. 10-11B). Repeat for a total of two to three times.
- Repeat these routines as needed with concentration at the SIJ(s) that is/are restricted.

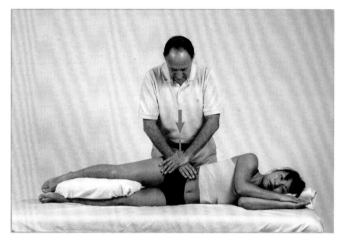

Figure 10-11B

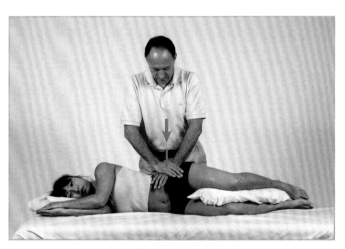

Figure 10-11A

ROUTINE 10-4: SACROILIAC JOINT SUPINE: COMPRESSION

Similar to prone and side-lying compressions, the SIJ can be mobilized with the client lying supine. In this position, pressure is placed bilaterally on the client's anterior superior iliac spines (ASISs), so both SIJs are mobilized at the same time.

The following are the steps to perform supine compression mobilization of the SIJ:

- The client is supine, and you are standing at either side of the table.
- Cross your arms, placing one hand on the client's right ASIS and your other hand on the client's left ASIS.
- The sacrum is stabilized from moving to either side by the pressure of your treatment hand on the other side ASIS.
- Gently lean in with body weight, adding compression force to the ASISs posteriorly (down toward the table/floor) and slightly laterally until you reach tissue tension at the end of passive range of motion.
- Now gently stretch the SIJs into their joint play by leaning in further with body weight, adding a small increased force on the ASISs (Fig. 10-12). *Note:* This mobilization motion causes external rotation of the ilium on each side and results in gapping of the anterior aspect of the SIJs.
- Hold for only a fraction of a second and then release.
- This joint mobilization of the SIJs may then be repeated for a total of three to five times.
- Repeat this routines as needed.

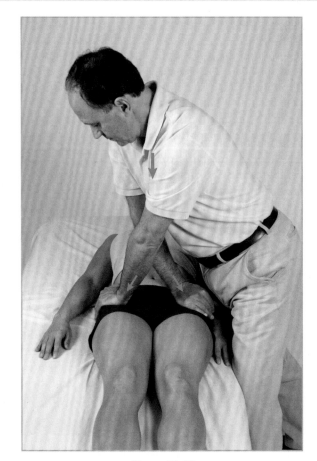

Figure 10-12

ROUTINE 10-5: SACROILIAC JOINT SUPINE: SINGLE KNEE TO CHEST

The SIJ can also be mobilized with the client supine by flexing the client's thigh and bringing the knee up to his chest. Via femoropelvic rhythm, thigh flexion couples with posterior tilt of the ilium on that side, so bringing the knee to the chest posteriorly tilts the same-side (ipsilateral) ilium. Because the pelvis remains on the table, the other (contralateral) ilium remains stable. When the ipsilateral ilium moves into the posterior tilt and the contralateral ilium remains stable, motion is introduced into the SIJs. This motion will be introduced first into the ipsilateral SIJ. As the ipsilateral ilium continues to posteriorly tilt and reaches the end range of its motion, the sacrum will move with it, and motion will then be introduced into the contralateral SIJ. Therefore, supine single knee to chest routine primarily mobilizes the same-side SIJ but can also mobilize the SIJ on the other side of the body. It is usual to perform this mobilization bilaterally to optimally mobilize both SIJs.

The following are the steps to perform supine single knee to chest mobilization of the right SIJ:

- The client is supine, and you are standing at the right side of the table.
- Flex the client's right hip and knee joints. Pressing on the posterior surface of the distal thigh, bring the client's knee/thigh toward his chest.
- For maximal stabilization of the sacrum, place your right knee on the anterior surface of the client's left thigh. Stabilizing his left thigh stabilizes his left ilium, which helps to stabilize his sacrum.
- Gently lean in with body weight, pressing the right thigh into flexion toward his chest until you reach tissue tension at the end of passive range of motion.
- Now gently stretch the right SIJ into its joint play by leaning in further with body weight, adding a small increased force on the posterior thigh (Fig. 10-13A). This will involve a very small excursion of posterior tilt of the ilium on that side.

- Hold for only a fraction of a second and then release.
- This joint mobilization of the SIJ may then be repeated for a total of three to five times.

- Repeat for the other side SIJ, switching which side of the table you are standing on (Fig. 10-13B).
- Repeat these routines as needed.

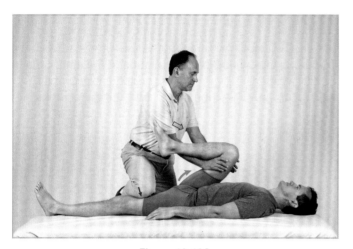

Figure 10-13A

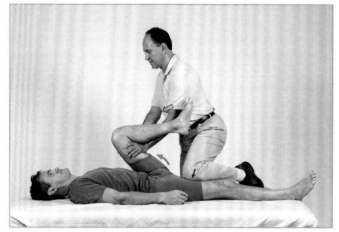

Figure 10-13B

10.3 PRACTICAL APPLICATION

Place Client's Foot on Your Clavicle and Watch the Orientation of the Stretch

An excellent alternative position for the therapist to perform supine single knee to chest mobilization is to place the client's foot on your clavicle. Body mechanics wise, this allows you to use your core to lean in and press the client's thigh into flexion against the chest. However, this position should not be used if the client's knee is unhealthy. To further improve body mechanics, position yourself on the table so that your core is in line with the client's lower extremity (**Fig. A**). Of course, do not climb onto the table if there is any doubt as to the table's ability to support both your weight and that of the client.

It is also important to pay attention to the orientation of the stretching force that you apply to the client's thigh. If you are not stabilizing the client's opposite-side

thigh with your knee, and you press horizontally (parallel with the table) in the cephalad (cranial) direction instead of down toward his chest, the client's pelvis will lift from the table and the mobilization to the SIJ will be lost because the opposite-side ilium and the sacrum will no longer be stabilized (**Fig. B**). It is important to also not compress the client's thigh too much into his chest because the client might experience discomfort or pain in the anterior hip joint region (groin). Optimal is to press as little into his chest as possible (i.e., as much horizontally parallel to the table in the cephalad/cranial direction as possible) and still keep his pelvis down on the table (see Fig. A). The balance between these two directions will vary from client to client.

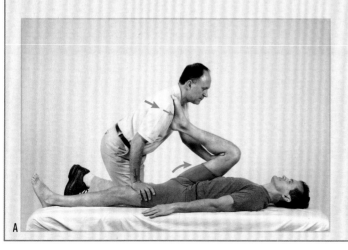

A

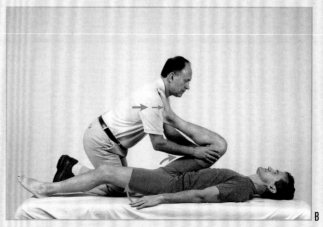

B

ROUTINE 10-6: SACROILIAC JOINT SUPINE: HORIZONTAL ADDUCTION

Similar to the single knee to chest mobilization, the SIJ can be mobilized by bringing the client's thigh into flexion and then across his body into horizontal adduction. Horizontal adduction adds a component of internal rotation of the ilium (to the posterior tilt of the ilium created by the thigh flexion), gapping the posterior aspect of the SIJ. Thus far, this routine is identical to the horizontal adduction stretch routine shown in Chapter 6 (see Routine 6-10, stretch #1), which stretches the lateral rotation musculature of the posterior buttock (and also stretches/mobilizes the SIJ). To augment the SIJ mobilization for this routine, you can use your hand to contact and add mobilization force to the PSIS of the ilium.

The following are the steps to perform supine horizontal adduction mobilization of the left SIJ:

- The client is supine, and you are standing at the (opposite) right side of the table.
- Flex the client's left hip and knee joints and then bring the client's thigh into horizontal adduction across his body by trapping the client's knee between your left arm and trunk.
- Curl the finger pads of your right hand around the medial side of the client's left PSIS.
- The sacrum is stabilized by body weight, so no stabilization hand is needed.
- Gently lean in with body weight, pressing the client's left thigh into horizontal adduction across his chest (and somewhat down into his chest to prevent the pelvis from lifting from the table) until you reach tissue tension at the end of passive range of motion.

- Now gently stretch the left SIJ into its joint play by leaning in further with body weight, adding a small increased force on the posterior thigh, while you simultaneously add a mobilization force to the PSIS with the finger pads of your right hand, gapping it away from the sacrum (Fig. 10-14A). *Note*: This mobilization motion causes posterior tilt of the ilium; it also causes internal rotation of the ilium on that side, resulting in gapping of the posterior aspect of the SIJ.
- Hold for only a fraction of a second and then release.

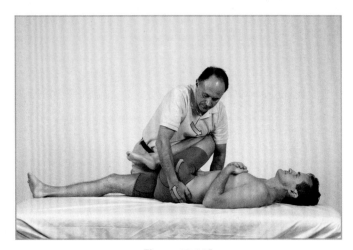

Figure 10-14A

- If the client experiences discomfort/pain at the anterior hip joint region, your hands can be used to traction the anterior proximal thigh away from the pelvis as the mobilization is performed (Fig. 10-14B). This often relieves the client's discomfort/pain. However, using the right hand to help traction the thigh means that it cannot be used to contact the PSIS and augment the mobilization. If the thigh can be tractioned with just the left hand, then the right hand can maintain the joint mobilization force on the PSIS.

- This joint mobilization of the SIJ may then be repeated for a total of three to five times.
- Repeat for the other side SIJ, switching which side of the table you are standing on (Fig. 10-14C).
- Repeat these routines as needed.

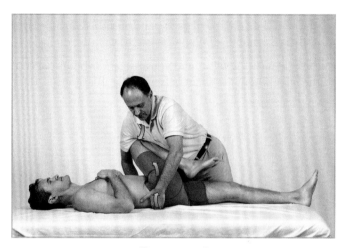

Figure 10-14C

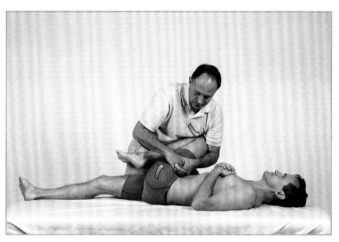

Figure 10-14B

| 10.4 | PRACTICAL APPLICATION |

Alternative Therapist Position

An alternative position for the therapist is to stand on the same side of the table as the thigh that is being horizontally adducted and pushing the thigh from that side (see accompanying figure). This position is easier to learn at first but has two disadvantages. It does not easily allow for a hand to be used to contact the PSIS to add to the mobilization force on the ilium. Also, if the client experiences discomfort/pain at the anterior hip region (see Practical Application Box 6.6), it does not as easily allow for a hand to be used to traction the anterior proximal thigh to relieve the discomfort/pain.

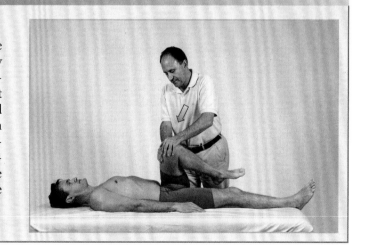

ROUTINE 10-7: SACROILIAC JOINT SIDE-LYING: HORIZONTAL ADDUCTION

Side-lying horizontal adduction is the most powerful mobilization of the SIJ. The therapist uses core body weight to bring the thigh into horizontal adduction while adding to the mobilization force by contacting the PSIS of the ilium. This gaps the SIJ by internally rotating the ilium.

The following are the steps to perform side-lying horizontal adduction mobilization of the left SIJ:

- The client is side-lying, and you are standing at the side of the table where the client is facing (Fig. 10-15A).

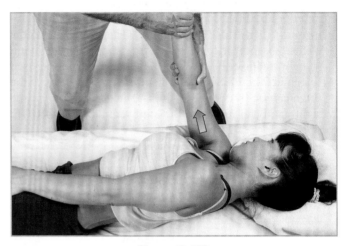

Figure 10-15B

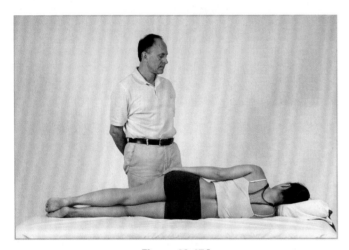

Figure 10-15A

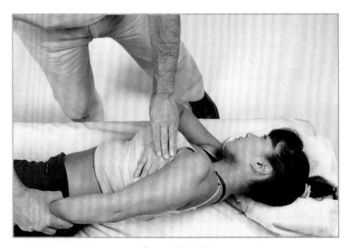

Figure 10-15C

10.8 THERAPIST TIP

How Close to the Side of the Table Do You Position the Client?

Knowing exactly how close to the side of the table the client should lie for side-lying mobilization comes with experience. Exactly where the client should be positioned will vary based on the size of the client and his or her flexibility. If the client is too far from the side, his or her thigh will hit the table as you horizontally adduct it; if the client is too close, you might not be able to control the client's body weight when performing the mobilization and the client might fall to the floor. If you start the procedure and realize that the client is too far or too close to the side, start over and reposition the client appropriately.

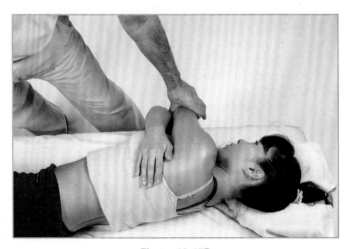

Figure 10-15D

- Bring the client onto the back of her right shoulder by gently pulling on the right arm (Fig. 10-15B).
  - Now place her right hand on the side of the upper trunk (Fig. 10-15C).
  - Let the client's other hand drape down off the side of the table (Fig. 10-15D).

■ Rotate the client's pelvis so that it is stacked, meaning that the PSISs are oriented in a vertical line (Fig. 10-15E). *Note*: Sometimes, especially for flexible clients, it is helpful to have the start position of the client's pelvis such that it is unstacked with the upper PSIS (the one away from the table) rotated back away from you. This way, when you perform the mobilization, the client ends up in a stacked position of the pelvis.

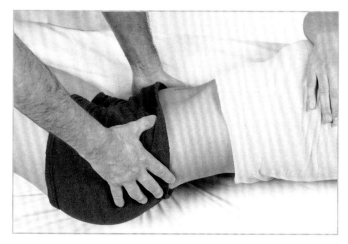

Figure 10-15E

■ Stabilize the client's upper body by placing your left hand on the client's right hand and pushing superiorly on her hand/trunk (Fig. 10-15F).

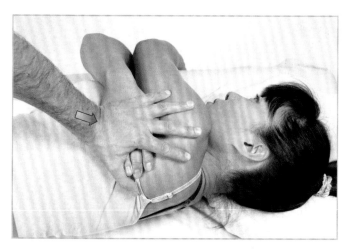

Figure 10-15F

■ Locate the client's left PSIS and place your finger pads on the medial side of it over the left SIJ (Fig. 10-15G).
■ Flex the client's left hip and knee joints using your right thigh until tension is felt with the finger pads of your right hand at the client's left SIJ (Fig. 10-15H).

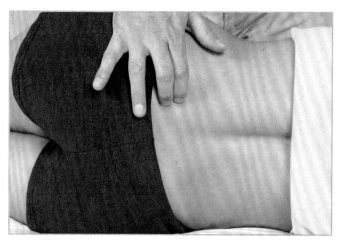

Figure 10-15G

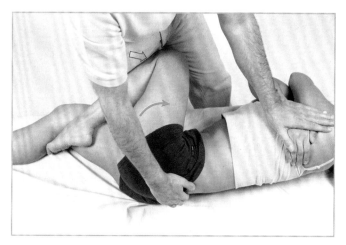

Figure 10-15H

■ Now climb up onto the anterolateral surface of the client's left thigh with the anterolateral surface of your right thigh (Fig. 10-15I).
  ■ This will require you to lift your right foot from the floor.
  ■ This step is often called **"pocket to pocket"** because you can think of bringing your pocket to the client's pocket (pockets are located anterolateral on each thigh).
  ■ It is important to maintain tension at the client's left SIJ by maintaining her hip joint flexion. This is accomplished by keeping friction against her leg and thigh as you climb up, bringing pocket to pocket.
  ■ *Note*: This is the most challenging step of this mobilization technique. Therefore, when first learning this protocol, it might be easier to perform the pocket to pocket step by doing it in three stages. Instead of trying to reach all the way to the client's "pocket" in one maneuver, achieve that position in multiple, perhaps three, steps. The first time, move up her thigh approximately ⅓ of the way and then bring your right foot back down to the floor until you are comfortably bal-

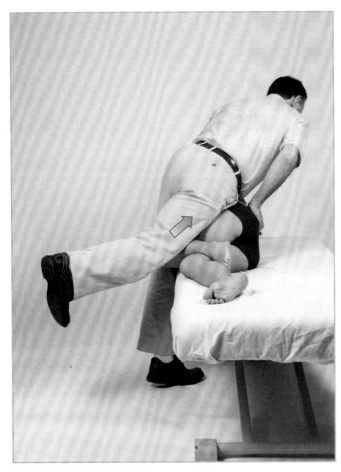

Figure 10-15I

anced and bearing weight on it. Repeat this again, moving farther up the client's thigh, and then return your right foot to the floor. Then perform it one more time, this time reaching all the way to the client's pocket.

■ Now reorient your right hand so that the thenar eminence is on the medial side of the client's PSIS (Fig. 10-15J).

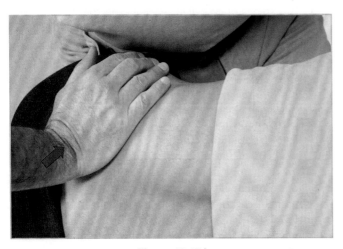

Figure 10-15J

■ Slowly bring your body weight down on the client's left thigh, horizontally adducting it and stretching the client's SIJ, maintaining contact and pressure as you lower your right foot back to the floor and until you are comfortably able to balance and bear weight on your right foot (Fig. 10-15K).

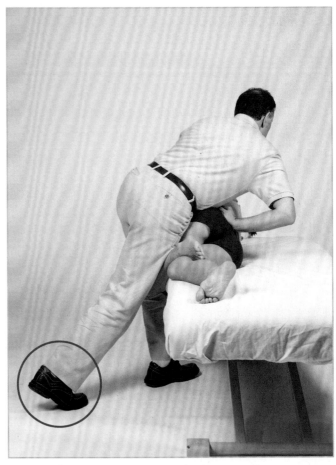

Figure 10-15K

■ It is important to maintain the tension at the left SIJ by maintaining the flexion of the client's thigh.

■ This motion can be facilitated by pressing on the medial side of the client's PSIS with your right hand.

■ Once you have completed bringing the client into this position, your sternum (i.e., the body weight of your upper trunk) should be on the posterior side of the client (Fig. 10-15L).

■ You should also have your body stable against the side of the table so that the client cannot fall off the table.

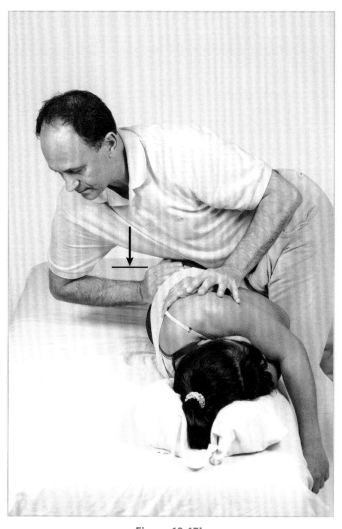

Figure 10-15L

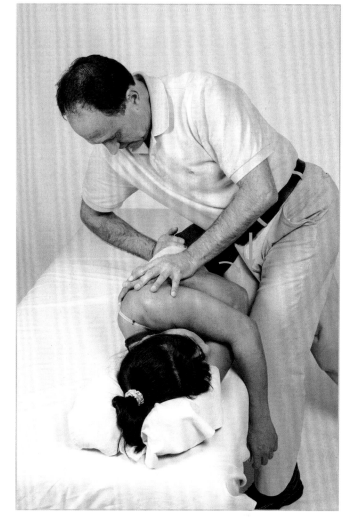

Figure 10-15M

- The opposite side ilium and sacrum are stabilized by body weight against the table, so no stabilization hand is needed for this purpose.
- Gently drop down against the client's left thigh with your right thigh and body weight, pressing the client's left thigh further into horizontal adduction until you reach tissue tension at the end of passive range of motion (Fig. 10-15M).
  - It is important that you leave enough room between your thigh and the table for the client's left thigh to further horizontally adduct down toward the floor.
- Now gently stretch the left SIJ into its joint play by leaning in further with body weight, adding a small increased force on the thigh, while you simultaneously add a mobilization force to the left PSIS with the thenar eminence of your right hand, gapping it away from the sacrum (Fig. 10-15N).
  - *Note*: Flexion of the thigh causes posterior tilt of the ilium; horizontal adduction causes internal rotation of the ilium on that side, causing gapping of the posterior aspect of the SIJ.

- Hold for only a fraction of a second and then release.
- This joint mobilization of the SIJ may then be repeated for a total of three to five times.
- Repeat for the other side SIJ, switching contact and stabilization hands and which side of the table you are standing on (Fig. 10-15O).
- Repeat these routines as needed.

Note: An alternative position for the client's left hand is to place it on her right hand as seen in Figure 10-15P instead of draping it over the side of the table as seen in Figure 10-15D. The advantage of this positioning is that it is easier to stabilize the client's upper body. The disadvantage is that it is easier to torque the client's spine if you press posteriorly on her hands/trunk.

 If you use this alternative hand positioning, be sure to not torque the client's spine. Torqueing the LSp can cause injury to the client.

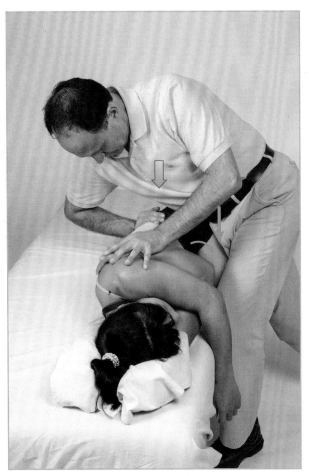

Figure 10-15N

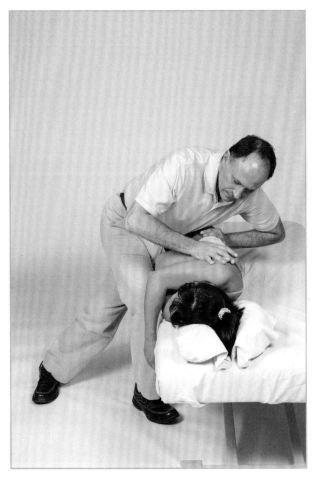

Figure 10-15O

Caution must be exercised with the side-lying horizontal adduction mobilization routine for the SIJ (and LSp; see Practical Application Box 10.6) because it is so powerful.

- *Side-lying horizontal adductions mobilization should not be performed if the client has a space-occupying lesion of the LSp (e.g., pathologic lumbar disc or bone spur).*
- *As with all joint mobilizations, never add a fast thrust when applying the stretch mobilization.*
- *It is also important to make sure that the client's spine is torqued/twisted as little as possible. This is accomplished by making sure that the stabilization hand on the upper trunk is pushing superiorly toward the client's head and not posteriorly. This is especially important if the alternative hand position is used (see Fig. 10-15P).*
- *If the apex of the sacrum is contacted (see Practical Application Box 10.5), be sure not to contact the client too inferiorly. If pressure is placed on the coccyx instead of the sacrum, a sprain of the sacrococcygeal ligament or fracture of the coccyx could occur.*
- *This is also the most challenging mobilization routine to learn and become proficient with. It is strongly recommended that you view the video on the DVD that accompanies this book, and if possible, attend an in-person low back joint mobilization workshop. It is also recommended that you practice this routine many times before employing it with clients.*

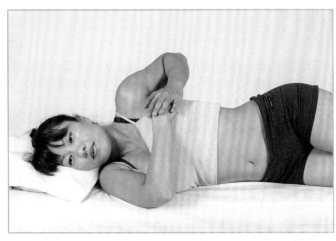

Figure 10-15P

10.5 PRACTICAL APPLICATION

Variations of the Sacroiliac Joint Side-Lying Horizontal Adduction Sacroiliac Joint Mobilization

There are variations on how the side-lying mobilization of the SIJ with horizontal adduction of the client's thigh can be performed.

With the PSIS contact, instead of pressing the client's PSIS directly anteriorly, which maximizes the internal rotation of the ilium and gaps the posterior aspect of the joint, the thenar eminence contact on the PSIS can press anteriorly and inferiorly to increase the posterior tilt motion of the ilium (**Fig. A**). It is also possible to press anteriorly and superiorly on the PSIS to add anterior tilt to the gapping of the SIJ (**Fig. B**). However, if this is done, it is important to lessen the flexion of the client's thigh (the reason for the thigh flexion was to cause posterior tilt of the ilium).

It is also possible to contact the sacrum instead of the PSIS with the thenar eminence of the contact hand. If this is done, the direction of the mobilization force can vary depending on what aspect of the sacrum is contacted. If the sacral base is contacted, the thenar eminence of the contact hand should be placed on the side of the base that is away from the table to mobilize the SIJ that is on that side of the client's body (the one that is away from the table) (**Fig. C**). The direction of the mobilization stretch is directed anteriorly, superiorly, and laterally (this is similar to the prone sacral mobilization seen in Fig. 10-10A in Routine 10-2). This mobilization will cause anterior tilt (nutation) of the sacrum as well as a nonaxial glide of the sacrum relative to the ilium. If the sacral apex is contacted, the direction of the mobilization stretch would be primarily anterior and inferior to create posterior tilt (counternutation) of the sacrum relative to the ilium (**Fig. D**) (this is similar to the prone sacral mobilization seen in Fig. 10-10B in Routine 10-2).

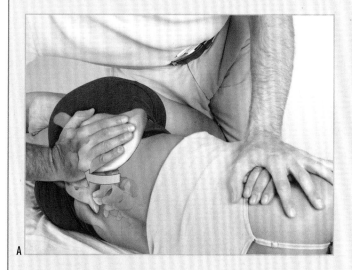
A

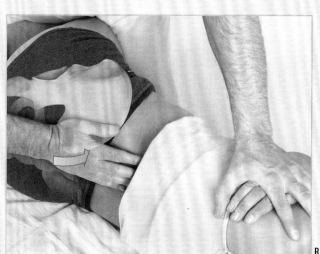
B

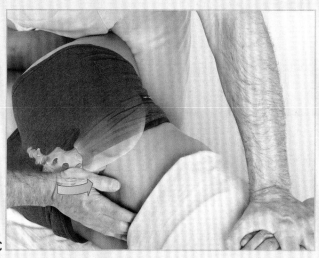
C

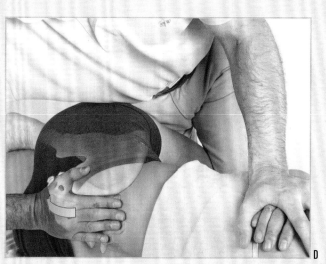
D

10.6   **PRACTICAL APPLICATION**

Transitioning Side-Lying Horizontal Adduction Mobilization from the Sacroiliac Joint to the Lumbar Spinal Joints

The side-lying horizontal adduction joint mobilization for the SIJ can be easily transitioned to be a mobilization of the LSp instead. Only two modifications are needed.

The first modification is that the client's thigh needs to be brought into more flexion so that tension is created in the LSp **(Fig. A)**; joint mobilization can only be done if the joint is first brought to tension. Via femoropelvic rhythm, thigh flexion causes posterior tilt of the ilium on that side, causing tension at the SIJ on that side. Increasing thigh flexion causes so much tension at the SIJ that the sacrum must now move (into posterior tilt/counternutation) with the ilium. As the sacrum moves, tension is created at the lumbosacral (L5-S1) joint. If the thigh is brought further into flexion, this tension moves up the LSp, allowing for effective joint mobilization at these lumbar joints.

The second modification is the placement of the contact treatment hand. Instead of contacting the PSIS of the ilium, the LSp must be contacted. Rotation mobilization is performed by contacting the vertebral SP on the side that is closer to the table. In other words, if the client is lying on the right side, the right side of the SP is contacted; the mobilization stretch force is added up against the SP, rotating the SP toward the left, resulting in right rotation of the vertebra (rotation is named for the direction that the anterior surface of the body orients) **(Fig. B)**. For lateral flexion mobilization, contact the SP/lamina on the side that is away from the table. In other words, when the client is lying on the right, the mobilization force is added against the left side SP/lamina and is directed down toward the table (anteriorly and medially) **(Fig. C)**.

As with side-lying SIJ horizontal adduction, side-lying mobilization for the LSp should then be performed for the other side, switching contact and support hands and which side of the table you are standing on.

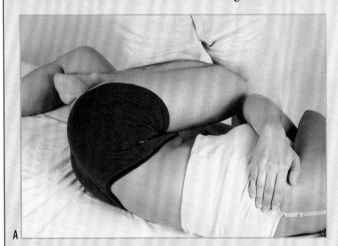

A

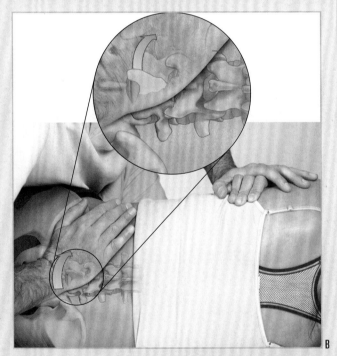

B

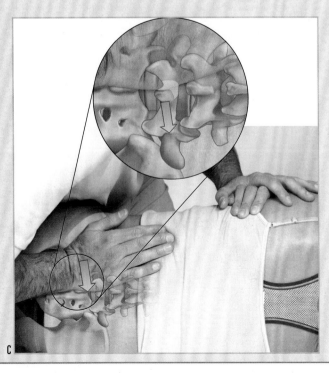

C

SECTION 2: LUMBAR SPINE JOINT MOBILIZATION ROUTINES

LSp mobilization introduces motion into the lumbar vertebrae. The motion that is introduced can vary depending on which lumbar vertebra is mobilized and in what direction. The most common contact for the mobilization hand is the SP because that is the easiest vertebral landmark to locate and access. However, contact against the lamina or mammillary/transverse processes is also sometimes done. Because of the lordotic curve of the LSp, it can sometimes be challenging to contact vertebral landmarks for LSp mobilization. The challenge is increased if the client has very well developed paraspinal musculature.

Depending on the position of the client, the use of a stabilization hand for LSp mobilization may or may not be necessary. Often, the client's body weight provides adequate stabilization. The goal of LSp mobilization is to stretch/mobilize the facet joint capsules, ligaments, and intrinsic muscles of the region.

Notes:

1. Seated mobilization routine was shown in the "Overview of Technique" section and Therapist Tip Box 10.2 that followed immediately thereafter. For this mobilization, please see Figures 10-2 and 10-3 and Therapist Tip Box 10.2.

2. Further, the most powerful mobilization for the LSp is side-lying horizontal adduction, which is a variant of the side-lying horizontal adduction mobilization for the SIJ (Routine 10-7), and transitioning this routine from the SIJ to the LSp was addressed in Practical Application Box 10.6. Please refer to Routine 10-7 and Practical Application Box 10.6 for the side-lying horizontal adduction LSp mobilization routine.

Seven LSp mobilization routines are presented in this chapter.

- Routine 10-8—LSp prone: extension compression
- Routine 10-9—LSp prone: lateral flexion and rotation
- Routine 10-10—LSp prone: flexion distraction
- Routine 10-11—LSp seated: mobilizations
- Routine 10-12—LSp side-lying: horizontal adduction
- Routine 10-13—LSp supine: towel traction/distraction
- Routine 10-14—LSp supine: manual traction/distraction

As a rule, lumbar joint mobilizations should not be done at the level of or nearby the level of segmental joints that have a space-occupying lesion, such as a pathologic disc or bone spur. Further, compression mobilizations are contraindicated in clients who have spondylolisthesis or osteoporosis. If there is any doubt as to the safety of lumbar joint mobilization, consult first with the client's chiropractic or medical physician. Joint mobilizations should never involve any type of fast thrust.

ROUTINE 10-8: LUMBAR SPINE PRONE: EXTENSION COMPRESSION

As with prone SIJ compression mobilization, prone compression mobilization of the LSp can also be performed. The direction of the mobilization force is posterior to anterior (down toward the table/floor) and mobilizes the lumbar vertebra(e) into extension.

The following are the steps to perform prone extension compression mobilization of the LSp:

- The client is prone, and you are standing at the left side of the table.
- Place your right hand on the client's LSp, with the SP of the vertebra you are mobilizing positioned in the intereminential groove of the hand.
- Support your right hand with the thumb web of your left hand. *Note*: The "support" left hand does not just support the contact hand. It can also function to add to the force of the mobilization by adding downward pressure through the contact hand into the client.
- Body weight stabilizes adjacent vertebrae, so no stabilization hand is needed.
- Gently lean in with body weight, adding compression force anteriorly until you reach tissue tension at the end of passive range of motion.

- Now gently stretch the lumbar vertebra into its joint play by leaning in further with body weight, adding a small increased compression force on the SP. This will involve a very small excursion of extension of that vertebra relative to the adjacent vertebrae (Fig. 10-16).

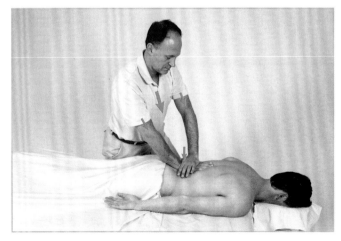

Figure 10-16

- Hold for only a fraction of a second and then release.
- This lumbar vertebral joint mobilization may then be repeated for a total of three to five times.
- Once the joint mobilization has been performed at one level, apply it at all the other levels of the LSp so that all LSp joints are mobilized into extension.
- Repeat these routines as needed with concentration at the lumbar vertebrae that are restricted.
- *Note*: This mobilization technique can be performed with the therapist standing on either side of the table. If you choose to stand at the other (right) side of the table, switch treatment and support hands.

10.7 PRACTICAL APPLICATION

Regaining the Lumbar Lordotic Curve

Prone compression of the LSp is indicated and beneficial to help regain the proper lumbar lordotic curve in clients who have a hypolordotic lumbar curve or a kyphotic (reverse) lumbar curve. Loss of the healthy normal lordosis often occurs in clients who stand or sit in excessive posterior pelvic tilt, causing the LSp to be kyphotic.

10.9 THERAPIST TIP

Lumbar Spine Prone Extension Compression

When performing prone extension compression mobilization to the LSp, the direction of the mobilization force does not have to be directly posterior to anterior. Depending on the degree of the client's lumbar lordotic curve and the level of the LSp that you are mobilizing, it can be beneficial to add a superior or inferior component to the mobilization stretch. In the upper LSp, it is usually preferable to press anteriorly and slightly superiorly to better match the orientation of the facets due to the lumbar curve at that level (**Fig. A**). In the lower LSp, it is usually preferable to press anteriorly and slightly inferiorly to better match the orientation of the facets due to the lumbar curve at that level (**Fig. B**). At the mid-LSp, pressure should usually be applied directly anteriorly because it is the middle of the lumbar curve.

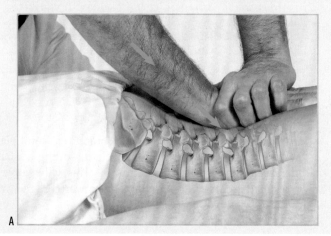

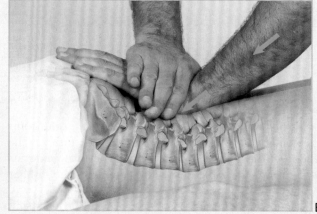

ROUTINE 10-9: LUMBAR SPINE PRONE: LATERAL FLEXION AND ROTATION

Routine 10-8 demonstrated posterior to anterior lumbar compression mobilization to create extension. An effective variation on this mobilization routine is to alter the vertebral contact and direction of the stretch mobilization force to introduce lateral flexion and/or rotation of the vertebra instead of extension.

Joint mobilization into lateral flexion stretches opposite-sided lateral flexor musculature, especially the smaller, deeper intrinsic muscles of the joint, and the ligamentous and joint capsular tissue on the other side of the joint being mobilized. Joint mobilization into rotation to one side stretches musculature that causes rotation to the other side as well as ligamentous and joint capsular tissue.

The following are the steps to perform prone (left) lateral flexion and (right) rotation mobilizations to the left side of the client's LSp:

- The client is prone, and you are standing at the left side of the table.
- For lateral flexion mobilization, place the ulnar side of your right hand on the client's LSp against the left side of the SP/lamina of the vertebrae you are mobilizing; this contact can be localized and made more specific by contacting and placing your pressure through the pisiform of your contact hand. Your pressure will be directed anteriorly toward the table/floor as well as laterally toward the other (right) side of the client's body (Fig. 10-17A). This will create left lateral flexion mobilization of the LSp.

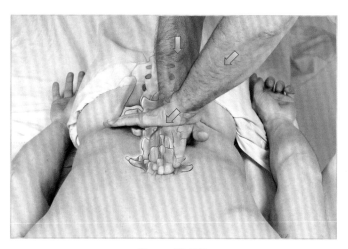

Figure 10-17A

- For rotation mobilization, place the ulnar side (or more specific contact of the pisiform) of your right hand on the client's LSp directly lateral to (to the left side of) the SP over the mammillary and transverse processes of the vertebrae you are mobilizing. Your pressure will be directly anterior (toward the table/floor) (Fig. 10-17B). This will create right rotation mobilization of the LSp (the SPs will rotate to the left, but the anterior bodies, for which rotation is named, will rotate to the right).

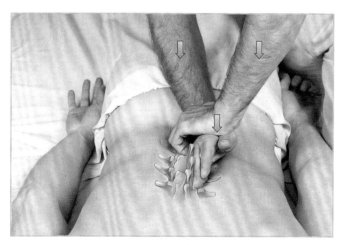

Figure 10-17B

- *Note:* For both mobilizations, because your hand contact is a fairly large and broad, it is usually not possible to isolate just one segmental vertebral level. Instead, two or three vertebrae are mobilized together.
- Support your right contact hand with the thumb web of your left hand.
- Body weight stabilizes adjacent vertebrae, so no stabilization hand is needed.
- Gently lean in with body weight, adding compression force in the appropriate direction until you reach tissue tension at the end of passive range of motion.
- Now gently stretch the lumbar vertebra into its joint play by leaning in further with body weight, adding a small increased compression force on the vertebrae.
- Hold for only a fraction of a second and then release.
- This lumbar vertebral joint mobilization may then be repeated for a total of three to five times.
- Once the joint mobilization has been performed at one level, apply it at all the other levels of the LSp so that all LSp joints are mobilized.
- Repeat for the other side, switching contact and support hands and which side of the table you are standing on.

■ Figure 10-18A illustrates (right) lateral flexion mobilization for the right side of the body. Figure 10-18B demonstrates the ulnar side contact for (left) rotation mobilization applied to the right side of the body.

■ Repeat these routines as needed with concentration at the lumbar vertebrae that are restricted.

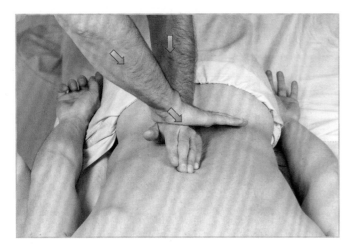

Figure 10-18A

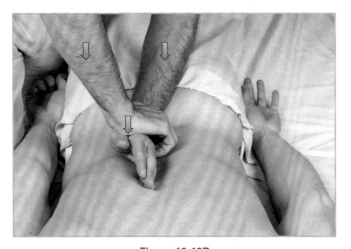

Figure 10-18B

Multiplane Prone Joint Mobilization into Extension and Lateral Flexion

Joint mobilization of the LSp can be performed in an oblique plane, in other words, across two or more cardinal planes. An effective oblique plane lumbar mobilization is to combine extension with lateral flexion. To perform this mobilization, set up as if you are doing a lateral flexion mobilization, contacting the client to one side of the SP. Now alter your stretch mobilization force so that it is more anterior in direction, introducing extension in addition to the lateral flexion motion (see accompanying figure). This can be performed on both sides.

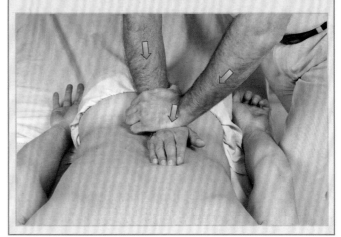

ROUTINE 10-10: LUMBAR SPINE PRONE: FLEXION DISTRACTION

Routines 10-8 and 10-9 demonstrated how to mobilize the LSp into extension, lateral flexion, and rotation. Mobilizing the LSp into flexion is more challenging because an effective contact for the stabilization hand would have to be located anteriorly on the spine; this is not possible because you cannot easily contact the anterior aspect of the spine through the anterior abdominal wall. It is also more challenging for the treatment hand contact that creates the mobilization force to push on a lumbar vertebra in the direction of flexion. For these reasons, it is not possible to create a strong flexion mobilization force. However, for clients whose LSp is greatly restricted into flexion, even small flexion mobilizations can be very beneficial.

Mobilizing the LSp into flexion can be done with prone flexion distraction mobilization technique. This mobilization is similar to SIJ prone sacrum compression with the mobilization force applied to the sacral apex, mobilizing it toward posterior tilt (counternutation) (see Figure 10-10B). However, to create a flexion mobilization of the LSp, a lumbar vertebra must also be contacted. This routine is described as flexion *distraction* because in addition to the flexion, there is also a small element of axial distraction. Axial distraction is also known as traction and is described in more detail in Routine 10-13.

The following are the steps to perform prone flexion distraction mobilization of the LSp:

- The client is prone with a pillow under his abdomen, and you are standing at the left side of the table.
- Place your treatment (right) hand on the client's LSp, with the SP of the vertebra you are mobilizing positioned in the intereminential groove of the hand.
- Place your stabilization (left) hand on the middle of the apex of the sacrum. Be careful to not contact so far inferiorly that you are on the coccyx instead. Pressure on the coccyx could cause injury to the sacrococcygeal ligament and/or the coccyx itself.
- Gently lean in with body weight, pressing in a superior direction on the lumbar SP with your right hand as your

left hand presses inferiorly on the sacral apex, until you reach tissue tension at the end of passive range of motion.

- Now gently stretch the lumbar vertebra into its joint play by leaning in further with body weight, adding a small increased force on the SP, as you slightly increase the force on the apex of the sacrum. This will involve a very small excursion of flexion of that vertebra relative to the adjacent vertebrae; it also creates a slight distraction/traction of the mobilized vertebra (as well as a slight distraction/traction of the entire LSp) (Fig. 10-19).
- Hold for only a fraction of a second and then release.
- This lumbar vertebral joint mobilization may then be repeated for a total of three to five times.
- Once the joint mobilization has been performed at one level, apply it at all the other levels of the LSp so that all LSp joints are mobilized into flexion and distraction.
- Repeat these routines as needed with concentration at the lumbar vertebrae that are restricted.
- *Note*: This routine can be performed from the other side of the table instead; simply switch treatment and stabilization hands.

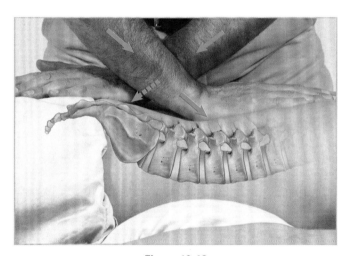

Figure 10-19

ROUTINE 10-11: LUMBAR SPINE SEATED: MOBILIZATIONS

Joint mobilization into left lateral flexion stretches right lateral flexor musculature, especially the smaller, deeper intrinsic muscles of the joint, and the ligamentous and joint capsular tissue on the right side of the joint being mobilized. Joint mobilization into left lateral flexion was demonstrated in the "Overview of Technique" section, Figures 10-2 and 10-3.

To perform right lateral flexion joint mobilization of the LSp, follow the directions given for left lateral flexion but switch for the right side of the body (Fig. 10-20). Joint mobilization into right lateral flexion stretches left lateral flexor musculature, especially the smaller, deeper intrinsic muscles of the joint, and the ligamentous and joint capsular tissue on the left side of the joint being mobilized.

To perform seated rotation mobilizations and seated extension mobilization for the LSp, follow the directions given in Practical Application Box 10.1.

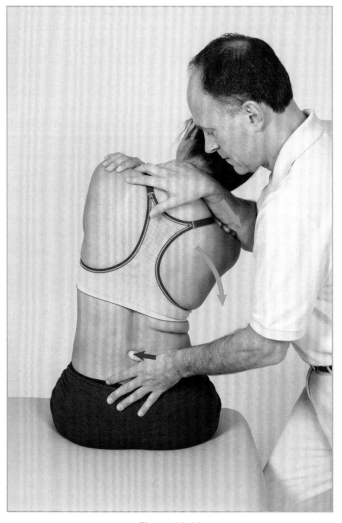

Figure 10-20

ROUTINE 10-12: LUMBAR SPINE SIDE-LYING: HORIZONTAL ADDUCTION

LSp side-lying horizontal adduction is the most powerful mobilization for the LSp and is a variant of the side-lying horizontal adduction mobilization for the SIJ (Routine 10-7). Transitioning from the SIJ to the LSp in side-lying position was addressed in Practical Application Box 10.6. Please refer to Routine 10-7 and Practical Application Box 10.6 for this LSp mobilization.

ROUTINE 10-13: LUMBAR SPINE SUPINE: TOWEL TRACTION/DISTRACTION

Distraction mobilization of the spine, also known as **axial distraction**, is usually called **traction**. In the LSp, it usually involves an inferior glide of a vertebra relative to the vertebra that is above it. Distraction lengthens and stretches all of the tissues that run vertically in the spine at the level(s) of distraction. When performed by hand, it is also called **manual traction**. When performed with the aid of a towel, it can be called **towel traction**. Towel traction of the LSp is demonstrated in this routine; manual distraction/traction of the LSp is shown in Routine 10-14.

The following are the steps to perform distraction/traction joint mobilization of the LSp using a towel:

- The client is supine with a towel or king-sized pillowcase wrapped around the distal legs as seen in Figure 10-21A. Place the towel over the distal anterior legs. Wrap the two sides of the towel back under and up through to the medial side of the legs, superior to the part of the towel that is lying anteriorly across the legs. The ends of the towel are now draped distally toward the feet.

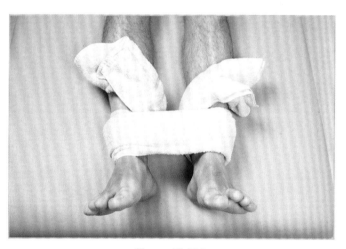

Figure 10-21A

- You are standing at the foot end of the table, in a sagittal plane stance with your body weight balanced on your forward foot (Fig. 10-21B).

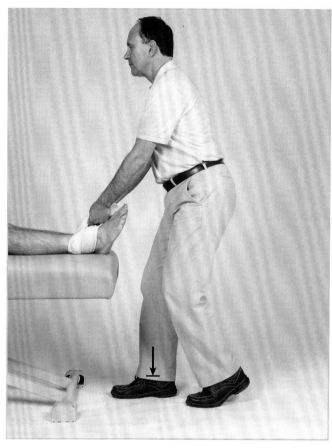

Figure 10-21B

■ Gently and gradually begin pulling on the towel directly inferiorly/distally (parallel with the table) as you slowly shift your weight back onto your rear foot (Fig. 10-21C). Continue pulling until you feel tissue tension.

■ Once tension is reached, perform the mobilization by gently leaning further back, increasing the traction force. This will cause a distraction force that tractions the pelvis away from the LSp, and sequentially as tension is increased, tractions each lumbar vertebra inferiorly away from the vertebra superior to it (Fig. 10-21D).

■ Hold for a second or so and then release.

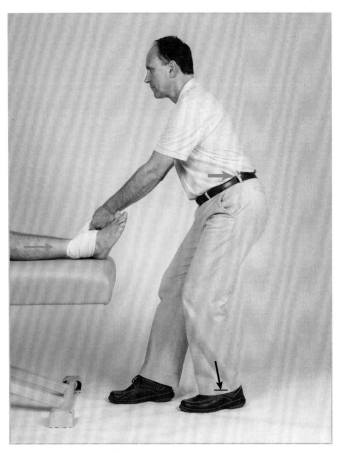

Figure 10-21C

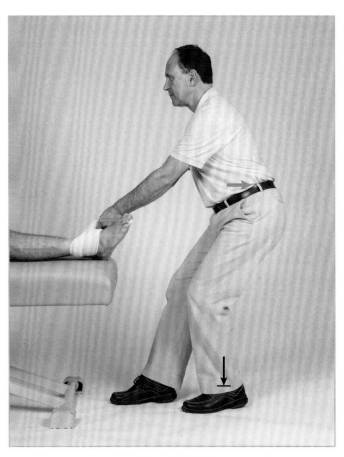

Figure 10-21D

■ With this distraction technique, the weight of the client's upper body will provide overall stabilization for the rest of the body, but it may not provide sufficient stabilization. If the client's body begins to slip on the table, the client can be asked to hold onto the upper table with his hands for further stabilization (Fig. 10-21E). Having flannel sheets or another similar fabric can help to stabilize the client's upper body by adding friction to minimize his sliding.

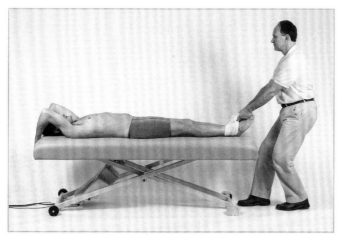

Figure 10-21E

■ Depending on how tight the client is, some of the traction force might travel farther up the spine to the thoracic and perhaps even the cervical spine. The tighter the client, the higher up the spine the traction will be felt. One way to focus the traction to the LSp is to stabilize the thoracic spine with a strap or seat belt. If this is done, for client comfort, it is important to place padding between the restraining belt and the client (Fig. 10-21F).

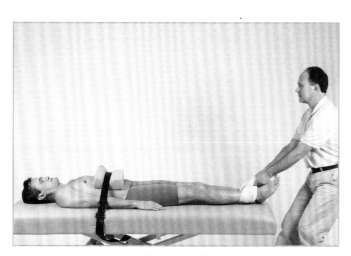

Figure 10-21F

■ This mobilization technique can be repeated for a total of three to five times.
■ In time, the position of traction stretch can be held for longer, perhaps 5 to 10 seconds or more.
■ To increase the traction tension on one side of the client's back, the client's legs can be brought to the other side (Fig. 10-21G). For body mechanics and balance, the therapist's feet position should be shifted toward more of a frontal plane stance.

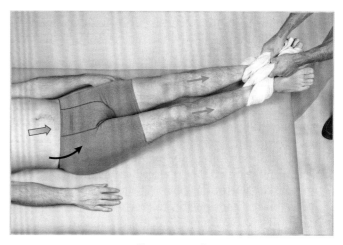

Figure 10-21G

10.9   PRACTICAL APPLICATION

Towel Distraction/Traction

Towel traction can be an extremely effective form of LSp joint mobilization distraction, and most clients enjoy it. However, choosing the proper towel is important. If the towel is too thick or too plush, it is difficult to grab the client's skin and difficult to hold on to. The optimal towel is a well-used, somewhat threadbare bath-sized towel (approximately 40 × 24 inches [100 × 60 cm]). A king-sized flannel pillowcase also works well. But if the fabric of the towel or pillowcase is too thin, the contact can be too narrow and feel uncomfortable to the client.

It is also important to emphasize that the direction of your pull should be as horizontal and parallel with the table as possible. Do not lift the client's feet up as you pull.

When using a towel on the legs to traction the client's spine, the traction force transfers through the client's knee, hip, and SIJs before the traction is felt in the LSp. If the client has a pathologic hip, knee, or SIJ, this mobilization technique might be contraindicated. If any of these joints are hypermobile/unstable, this technique is contraindicated. On the other hand, if the hip or SIJ is hypomobile/restricted, this traction technique might actually be indicated for these joints as well as the LSp joints.

ROUTINE 10-14: LUMBAR SPINE SUPINE: MANUAL TRACTION/DISTRACTION

Manual traction/distraction joint mobilization of the LSp can also be effectively performed. In fact, the manual traction technique routine presented here is generally more effective than towel traction technique placed at the legs (Routine 10-13). Because the thigh is used as the lever to pull and traction the LSp, the knee joints are spared involvement. However, the hip and SIJs are still involved (see the caution regarding possible contraindications for this routine if these joints are unhealthy).

The following are the steps to perform manual distraction/traction joint mobilization of the LSp using the client's right thigh:

- The client is supine with her left lower extremity straight on the table, her right hip and knee joints flexed, and her right foot flat on the table.
- You are sitting toward the foot end of the table, on the client's right side. Your right (lower) leg and foot are under the client's right knee; your left thigh and knee joints are flexed, and your left foot is placed on the top of the table, to the right side of the client. The fingers of your hands are interlaced, and you are grasping the anterior proximal right thigh of the client (Fig. 10-22A). It is important to be as proximal on the client's thigh as possible. *Note:* The therapist can choose to either wear or not wear his or her shoes when on the table. If shoes are not worn, be sure to check that health codes allow this. Also, it can be difficult to grab with traction with stocking feet.

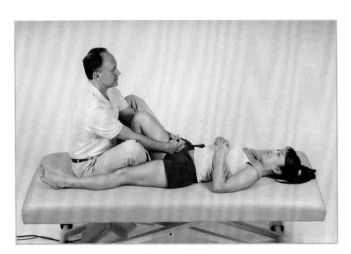

Figure 10-22A

- Gently and gradually begin pulling on the client's right thigh as you slowly shift your weight back on the table. Press onto the table with your left foot to help stabilize your body as you lean back (Fig. 10-22B). The direction of your pull on the client's thigh should be as horizontal and parallel with the table as possible. Continue pulling until you feel tissue tension.

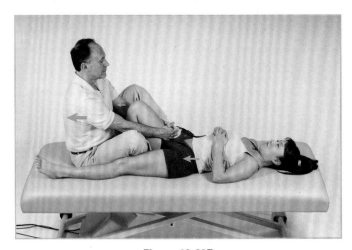

Figure 10-22B

- Once tension is reached, perform the mobilization by gently leaning further back, increasing the traction force. This will cause a distraction force that tractions the pelvis away from the LSp and, sequentially as tension is increased, tractions each lumbar vertebra inferiorly away from the vertebra superior to it (Fig. 10-22C).

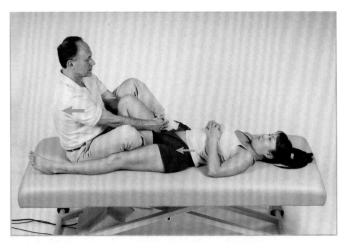

Figure 10-22C

- Hold for a second or so and then release.
- As with the towel traction routine, the weight of the client's upper body will provide overall stabilization for the rest of the body. If the client's body begins to slip on the table, the client can be asked to hold onto the upper table with her hands for further stabilization (see Fig. 10-21E). Having flannel sheets or another similar fabric can help to stabilize the client's upper body by adding friction to minimize her sliding. And as with the previous routine, a strap or seat belt can be used to better stabilize the client's upper body (see Fig. 10-21F).
- This mobilization technique can be repeated for a total of three to five times. In time, the position of traction stretch can be held for longer, perhaps 5 to 10 seconds or more.

10.10 THERAPIST TIP

Manual Lumbar Traction Mobilization

Using the client's thigh to traction the LSp has the advantage of skipping the knee joints and not involving them in the technique. If an unhealthy or painful hip joint of the client precludes using that thigh to traction the spine, simply sit on the other side of the client and use the client's other thigh instead, assuming it is healthy. It is also possible to traction the client's LSp by contacting directly on the client's pelvis, thereby skipping the hip joints altogether, as seen in the accompanying figure. This can also be performed with the client lying at the end of the table so that the therapist can stand at the end of the table for a better base of support.

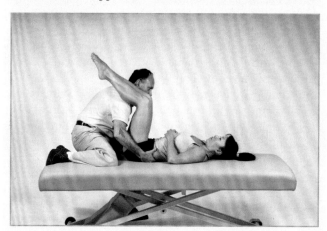

CHAPTER SUMMARY

Joint mobilization is a valuable advanced technique in the therapist's array of treatment options. In essence, it is a very specific form of pin and stretch in which the therapist pins (stabilizes) one vertebra while moving (mobilizing/stretching) the adjacent vertebra. For clients with segmental hypomobility (a soft tissue restriction that is limited to one or a few spinal joint levels of the LSp), joint mobilization is often the only treatment technique that is effective at loosening the taut tissues. It is especially effective for stretching the smaller, deeper intrinsic muscles and the ligaments and joint capsules of the joint being mobilized. As with any stretching technique, joint mobilization is usually most effective when performed after the client's tissues are first warmed up, whether through massage, heat, or physical activity. Although it is important to practice and hone your skills with all new treatment techniques before using them with your clients, because joint mobilization of the LSp is such a powerful technique, particular care needs to be paid to practicing this technique before incorporating it into your treatment regimen.

CASE STUDY

ALICIA

■ **History and Physical Assessment**

A new client, Alicia Alexander, age 32 years, comes to your office complaining of low back pain and stiffness. She describes the pain as a 5 to 7 on a scale of 0 to 10. She tells you that her condition has been progressing for about a year and that she believes it is a result of the increased time she has been spent sitting. She first noticed the discomfort late last year after an 8-hour car ride back from vacation. Since then, she has had many deadlines at work that require her to spend a lot of time seated at the computer; she is a graphic artist.

You perform a thorough client history, which reveals no trauma. She reports that her discomfort is localized to the lower left side of her low back. There is no referral into either of the lower extremities. She tells you that she has seen a massage therapist once a week for the past 4 weeks, with treatment consisting of heat, deep tissue work, as well as standard and contract relax stretching, but that the pain and tightness have only improved slightly. She has also been walking more, hoping that it would help to loosen her low back; it seems to help for a couple of hours but then the discomfort and pain return. She describes the discomfort/pain as a deep dull ache and stiffness.

You perform the passive and active straight leg raise, and you ask her to perform the cough and slump tests and the Valsalva maneuver, the results of which are all negative.

Your assessment shows that her LSp gross ranges of motion are all normal, although she describes feeling slightly stiff when moving into flexion and right lateral flexion. Upon palpation, you find a mild to moderate muscle spasming in the left low back/pelvis region, specifically at the left lumbosacral paraspinal muscles, the superomedial fibers of the left gluteus maximus, and the left piriformis. When you ask her to indicate where her pain and tightness are located, she points to the medial side of the left PSIS. Upon joint play/motion palpation of the LSp and SIJs, all joints are moving well except that you find a marked hypomobility in her left SIJ. (For a review of assessment procedures, see Chapter 3.)

■ **Think-It-Through Questions:**

1. Should an advanced technique such as joint mobilization be included in your treatment plan for Alicia? Why, or why not?

2. Is joint mobilization safe to use with Alicia? If yes, how do you make that determination?

3. If you do joint mobilization, which specific joint mobilization routines should you use? How and why would you choose those particular routines?

Answers to these Think-It-Through Questions and the Treatment Strategy employed for this client are available online at thePoint.lww.com/MuscolinoLowBack

Page numbers followed by *b, f,* and *t* denotes boxes, figures, and tables, respectively. Page numbers in italics denote online chapters.